Veterinary Microbiology and Microbial Disease

Veterinary Microbiology and Microbial Disease

Editor: Andrea Santoro

Callisto Reference
www.callistoreference.com

Callisto Reference,
118-35 Queens Blvd., Suite 400,
Forest Hills, NY 11375, USA

Visit us on the World Wide Web at:
www.callistoreference.com

ISBN: 978-1-64116-771-0 (Hardback)

Cataloging-in-Publication Data

Veterinary microbiology and microbial disease / edited by Andrea Santoro.
p. cm.
Includes bibliographical references and index.
ISBN 978-1-64116-771-0
1. Veterinary microbiology. 2. Animals--Diseases. 3. Veterinary medicine. I. Santoro, Andrea.
SF780.2 .V48 2023
636.089 690 41--dc23

Table of Contents

Preface

Veterinary microbiology refers to a field of study that is primarily focused on the microbes that cause diseases in animals. It studies the microbial diseases of domesticated animals used for food production and other useful purposes. It also addresses the microbial diseases of wild animals in relation to their interactions with domesticated animals. Microorganisms that can cause diseases include protozoa, bacteria, fungi, viruses along with a few different kinds of worms. Some of the common diseases caused by microorganisms include rabies, cholera, histoplasmosis, and malaria. Different kinds of antibiotics such as beta-lactams, macrolides, fluoroquinolones and aminoglycosides can be used to treat bacterial diseases in animals. This book contains some path-breaking studies in veterinary microbiology. It is appropriate for students seeking detailed information on the microbial diseases studied within this field. Researchers and students in this field will be assisted by this book.

The information contained in this book is the result of intensive hard work done by researchers in this field. All due efforts have been made to make this book serve as a complete guiding source for students and researchers. The topics in this book have been comprehensively explained to help readers understand the growing trends in the field.

I would like to thank the entire group of writers who made sincere efforts in this book and my family who supported me in my efforts of working on this book. I take this opportunity to thank all those who have been a guiding force throughout my life.

Editor

1

Investigation of Pre- and Post-Weaning Mortalities in Rabbits Bred in Egypt, with Reference to Parasitic and Bacterial Causes

Saeed El-Ashram [1,2,*], Shawky M. Aboelhadid [3,*], El-Sayed M. Abdel-Kafy [4], Shymaa A. Hashem [4], Lilian N. Mahrous [3], Eman M. Farghly [4] and Asmaa A. Kamel [3]

1 College of Life Science and Engineering, Foshan University, 18 Jiangwan street, Foshan 528231, China
2 Faculty of Science, Kafrelsheikh University, Kafr el-Sheikh, 33516, Egypt
3 Parasitology Department, Faculty of Veterinary Medicine, Beni Suef University, Beni-Suef 62511, Egypt; dr.lilian_nagy@yahoo.com (L.N.M.); drasmaaalaa@yahoo.com (A.A.K.)
4 Animal Production Research Institute, Agricultural Research Center, Dokki, Giza 12651, Egypt; sayedabdkaffy@yahoo.com (E.-S.M.A.-K.); shaimaaahmedparavet@yahoo.com (S.A.H.); hawk18922@gmail.com (E.M.F.)
* Correspondence: saeed_elashram@yahoo.com (E.-A.S.); shawky.abohadid@vet.bsu.edu.eg (S.M.A.)

Simple Summary: Pre- and postweaning stages are critical in the management of rabbits due to the increased risk of mortalities. Mortality rates during pre- and postweaning periods were 67.10% and 31.90%, respectively. The preweaning mortality was mainly due to causes related to does (95.23%) and infectious agents, including *Escherichia coli*, and *Salmonella* (4.77%). The postweaning mortality was mainly referred to managemental factors and infectious causes, including *Eimeria* species, *E. coli*, and *Salmonella*.

Abstract: This study was conducted to investigate the causes of mortality in young rabbits. A total of 110 V-Line breed female rabbits aged 5 m were used in this study. Rabbit kits were examined daily in pre- and postweaning stages to detect clinical disorders that caused death. The postmortem examination was carried out on dead kits. Furthermore, rabbits were examined for the probable bacteriological and parasitological causes of death. Fecal samples were collected from each dead kit and examined by standard microbiological procedures for bacterial pathogens and macroscopically and microscopically for the presence of endo- and ectoparasites. Throughout two breeding seasons, 2238 newborns were obtained, of which 1736 died, accounting for a 77.57% mortality rate. During preweaning (1st month of age) and postweaning (up to 3 months of age), 1501 (67.10%) and 235 (31.90%) deaths were recorded, respectively. A postweaning fecal examination revealed that 198 out of 229 (86.50%) were diarrheic rabbits due to *Eimeria* infection. *Cittotaenia* spp. eggs were detected in 4.37% of fecal samples, and mites (*Sarcoptis scabiei*) were present in 6.55%. *E. coli* was detected in 100% of examined animals during pre- and postweaning periods; however, *Salmonella* spp. were 97.22% and 43.67, respectively. Managemental risk factors were the main causes in preweaning mortality, including insufficient milk supply (37.37%), cannibalism (26.38%), mange infestation of a rabbit doe (22.20%), mastitis (4.30%), lack of doe care (5.00%), bronchopneumonia (2.13%), and enteritis (1.80%). However, risk factors in postweaning mortality included sudden death with general septicemia (13.80%), enteritis (9.63%), bronchopneumonia (5.43%), mange infestation (2.04%), and malnutrition (0.81%). In conclusion, the etiology of preweaning mortality in kits was related mainly to the doe, especially managemental risk factors. However, a combination of multiple pathogenic agents (parasites and bacteria) and managemental factors was reported in the postweaning stage. Careful attention must be paid to avoid these causes.

Keywords: pre- and postweaning; rabbits; mortality; *Eimeria*; *Salmonella*; *E. coli*; management

1. Introduction

Rabbits play a significant role in solving the problem of protein shortage in many parts of the world due to their high fertility, prolificity, and rapid growth. However, pre- and postweaning mortalities could seriously damage the domestic rabbit industry, which affects lower-income families [1]. Weaning, which is a crucial period in the productive cycle of rabbits, has been associated with increased stress and susceptibility to diseases [2]. Moreover, establishing causes of pre- and postweaning mortalities remain difficult because multiple causes included either pathogenic agents (parasites, bacteria or viruses) or managemental factors in addition to adverse climatic conditions [3,4]. While 50% of mortality causes in rabbits are still unknown, parasites (*Eimeria* spp.) and bacteria (enteropathogenic *Escherichia coli*) remain the primary cause of nest mortality [5]. Coccidiosis is responsible for high losses in rabbit production and is considered a risk factor for intestinal disorders in the early postweaning period [6] and for liver condemnations as a result of hepatic coccidiosis [7]. Otherwise, sarcoptic mange infestation is one of the most common and major problems in the rabbit industry [8,9]. Sarcoptic mange mites are highly contagious and spread from rabbit to rabbit by direct skin contact or indirectly through fomites [9]. Severe sarcoptic mange infestations especially in young or debilitated rabbits cause high mortality [10]. The causes, such as infanticide, insufficient milk, birthing outside the nest box, mastitis, abscesses, genital infections, and death of dam may result in nest mortality. In addition, genetic and environmental factors may affect growth variation [4,11]. The aim of this study was to investigate the main parasitic, bacterial, and managemental causes of mortality in young rabbits during pre- and postweaning stages.

2. Materials and Methods

2.1. Study Location and Ethics

This study was conducted in Sids station for animal breeding in Beni-Suef, Egypt, which belongs to the Animal Production Researches Institute (APRI), Agriculture Research Center (ARC), Ministry of Agriculture. The ethical rules for animal regulations were followed and approved by Beni-Suef University committee in January 2017 (BSU-19-2017).

2.2. Period of the Study

This study was carried out continuously for two consecutive breeding seasons (2017–2019). Mortality rates were recorded for each season to assess the effect of infectious agents and managemental factors on the newborn survival rate. No births were recorded during summer as there was no breeding during the hot season.

2.3. Rabbit Husbandry and Management

A total of 110 V-Line breed adult female rabbits (first-time mothers) aged 5 m was each kept in wire mesh cages (1 rabbit/cage), with natural ventilation, lighting, and ambient temperatures. Animals were fed ad libitum on commercial rabbit pelleted diet (not contain anticoccidial agents) in galvanized steel feeding hoppers and were provided water by automatic nipple drinkers. Each doe was identified by a numbered ear tag. About 3 d before birth, a nest box containing hay-straw bedding was placed in each cage. Does and their newborn kits were daily observed after birth, mainly for 3 d.

2.4. Recording of Production Data

A record sheet was prepared for each doe and kit on which to record all the detailed information, including doe number; date of birth; number of delivered; total litter size/birth; and maternal and newborn conditions, such as milk yield, disease conditions, mange infestation, abscessation of mammary glands, respiratory and digestive infections, and cannibalism signs.

2.5. *Reporting Causes of Pre-and Postweaning Mortalities*

2.5.1. Preweaning Stage

About 2238 kits were born in two consecutive breeding seasons. Does were daily examined for maternal behavior and a swollen and whitish belly as a sign of initial milk feeding, while kits were observed for an increase in body mass as an indicator to normal growth. Dead kits were daily collected for postmortem (PM) examination. Furthermore, affected organs, including liver, lungs, trachea, kidneys, and alimentary tract, in addition to cecal content were collected from dead kits for microbiological and parasitological examinations to identify the causative agents that may be associated with mortality. The does were inspected for any disorders that affected newborn.

2.5.2. Postweaning Stage

A total of 737 rabbits weaned at 35 days of age were separated from their does and transferred to new cages after inspection for postweaning disorders. Weaned rabbits were daily examined for clinical disorders associated with mortality in rabbits, including bloating, diarrhea, nasal discharges, and mange infestation. Dead rabbits were collected for postmortem (PM) examination, and organs with macroscopic lesions were sampled and sent to the laboratory for bacterial and parasitological examination.

2.6. *Investigation of Pathogenic Causes of Pre-and Postweaning Mortalities in Rabbits*

2.6.1. Parasitological Examination of Fecal Samples

A total of 301 fecal samples were obtained from young rabbits suffering from diarrhea. The samples represented 72 kits in the preweaning stage and 229 rabbits in the postweaning stage. Fecal samples were placed in separate labeled clean plastic cups to prevent potential cross contamination between samples and were transported on ice to the laboratory. Fecal samples were examined macroscopically and microscopically (Labomed Inc., New York, NY, USA) for their physical appearance and parasites, respectively [12]. A direct fecal smear was prepared from each fecal sample and examined for protozoal vegetative forms, cysts, and helminth eggs. The salt flotation technique was used to detect *Eimeria* oocysts [13]. The obtained *Eimeria* oocysts from fecal samples were separately stored into 2.5% potassium dichromate solution at 27 °C and 60%–80% humidity for 7 d [14]. Sporulated oocysts were collected after centrifugation (Centurion, Hoddesdon, UK), washed using distilled water, and identified under a microscope.

2.6.2. Mange Examination

Scabs were obtained from the edges of skin lesions by a scalpel from 15 postweaning rabbits suffering from mange clinical signs, were placed into plastic tubes, and were transferred to the laboratory. Scabs were placed in Petri dishes, incubated at 35 °C for 30 min in a biochemical oxygen demand (BOD) incubator (Velp, Usmate Velate MB, Italy), and examined microscopically for the presence of mites [15].

2.6.3. Bacteriological Examination

A total of 301 young rabbits (72 from preweaning and 229 from postweaning) were found dead and examined for clinical signs. Affected organs, including liver, lungs, trachea, kidneys, and alimentary tract, that showed congestion, enlargement, and inflammation were collected in sterile plastic bags and kept in the ice box for examination. Tissue samples were screened for the presence of *Staphylococcus*, *Salmonella*, and *E. coli*. Bacterial colonies were identified according to previously described standard procedures [16–19]. Polymerase chain reaction (PCR) experiments were carried out following procedures previously published to confirm the identification of the isolates (Labnet Gradient PCR, Edison, NJ, USA) [20].

2.7. Statistical Analysis

All data were coded, entered, and analyzed using the statistical package SPSS version 22 (IBM Corp. Released 2013. IBM SPSS Statistics for Windows, Version 22.0., Armonk, NY, USA). Quantitative value data were summarized and described as frequencies and percentages. The relations between data grouped were tested by the Chi-square test for quantitative variables, and p-values were calculated if less than or equal to 0.05 ($p \leq 0.05$) were considered significant.

3. Results

3.1. Mortality Rates

In the two consecutive breeding seasons (the combined effects of two consecutive breeding seasons), 2017–2018 and 2018–2019, a total of 2238 kits were born from 110 does. The total kit mortality rate was 77.57% (1736/2238), including preweaning (67.07%, 1501/2238) and postweaning (31.89%, 235/737) periods (Figure 1).

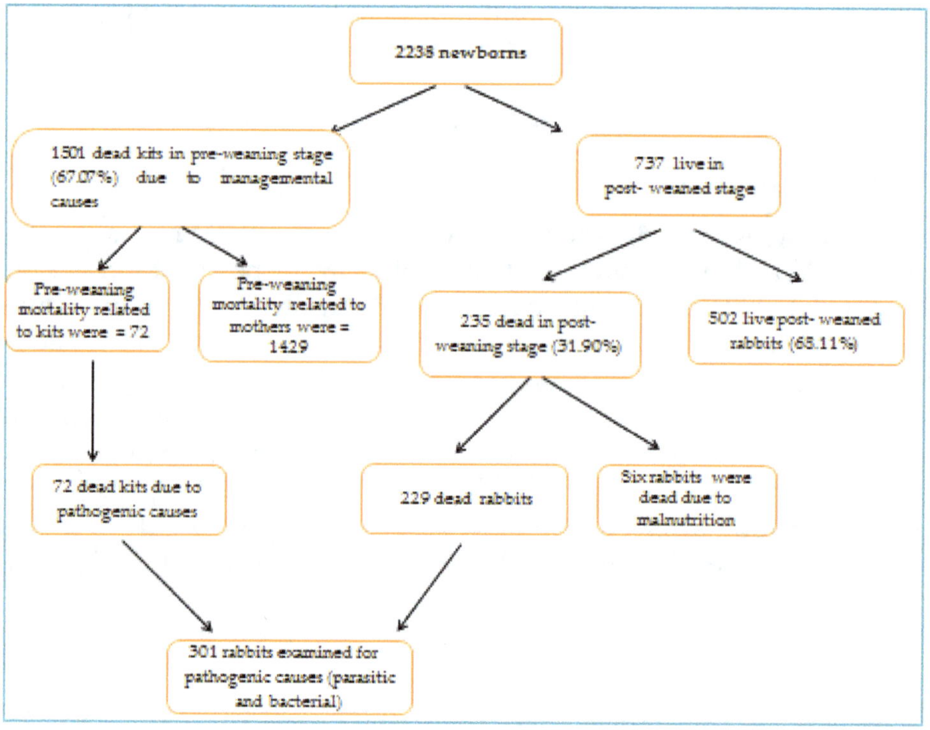

Figure 1. Flow chart showing the causes of newborn deaths in pre-and postweaning stages.

3.2. Managemental Causes of Preweaning Mortality

The preweaning mortality rate was 67% over the two consecutive seasons. Causes of mortality related to does (1429/1501) were insufficient milk supply within the first few days after birth (37.37%), cannibalism (26.38%), mange infestation of does (22.20%), and mastitis (4.30%). Moreover, some does neglected their kits, which led to death of the whole litter (5.00%). Mortality rates related to the kits (72/1501) were bronchopneumonia (2.13%) and enteritis (1.80%). Sudden death without obvious causes was recorded in few cases 0.90% (Table 1). There was a significant difference ($p < 0.05$) between different managemental causes of preweaning mortality.

Table 1. Managemental causes of preweaning mortality related to mothers and kits.

Causes of Kit's Death	Mortality Related to Mothers	Mortality Related to Kits	SEM	p *
Insufficient milk supply	561(37.37%)	0		
Infanticidal does (cannibalism)	396 (26.38%)	0		
Mange infested does	333 (22.20%)	0		
Mastitis	64 (4.30%)	0		
Lack of mothering	75 (5.00%)	0	1.109	0.000
Bronchopneumonia in litters	0	32 (2.13%)		
Enteritis in litters with diarrhea	0	27 (1.80%)		
Sudden death in litters	0	13 (0.90%)		
Total	1429 (95.23%)	72 (4.83%)		

SEM: standard error of mean. * $p < 0.05$ is significant.

3.3. Pathogenic Causes of Preweaning Mortality in Rabbits

Bacteriological Causes of Preweaning Mortality

Examination of 72 dead kits in the preweaning stage revealed the presence of *E. coli* in all the 72 animals. Moreover, *Salmonella* was found in 97.22% of preweaned rabbits. PCR assay confirmed the identification of *Salmonella* species (Figure 2A). No parasitic causes were determined in the preweaning stage.

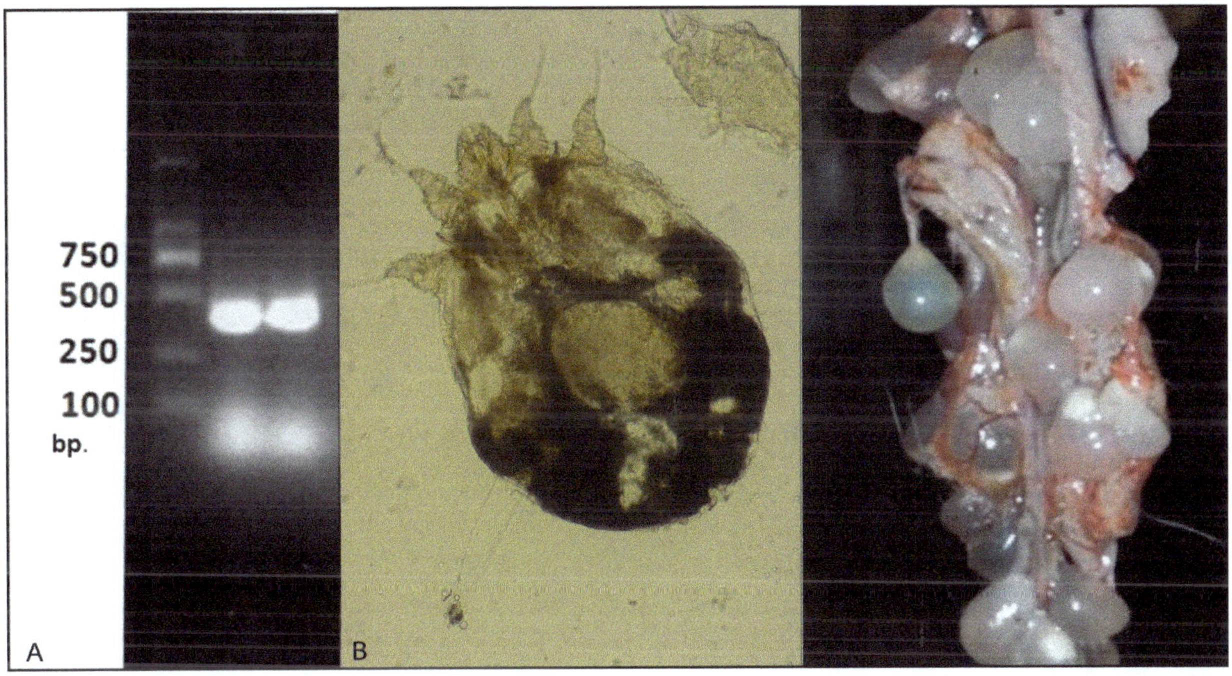

Figure 2. (**A**) *Cysticercus pisiformis* from the peritoneal cavity of rabbits, (**B**) *Sarcoptes scabiei* from the rabbit skin, and (**C**) analysis of *Salmonella* pure culture with the primer set: ST11-ST15. Lane 1 and Lane 2: *Salmonella*.

3.4. Seasonal Prevalence of Preweaning Mortality

Prevalence of preweaning mortality was highest during winter (36.5%) followed by autumn (32.6%) and spring (30.9%). In winter, the mortality as a result of insufficient milk supply, cannibalism, bronchopneumonia, and sudden death were recorded at the highest rates comparing to other seasons (Table 2). Meanwhile, mastitis and enteritis were the highest prevalence in spring. However, autumn showed the highest rate of mortality due to lack of mothering care (Table 3). The seasonal effect on preweaning mortality showed a significant difference ($p < 0.05$) between different seasons.

Table 2. Seasonal prevalence of preweaning mortality.

Causes of Kit's Death.	Total No. of Dead Kits	Autumn	%	Winter	%	Spring	%	SEM	p *
Insufficient milk supply	561	149	26.6	254	45.28	158	28.16		
Mange infested does	333	213	63.96	48	14.41	72	21.62		
Infanticidal does	396	47	11.87	201	50.76	148	37.37		
Mastitis in lactating females	64	-	0	18	28.1	46	71.9	0.751	0.000
Lack of mothering	75	65	86.7	-	0	10	13.3		
Bronchopneumonia	32	5	15.6	15	46.9	12	37.5		
Enteritis	27	7	25.9	6	22.2	14	51.9		
Sudden death	13	3	23	6	46.15	4	30.8		
Total	1501	489	32.6	548	36.5	464	30.9		

SEM: Standard error of mean. * $p < 0.05$ is significant.

Table 3. Prevalence of postweaning mortality related to the cause of death.

Causes of Death	Number of Dead Kits/737	%	SEM	p *
Sudden death with Septicemia	103	13.80		
Diarrhea (enteritis)	71	9.63		
Bronchopneumonia	40	5.43	0.725	0.000
Mange infestation	15	2.04		
Malnutrition	6	0.81		
Total	235	31.90		

SEM: Standard error of mean. * $p < 0.05$ is significant.

3.5. Managemental Causes of Postweaning Mortality

The prevalence of postweaning mortality rate was 31.90% (235/737) (Figure 1). Sudden death with symptoms of general septicemia in the muscles and internal organs was 13.80% followed by enteritis (9.63%), while the prevalence of bronchopneumonia was 5.43%. Moreover, the prevalence of mange mites was 2.04% and of malnutrition was 0.81% (Table 3). There was significant difference ($p < 0.05$) between different causes of postweaning mortality.

3.6. Pathogenic Causes of Postweaning Mortality in Rabbits

3.6.1. Parasitological Findings of Postweaning Mortality

Examination of 229 fecal samples from diarrheic rabbits revealed that 86.50% (198/229) of rabbits were positive for *Eimeria* spp. Microscopic identification of eimerian oocysts revealed the presence of seven *Eimeria* species including (*E. media*, *E. perforans*, *E. intestinalis*, *E. magna*, *E. coecicola*, *E. exigua*, and *E. flavescens*). *E. media* was the most prevalent species (Figure 3). Furthermore, *Cittotaenia spp.* eggs were detected in 4.37% of fecal samples (Table 4). Mites (*Sarcoptes scabiei*) were detected in 6.55% (15/229 postweaning rabbits) (Table 4, Figure 2B). There were significant differences ($p < 0.05$) between the frequencies of different parasitic causes in the postweaning period.

Table 4. Prevalence of pathogenic causes in postweaning periods in rabbits.

Pathogenic Agents	Postweaning Mortality (n = 229)	Prevalence %	SEM	p *
Eimeria spp. Oocysts	198	86.50		
Cittotaenia spp. Eggs	10	4.37		
Sarcoptes scabiei	15	6.55		
E. coli	229	100	1.26	0.000
Salmonella	100	43.67		
Eimeria spp. + *E. coli*	198	86.50		
Eimeria spp. + *Salmonella*	100	43.67		

SEM: Standard error of mean. * $p < 0.05$ is significant.

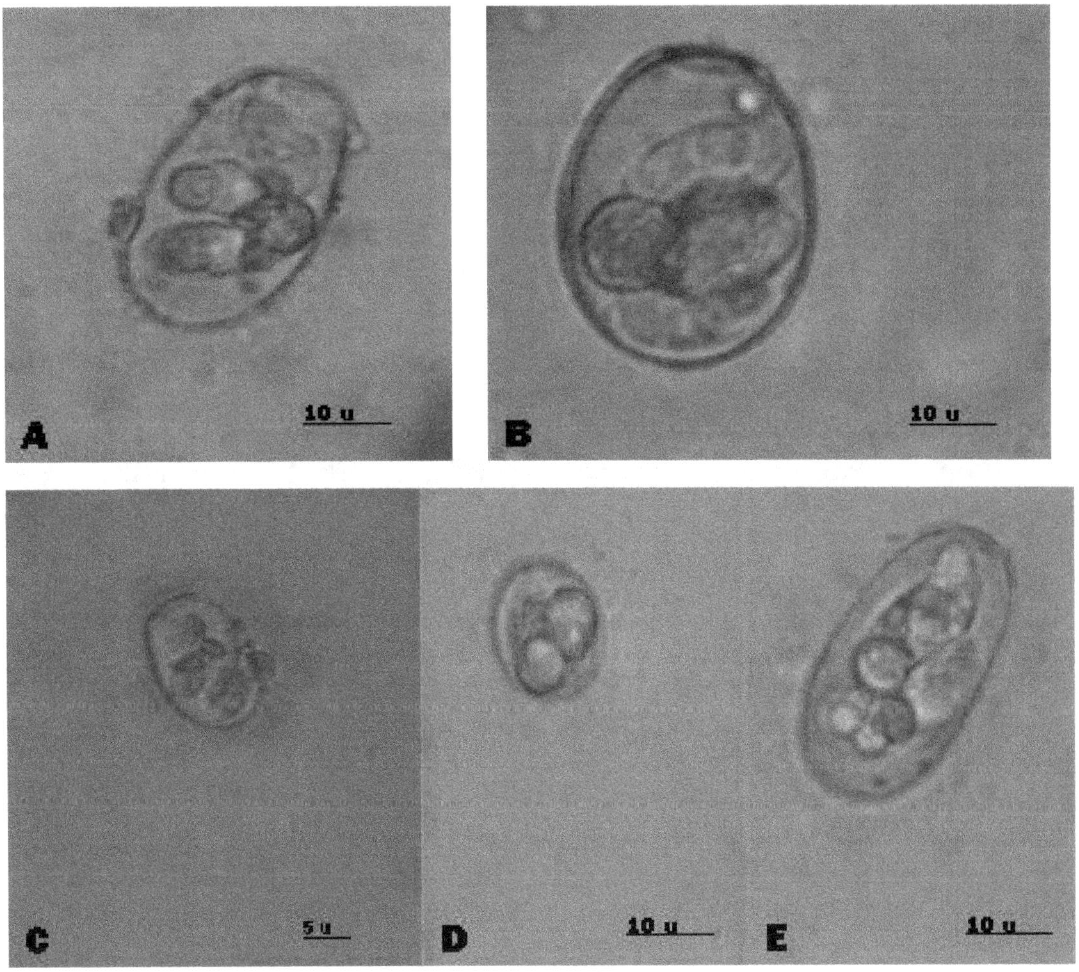

Figure 3. Sporulated oocysts of different species of *Eimeria* isolated from rabbits: (**A**) *E. media*, (**B**) *E. intestinalis*, (**C**) *E. magna*, (**D**) *E. exigua*, and (**E**) *E. coecicola*.

3.6.2. Bacteriological Causes of Postweaning Mortality

E. coli was found in all 229 animals. Moreover, *Salmonella* was found in 43.67% of postweaning animals (Table 4). Significant differences ($p < 0.05$) were found between the frequencies of different bacterial causes of postweaning mortality.

3.7. *PostMortem Lesions of Postweaning Mortality*

All necropsied rabbits carried *Eimeria* spp., pointing to coccidiosis as a probable cause of the death. Necropsied carcasses showed tinged blood and mucoid content in different parts of the intestinal tract with severe congestion and swelling. Furthermore, *Taenia pisiformis* cysts were attached to the peritoneal membrane in 4.37% (10/229) of dead rabbits (Figure 2C).

3.8. *Seasonal Prevalence of Postweaning Mortality*

In the postweaning stage, the highest mortality rate was recorded in spring (48.9%) followed by winter (37.9%) while the lowest mortality rate was occurred in autumn (13.2%). No births were recorded in summer as breeding was stopped to avoid heat stress (Table 5). The seasonal effect on postweaning mortality showed a significant difference ($p < 0.05$) between different seasons.

Table 5. Seasonal prevalence of postweaning mortality.

Season	Postweaning Mortality	%	SEM	p *
Autumn	31	13.2	0.638	0.008
Winter	89	37.9		
Spring	115	48.9		
Total	235	31.90		

SEM: Standard error of mean. * $p < 0.05$ is significant.

4. Discussion

Data on causes and rates of mortality are crucial for determining profitability and net income in commercial rabbit farming. However, studies on causes and rates of mortality on rabbit farms during pre- and postweaning stages are limited. This study investigated causes of pre- and postweaning mortality in 110 does during two consecutive breeding seasons. The overall mortality during preweaning was 67.07%. Similar findings were obtained by Ahmed et al. and Tameem et al. [11,21], who recorded 49.074% to 62.13% mortality rate in Egypt. However, the preweaning mortality rate in this study was higher than that recorded by Karu et al. [22], who observed that the preweaning mortality varies from 2.34% to 15.23% in New Zealand white kits. This variation could be attributed to the different causes of mortality affecting young rabbits including parasitic, bacterial, or managemental. The deaths during weaning in rabbits were very high due to many diseases affecting young kits at pre- and postweaning ages [23]. Interestingly, mother does have a major role in the mortality rate (95.23%) during the preweaning stage. Concerning the managemental causes related to mothers led preweaning mortality, the main cause of mortality was insufficient milk supply, which was associated with 37.37% of mortality. Mortality due to inadequate milk supply was more prominent in does that had large litter sizes which resulted in greater competition for doe teats during suckling and higher consumption of milk for fitter kits, which did not allow smaller and weaker kits to consume enough milk with resultant starvation and death. These findings are in line with those recorded by [24–30]. Prevalence of preweaning mortality due to insufficient milk supply and large litter size was the highest in winter (45.28%) while the lowest was in autumn (26.6%). Similar results were obtained by [31,32]. The prevalence of preweaning mortality because of cannibalism was 26.38%. This finding agrees with [33,34], who suggested that does tend to eat their young kits due to insufficient drinking water around parturition time. The prevalence of preweaning mortality due to mite infestation in mothers was 22.20%. Moreover, sarcoptic manage contributed to high mortality because does became clinically aggressive due to severe irritation and restlessness, which were made worse with low feed intake resulting in inappetence and loss of body weight with poor growth for young rabbits. Similar findings were reported by several studies [35–38]. *Sarcoptes scabiei* was detected in all mite-infected rabbits in the current study, and the highest prevalence of infestation was in autumn (63.96%) while the lowest was in winter (14.41%), which is consistent with previous findings [23,39]. Warm conditions and the high humidity may have favored rapid mite reproduction, spread, and infestation among rabbits [9]. Furthermore, mastitis was observed in 4.30% of does. Mastitis interferes with suckling and may lead to complete breast dryness and milk cessation. These findings are supported by [34,40]. The highest prevalence of mastitis was recorded in late spring (71.9%) while, in winter, was (28.1%) consistent with results previously reported by [41]. Concerning the pathogenic causes of preweaning mortality, *E.coli* and *Salmonella* were identified as bacterial causes of mortality with prevalence of 100% and 97.22% of preweaned rabbits. Similar findings were reported by [42]. It is worthy to mention that no parasitic causes were determined in preweaning stage. Our findings revealed that the highest prevalence of pre-weaning mortality was recorded in winter (36.5%) due to cold or lower temperatures, inadequate warming, and insufficient heat insulation, which led in decreased feed intake, reduced vitality, and poor body conditions. The lowest prevalence was recorded in spring (30.9%). However, preweaning mortality increased with the increase of ambient temperature that could be attributed to the heat stress and reduction of dam's milk [40].

The prevalence of postweaning mortality was 31.90% (235/737); these results revealed that mortality decreased with growing age in accordance with previous studies [1,11,43]. Also, most of mortality causes were related to pathogenic agents. Differences in pre- and postweaning mortality may be attributed to several factors, including pathogenic, genetic, environmental and managemental conditions, and the maternal ability of mothers does as suggested by Rashwan [34]. Regarding the parasitic causes of mortality, oocysts of coccidia were a prominent cause of young rabbit mortality in this investigation. Different species of *Eimeria*,, including *E. media*, *E. perforans*, *E. intestinalis*, *E. magna*, *E. coecicola*, *E. exigua*, and *E. flavescens*, were detected in line with previous studies [6,7,44] which revealed that rabbit coccidiosis was an important cause of mortality within the first three to four days after birth in rabbits and that the main source of *Eimeria* spp. for young rabbits was *Eimeria* oocysts shed by adult rabbits. Sarcoptic mange (*Sarcoptes scabiei*) was also an important parasitic cause of mortality, which is in agreement with previous studies showing that sarcoptic mange was a highly contagious infectious disease, rapidly spreading parasitic disease in Egypt, and next to coccidiosis in the economic importance [9,37]. Furthermore, *E. coli* and *Salmonella* spp. were identified as probable bacterial causes of mortality as they were detected in 100% and 43.67% of rabbits, respectively. Similar findings were reported by Eid [42]. Necropsied rabbits revealed a number of lesions including enteritis 9.63% and bronchopneumonia (5.43%), which may have contributed to mortality. Pneumonia and enteritis may have been induced by parasitic and bacterial organisms. Both pneumonia and enteritis are major problems causing high mortalities in rabbitries [45]. Seasonal variations and climatic conditions play a vital role in rabbit survival due to the direct effect of ambient temperature on does and the young. The highest prevalence of postweaning mortality (48.9%) was recorded in late spring with the gradual rise in ambient temperature, whereas the lowest prevalence was in autumn (13.2%). Similar results were obtained previously in other studies [45–47], which reported that high ambient temperatures reduce the feed intake of lactating does from 25% to 50% leading to reduction energy and deterioration of doe vitality, body condition, and productivity.

5. Conclusions

In conclusion, doe and kit health can be achieved by reducing preweaning mortality through adjustment of the rabbitry's climatic conditions, by improving the managemental conditions, and by avoiding food and water contamination. Nevertheless, the results were based on a limited sample size (the combined effects of two consecutive breeding seasons), and larger well-designed studies (5 consecutive breeding seasons) are expected to confirm these preliminary findings.

Author Contributions: Conceptualization, S.M.A., S.E.-A., and E.-S.M.A.-K.; Formal analysis, S.E.-A.; Investigation, L.N.M., A.A.K., and S.A.H.; Methodology, S.A.H. and A.A.K.; Supervision, S.M.A., E.-S.M.A.-K., and E.M.F.; Writing—review and editing, S.E.-A. and S.M.A. All authors have read and agreed to the published version of the manuscript.

Funding: Startup Research Grant Program provided by Foshan University, Foshan city, Guangdong province for distinguished researchers, Guangdong Science and Technology Plan Project (grant No:1244 0600 4560 7389XC), and School of Life Science and Engineering fund (grant No: KLPREAD201801-02). This work was supported by the National Natural Science Foundation of China (No. 31502071); Youth Innovative Talents Project of Guangdong province Education Department (No. 2017KQNCX212); Guangdong province (2017GDK07); Startup Research Grant Program provided by Foshan University, Foshan city, Guangdong province for distinguished researchers, Guangdong Science and Technology Plan Project (grant No:1244 0600 4560 7389XC); and School of Life Science and Engineering fund (grant No: KLPREAD201801-02).

Acknowledgments: The authors greatly appreciate the help of the staff of Sides Station for animal production during the field work.

References

1. Rashwan, A.A.; Ahmed, S.A. Growing rabbit management, housing system, reduction of eating time and feeder space. In Proceedings of the 6th World Rabbit Congress, Toulouse, France, 9–12 July 1996.
2. Millar, J.S. Nest mortality in small mammals. *Ecoscience* **2007**, *14*, 286–291. [CrossRef]
3. Heppell, S.S.; Caswell, H.; Crowder, L.B. Life histories and elasticity patterns: Perturbation analysis for species with minimal demographic data. *Ecology* **2000**, *81*, 654–665. [CrossRef]
4. Oli, M.K.; Dobson, F.S. The relative importance of life-history variables to population growth rate in mammals: Cole's prediction revisited. *Am. Nat.* **2003**, *161*, 422–440. [CrossRef] [PubMed]
5. Licois, D. Domestic rabbit enteropathogens. In Proceedings of the 8th World Rabbit Congress, Puebla, Mexico, 7–10 September 2004.
6. El-Ashram, A.S.; Aboelhadid, S.M.; Abdel-Kafy, E.M.; Hashem, S.A.; Mahrous, L.N.; Farghly, E.M.; Moawad, U.K.; Kamel, A.A. Prophylactic and Therapeutic Efficacy of Prebiotic Supplementation against Intestinal Coccidiosis in Rabbits. *Animals* **2019**, *9*, 965. [CrossRef]
7. Pakandl, M. Coccidia of rabbit: A review. *Folia Parasitol.* **2009**, *56*, 153–166. [CrossRef]
8. Darzi, M.M.; Mir, M.S.; Shahardar, R.A.; Pandit, B.A. Clinicopathological, histochemical and therapeutic studies on concurrent sarcoptic and notoedric acariosis in rabbits *(Orytolagus cuniculus). Vet. Orhiv.* **2007**, *77*, 167–175.
9. Aboelhadid, S.M.; Mahrous, L.N.; Hashem, S.A.; Abdel-Kafy, E.M.; Miller, R.J. In vitro and in vivo effect of Citrus limon essential oil against sarcoptic mange in rabbits. *Parasitol. Res.* **2016**, *115*, 3013–3020. [CrossRef]
10. Bornstein, S.M.T.; Samuel, W.H. *Parasitic Diseases of Wild Mammals*; Iowa state University Press: Ames, IA, USA, 2001; pp. 107–119.
11. Tameem Eldar, A.A.; Elamin, K.M.; Yousif, I.A.; Hassan, H.E.; Musa, A.M. Growth and Mortality in Pre-and Post-Weaning Rearing Periods for Sudanese Local Rabbits. *J. Anim. Prod. Adv.* **2012**, *2*, 214–220.
12. Soulsby, E.J.L. *Helminths, Arthropods and Protozoa of Domesticated Animals*, 7th ed.; Baillere Tindall: London, UK, 1986; pp. 593–614.
13. Zajac, A.M.; Conboy, G.A. *Veterinary Clinical Parasitology*; Blackwell Publishing: Malden, MA, USA, 2006.
14. Huang, G.; Zhang, S.; Zhou, C.; Tang, X.; Li, C.; Wang, C.; Tang, X.; Suo, J.; Jia, Y.; El-Ashram, S.; et al. Influence of *Eimeria falciformis* infection on Gut Microbiota and Metabolic Pathways in Mice. *Infect. Immun.* **2018**, *86*, e00073-18. [CrossRef]
15. Fichi, G.; Flamini, G.; Zaralli, L.; Perrucci, S. Efficacy of an essential oil of *Cinnamomum Zeylanicum* against *Psoroptes cunicul. Phytomedicine* **2007**, *14*, 227–231. [CrossRef] [PubMed]
16. Holt, J.G.; Krieg, N.R.; Sneath, P.H.; Staley, J.T.; Williams, S.T. *Bergey's Manual of Determinate Bacteriology*, 9th ed.; Williams and Wilkins: Baltimore, NY, USA, 1994.
17. ISO 6888-2:1999. *International Organization for Standardization. Microbiology of Food and Animal Feeding Stuffs—Horizontal Method for the Enumeration of Coagulase-Positive Staphylococci (Staphylococcus aureus and other species) e Part 2: Technique Using Rabbit Plasma Fibrinogen Agar Medium*; International Organization for Standardization: Geneva, Switzerland, 1999.
18. ISO 6579:2002. *International Organization for Standardization. Horizontal Method for the Detection of Salmonella spp. Microbiology of Food and Animal Feeding Stuffs*; International Organization for Standardization: Geneva, Switzerland, 2002.
19. Lee, M.; Arp, L. Colibacillosis. In *A Laboratory Manual for the Isolation and Identification of Avian Pathogens*, 4th ed.; Swayne, D.E., Ed.; American Association of Avian Pathologists: Jacksonville, FL, USA, 1998; pp. 14–16.
20. Soumet, C.; Ermel, G.; Rose, V.; Rose, N.; Drouin, P.; Salvat, G.; Colin, P. Identification by a multiplex PCR-based assay of *Salmonella typhimurium* and *Salmonella* enteritidis strains from environmental swabs of poultry houses. *Lett. Appl. Microbiol.* **1999**, *29*, 1–6. [CrossRef]
21. Ahmed, S.; Marai, I.F.M. Milk yield and litter traits of rabbits as affected by breed, parity, number of nipples, and aminazine injection, under Egyptian sub-tropical conditions. In Proceedings of the First International Conference for Animal Production and Health in Semi-Arid Area, El-Arish, Egypt, 5–9 December 1998.
22. Karu, P.; Muthusamy, P.; Gopi, H.; Balasubramanyam, D.; Babu, M. Survivability in New Zealand White breed of rabbits under farming condition in Tamilnadu. *Int. Sci. Environ. Technol.* **2014**, *3*, 1772–1777.
23. Mohammed, H.A.; Eid, A.A.M.; El-Bakrey, R.M.M. A review of rabbit diseases in Egypt. *Wartazoa* **2013**, *23*, 185–194. [CrossRef]

24. Drummond, H.; Vázquez, E.; Sánchez–Colón, S.; Martinez–Gómez, M.; Hudson, R. Competition for milk in the domestic rabbit: Survivors benefit from littermate deaths. *Ethology* **2000**, *106*, 511–526. [CrossRef]
25. Poigner, J.; Szendrộ, Z.; Lèvai, A.; Radnai, I.; Birό-Nemeth, E. Effect of birth weight and litter size at suckling age on reproductive performance in does as adults. *World Rabbit Sci.* **2000**, *8*, 103–109. [CrossRef]
26. Castellini, C.; Dal Bosco, A.; Mugnai, C. Comparison of different reproduction protocol for rabbit does: Effect of rabbit production in tropical and sub-tropical agricultural system. *J. Amin. Sci.* **2003**, *63*, 1581.
27. Bautista, A.; Mendoza-Degante, M.; Coureaud, G.; Martinez-Gómez, M.; Hudson, R. Scramble competition in newborn domestic rabbits for an unusually restricted milk supply. *Animal Behav.* **2005**, *70*, 1011–1021. [CrossRef]
28. Hudson, R.; Trillmich, F. Sibling competition and cooperation in mammals: Challenges, developments and prospects. *Behav. Ecol. Sociobiol.* **2008**, *62*, 299–307. [CrossRef]
29. Gotz, A.A.; Wolf, M.; Stefanski, V. Psychosocial maternal stress during pregnancy: Effects on reproduction for F0 and F1 generation laboratory rats. *Physiol. Behav.* **2008**, *93*, 1055–1060. [CrossRef]
30. Rodel, H.G.; Prager, G.; Stefanski, V.; von Holst, D.; Hudson, R. Separating maternal and litter size effects on early postnatal growth in two species of altricial mammals. *Physiol. Behav.* **2008**, *93*, 826–834. [CrossRef] [PubMed]
31. Bhatt, R.S.; Sharma, S.R.; Singh, U.; Kumar, D.; Bhasin, V. Effect of different season on the performance of grey giant rabbits under sub-temperate Himalayan conditions. *Asian-Australian J. Anim. Sci.* **2002**, *15*, 812–820. [CrossRef]
32. Kumar, D.; Singh, U.; Bhatt, R.S.; Risam, K.S. Reproductive efficiency of female German Angola under Indian sub- temperate climatic conditions. *World Rabbit Sci.* **2005**, *13*, 113–122.
33. Rodel, H.G.; Starkloff, A.; Bautista, A.; Friedrich, A.C.; von Holst, D. Infanticide and maternal offspring defence in European rabbits under natural breeding conditions. *Ethology* **2008**, *114*, 22–31. [CrossRef]
34. Rashwan, A.A.; Marai, I.F.M. Mortality in young rabbits: A review. *World Rabbit Sci.* **2000**, *8*, 111–124.
35. Rashed, E.A.O. Survey on Parasitic Diseases of Rabbits. Master Thesis, Zagazig University, Zagazig, Egypt, 1993.
36. Dagleish, M.P.; Ali, Q.; Powell, R.K.; Butz, D.; Woodford, M.H. Fetal *Sarcoptes scabiei* infection of blue sheep *(Pseudoisnayaur)* in Pakistan. *J. Wildl. Dis.* **2007**, *43*, 512–517. [CrossRef] [PubMed]
37. Bonanno, A.; Mazza, F.; Di Grigoli, A.; Alicata, M.L. Body condition score and related productive responses in rabbit does. In Proceedings of the 9th World Rabbit Congress, Verona, Italy, 10–13 June 2008.
38. Rodel, H.G.; Starkloff, A.; Seltmann, M.W.; Prager, G.; von Holst, D. Causes and predictors of nest mortality in a European rabbit population. *Mamm. Biol.* **2009**, *74*, 198–209. [CrossRef]
39. EL-Zemity, S.R.; Rezk, H.A.; Zaitoon, A.A. Acaricidal activity of some essential oils and their monoterpenoidal constituents against the parasitic Bee mites *Varroa destructor* (Acari: Varroidae). *J. Appl. Sci. Res.* **2006**, *2*, 1032–1036.
40. Rosell, J.M.; de la Fuente, L.F. Culling and mortality in breeding rabbits. *Prev. Vet. Med.* **2009**, *88*, 120–127. [CrossRef]
41. Sánchez, J.P.; de la Fuente, L.F.; Rosell, J.M. Health and body condition of lactating females on rabbit farms. *J. Anim. Sci.* **2012**, *90*, 2353–2361. [CrossRef]
42. Eid, A.A.M.; Ibraheem, O.K. Sudden death among rabbits in Sharkia Province, Egypt. *Zagazig Vet. J.* **2006**, *34*, 108–119.
43. Peeters, J.E. Recent advances in intestinal pathology of rabbits and further prespectives. In Proceedings of the 4th World Rabbit Congress, Toulouse, France, 9–12 July 1996.
44. Shahin, A.M.; Lebdah, M.A.; Ali, G.R.M. *Escherichia coli* as an etiological agent of mucoid enteropathy in rabbits. *Researcher* **2011**, *3*, 8–16.
45. Habeeb, A.A.M.; Marai, I.F.M.; El-Maghawry, A.M.; Gad, A.A. Growth rabbits as effected by salinity in drinking water under winter and hot summer conditions of Egypt. *Egyptian J. Rabbit Sci.* **1997**, *7*, 81–94.
46. Shehata, A.S.; Sarhan, M.A.; El-Gendy, K.M. Digestibility, thyroid function and growth performance of New Zealand White rabbits as affected by season of the year and age. *Egyptian J. Rabbit Sci.* **1998**, *8*, 141–156.
47. Fortun-Lamothe, L. Energy balance and reproductive performance in rabbit does. *Anim. Reprod. Sci.* **2006**, *93*, 1–15. [CrossRef] [PubMed]

2

Epidemiological and Histopathological Investigation of Sarcoptic Mange in Camels

Marwa A. Ahmed [1,†], Ehab Kotb Elmahallawy [2,3,*,†], Ahmed Gareh [4], Abdelbaset Eweda Abdelbaset [5,6], Fatma A. El-Gohary [7], Nagwa M. Elhawary [8], Ahmed K. Dyab [9], Elzahara Elbaz [10] and Mostafa F. N. Abushahba [11,12]

1 Department of Pathology, Faculty of Veterinary Medicine, Aswan University, Aswan 24101, Egypt; marwaahmed78@yahoo.com
2 Department of Biomedical Sciences, University of León (ULE), 24071 León, Spain
3 Department of Zoonoses, Faculty of Veterinary Medicine, Sohag University, Sohag 82524, Egypt
4 Department of Parasitology, Faculty of Veterinary Medicine, Aswan University, Aswan 24101, Egypt; ahmedgareh86@gmail.com
5 National Research Center for Protozoan Diseases, Obihiro University of Agriculture and Veterinary Medicine, Obihiro 080-8555, Japan; abdelbaset2006@hotmail.com
6 Clinical Laboratory Diagnosis, Department of Animal Medicine, Faculty of Veterinary Medicine, Assiut University, Assiut 71515, Egypt
7 Department of Hygiene and Zoonoses, Faculty of Veterinary Medicine, Mansoura University, Mansoura 35516, Egypt; dr.fatmagohary@gmail.com
8 Department of Parasitology, Faculty of Veterinary Medicine, Kafrelsheikh University, Kafr El Sheikh 33511, Egypt; nagwaelhawary@yahoo.com
9 Department of Parasitology, Faculty of Medicine, Assiut University, Assiut 71515, Egypt; ahmedsaf2001@yahoo.com
10 Department of Internal Medicine and Infectious Diseases, Faculty of Veterinary Medicine, Mansoura University, Mansoura 35516, Egypt; dr.alzhraa.6712@gmail.com
11 Department of Medicine, Division of Infectious Diseases, School of Medicine, Washington University, St. Louis, MO 63110, USA; mateya@aun.edu.eg
12 Department of Zoonosess, Faculty of Veterinary Medicine, Assiut University, Assiut 71515, Egypt
* Correspondence: eehaa@unileon.es
† These authors are contributed equally in the manuscript.

Simple Summary: Sarcoptic mange is an important zoonotic parasite affecting camel production. Mange zoonosis in camels is complicated by scarcity of available data. One of the main strategies for disease control is early detection of the parasite combined with prevention/control of the major risk factors associated with the infection. The present study focused on the prevalence of sarcoptic mange in camels from Egypt together with a histopathological examination of the parasite and association of the major risk factors, to describe the epidemiological pattern of the disease. Our data demonstrate that 47.6% of the camels harbored sarcoptic mange infections. In addition, the animals exhibited obvious clinical signs of mange and numerous histopathological findings that are consistent with sarcoptic mange. The camel's age, gender and sampling season were found to be the most significant risk factors associated with the disease. Taken together, our epidemiological and histopathological data are consistent with sarcoptic mange being widespread among camels in the studied area. Our study suggests further research is needed for management of this zoonotic disease in Egypt.

Abstract: Mange has been considered one of the most common parasitic infestations among camels. It adversely impacts animal productivity and poses a risk to human health. Given the scarcity of available data about mange in camels, the current study focused on the prevalence of camel mange and its associated risk factors in Aswan Governorate, Egypt. Towards this end, a general visual inspection was conducted on camels (N = 210) in different markets and slaughterhouses in Aswan Governorate.

Skin scrapings from suspect infected camels were also examined microscopically. Importantly, these findings were further checked and confirmed by histopathology on samples from suspected cases collected post-slaughter in abattoirs. The possible risk-associated factors, which include the camel's age, sex and sampling season, were recorded and statistically analyzed. Interestingly, the data showed that a total of 100 camels (47.6%) were found exclusively infested by sarcoptic mange. Furthermore, the predominant histopathological changes included burrowing tunnel of mites in the skin, hyperkeratosis and acanthosisconsis of the epidermis, while the dermis showed hemorrhage, mononuclear inflammatory cell infiltration around the blood vessels and perifolliculitis. These major histopathological findings are consistent with sarcoptic mange. Furthermore, the statistical analysis of the possible associated risk factors, camel's age ($p = 0.006$), gender ($p = 0.032$) and sampling season ($p = 0.004$), were all found to be significantly affected and related to the disease. In this regard, camels $\geq$2 years old were found at higher risk of infection (odds ratio (OR) = 2.75; 95% confidence interval (CI), 1.345 to 5.604) versus younger animals (OR = 0.36; 95 CI, 0.1784 to 0.743). Females had higher odds of exposure (OR = 2.02; 95% CI, 1.096 to 3.708) compared to males (OR = 0.50; 95% CI, 0.269 to 0.912). Moreover, the exposure to infection was reported higher in winter (OR = 2.30; 95% CI, 1.297 to 4.098) than in summer (OR = 0.43; 95% CI, 0.244 to 0.771). Collectively, our data provide novel epidemiological and histopathological support for sarcoptic mange being widespread among camels in the studied area. Sarcoptic mange is extremely contagious and zoonotic. Therefore, our baseline investigation indicates an urgent need for additional multicenter-studies to investigate the occurrence of this disease in camels and humans combined with the appropriate control measures of camel importation for combating this disease.

Keywords: camel; Egypt; histopathology; prevalence; sarcoptic mange; zoonosis

---

1. Introduction

The one-humped camel (*Camelus dromedarius*) or Arabian camel possesses a myriad of unique adaptive physiological and anatomical traits, making them an important component of the desert and non-desert ecosystems [1–3]. In addition, the use of camels in work and as a source of milk and meat has been drastically increased by Egyptians in the recent years [4]. In Egypt, camel production is practiced on a small scale and the country demands are met by importation, particularly from Sudan [5]. However, the economic impact of camel production is hampered by highly contagious and zoonotic diseases, inappropriate veterinary services and feed insufficiency [6,7]. Of particular concern, mange was found to be the second most common parasitic disease infesting camels, preceded only by trypanosomiasis, and its zoonotic potential has been documented in several studies [8–13]. Clearly, mange is considered a substantial infectious and debilitating skin disease affecting camels [13–15]. Importantly, sarcoptic mange is considered the most common identified mange in camels, while chorioptic mange is rare [13,14]. The causative agent of sarcoptic mange in camels is *Sarcoptes scabiei* var. *cameli*, which is a tiny rounded parasite, whereas the dimensions of the female and male is 330 to 600 μm × 250 to 400 μm and 200 to 240 μm × 150 to 200 μm, respectively [16,17]. Mange is tenacious and not susceptible to common chemicals, making eradication quite difficult [18]. Besides the contagious nature of sarcoptic mange, it is also significant from a zoonotic point of view [15,19,20]. Humans contract the infection through direct contact with infected animals while inter-animal transmission occurs through direct contact or via infected fomites, such as trees, rugs and luggage [21,22].

It should be stressed that sarcoptic mange in camels is recurrent, abrupt in onset and repeatedly starts on the medial parts of the thigh or inguinal area, the neck or the flanks [23]. Its incidence is regularly connected with hygienic practices and nutrition and, therefore, high infection risk has been recorded in in camels with reduced hygiene management or malnutrition [24]. In affected animals, the lesions gradually progress from pruritic nodules that lead to scratching and eventually render the skin hairless, crusty and wrinkled, especially on the thighs, hocks and axillae [25]. The clinical picture of sarcoptic mange in camels includes intense pruritus, exudative dermatitis, parakeratotic scaly crust formation, alopecia, and dark, thickened skin [24]. Fissures develop in the crust and underlying epidermis, resulting in hemorrhages. Emaciation, debilitation, anemia and subcutaneous edema are common signs of mange in camels [26]. During the development of mange, itchiness distracts the animals from eating so that they often become emaciated [26,27]. Given the fact that the Aswan Governorate is considered a primary station for imported camels in Egypt, as well as the veterinary and public health significance of camel mange, the current study was undertaken to explore the prevalence of the disease in camels and the associated risk factors. The present study represents an epidemiological overview about mange in camels in Egypt and provides novel data on this topic. The present work also involved studying the histopathological changes in camel skin due to sarcoptic mange as a confirmatory tool for verification of the parasitological and epidemiological findings.

2. Material and Methods

2.1. Ethical Considerations

The study protocol was carefully reviewed and approved by the local guidance body on Research, Publication and Ethics of the Faculty of Veterinary Medicine, Mansoura University, Egypt, which complies with all the relevant Egyptian laws.

2.2. Study Area and Animal Data

The present study was conducted on camels showing skin lesions in different regions in the body. Those animals were from different geographical areas (Idfu, Kawm-Umbo and Abu-Simbel) in Aswan Governorate, Egypt, between June 2019 and March 2020. Aswan Governorate is located in the southernmost part of Upper Egypt located close to the Sudanese border. Imported Sudanese camels are normally quarantined for 10–15 days in the Abu Simbel or Shelateen facilities in Aswan before their release to different markets and slaughterhouses. A total of 210 dromedary camels of different age and sex (60 females and 150 males) were recruited in this current study. These camels were primarily imported from Sudan for the purposes of work, breeding and/or slaughtering. Sampling was conducted during different seasons to record the seasonal variations of the disease in camels.

2.3. Collection of Skin Scrapings

Following a general visual inspection of the animals, the suspected camels with skin lesions were clinically scored according to a system previously applied to horses with chorioptic mange [28], as follows: 0: no clinical signs; 1: mild signs; 2: moderate signs; and 3: severe signs. For sample collection, suspected camels with cutaneous lesions were restrained properly and the hairs were clipped from the margins of the lesions with the help of scissors. After sterilization of the skin, profound skin scraping was completed in different body areas, including the head, neck, flanks, front and posterior limbs of the affected animals, with the aid of a scalpel blade [21]. In the slaughterhouses, deep skin scrapings from the ends of the examined lacerations of the slaughtered camels were collected in petri plates and transported to the parasitology laboratory at Assiut University for further processing and examination, which included additional parasitological and histopathological investigations [29].

2.4. Clincal Manfestations

The lesions observed on the examined camels were recorded and ranged from mild to severe and scored on a scale from 1 to 3. Skin samples from animals showing mild clinical signs were given a score of 1, which include localized alopecia, crusting, scaling or lichenification, thickening and corrugation of skin, scab formation, pruritic dermatitis and intense itching. In turn, moderate symptoms (a score of 2) were represented by extensive alopecia, crusting, scaling or lichenification with or without mild excoriation. On the other hand, severe signs (a score of 3) were observed as severe excoriations in addition to other signs, such as debilitation, anemia and subcutaneous edema.

2.5. Parasitological Examination

The parasitological examination of mange was done using a previously published protocol [30]. Briefly, the collected skin scraping was mixed with a small amount of 10% potassium hydroxide solution and heated till just boiling or left to stand for 0.5–1 h until the skin particles have partly disintegrated. Briefly, skin scrapings from the edges of the clinical lesions were collected in labeled Petri dishes, the edges of which were smeared with Vaseline so as to prevent the mites from escaping. The collected skin scrapings were transferred to test tubes and mixed with a small amount of 10% potassium hydroxide solution and heated till just boiling or left to stand for 0.5–1 h until the skin particles have partly disintegrated. The tubes were centrifuged at 3000 revolutions per minute. The supernatant fluid was discarded, and a drop of sediment was investigated under a stereoscopic microscope (Olympus, Life Science Solutions, Tokyo, Japan) for the detection of the various stages of sarcoptic mites and their eggs.

2.6. Histopathological Examination

Skin samples from different areas of the body with lesions (neck, forelegs, hind legs, back, flank and abdomen) were also collected from Dromedary camels (N = 20) slaughtered in abattoirs with suspicion of mange for diagnostic purposes. As shown in Table 1, out of those twenty samples randomly collected for the histopathological examination, four animals showed mild clinical signs and six camels showed moderate clinical signs; the remaining samples had severe clinical signs (N = 10). These randomly selected samples were fixed in 10% neutral buffered formaldehyde. Samples were then processed by sectioning where the paraffin-embedded tissues were sectioned to a 4–5 μm thickness. Sections were mounted on slides, stained by hematoxylin and eosin (H&E) and then examined under light microscopy for the presence of mange mites and any associated histopathological changes [31,32]. The resulting histopathological changes were then ranked according to their degree of severity into three categories: mild, moderate and severe histopathological findings, as described elsewhere [33].

Table 1. Macroscopic and microscopic scoring of infected camels.

Clinical Signs Score	Number of Infected Animals	Selective Samples for Histopathology	Score of Histology		
			Mild Lesions (1)	Moderate Lesions (2)	Sever Lesions (3)
Mild (1)	15	4	3	1	0
Moderate (2)	40	6	0	4	2
Severe (3)	45	10	0	2	8

2.7. Statistical Analysis

Fisher's exact tests and odds ratios with 95% confidence intervals (95% CI) were used in our study to analyze the impact of the different variables (age, sex and season) on the disease prevalence in camels. GraphPad Prism software (JMP, Cary, NC, USA) was used to compute the data. A p value < 0.05 was considered significant.

3. Results

3.1. Epidemological Data and Clinical Mainfestations

The present study showed that all camels are remarkably exposed to mange caused by sarcoptic mites. The prevalence of mange in the population of this study was 47.6% (100/210). The highest prevalence of mange was reported among animals of more than two years of age (52.7%). Furthermore, a higher infection rate (60%) was recorded in female camels compared to males. Additionally, the highest prevalence of mange was detected in the winter season (55.4%). Analysis of the results revealed statistically significant differences related to the age, sex and season categories of the studied camels ($p < 0.05$), which are shown in Table 2.

Table 2. Prevalence of camel mange adjusted for age, sex and season.

Variable		No. Examined	Positive No. (%)	Negative No. (%)	Odds Ratio (95% CI), *p* Value
Age	≤2 year	45	13 (29)	32 (71)	2.75 (1.34 to 5.60) $p = 0.006$
	>2 year	165	87 (52.7)	78 (47.3)	
Sex	Female	60	36 (60)	24 (40)	2.02 (1.10 to 3.71) $p = 0.032$
	Male	150	64 (42.7)	86 (57.3)	
Season	Summer	80	28 (35)	52 (65)	2.30 (1.30 to 4.10) $p = 0.0045$
	Winter	130	72 (55.4)	58 (44.6)	
Total		210	100 (47.6)	110 (52.4)	

In accordance with the clinical manifestations, the infected animals showed various clinical signs, which are reported in Figure 1. The skin of some affected camels often became discolored to a slate grey color. These lesions were distributed in various areas of the body, particularly the areas with thin skin, including the neck, abdomen, prepuce and flank. As result of the infection, some animals were emaciated and exhibited erythema and numerous small vesicles combined with itching and then scratching against hard objects, such as walls, leading to redness and scab formation in the affected areas. Out of 100 positive skin scrapings, 15 skin samples originated from animals showing mild clinical signs (a score of 1), 40 from animals with moderate signs and 45 from animals with severe signs.

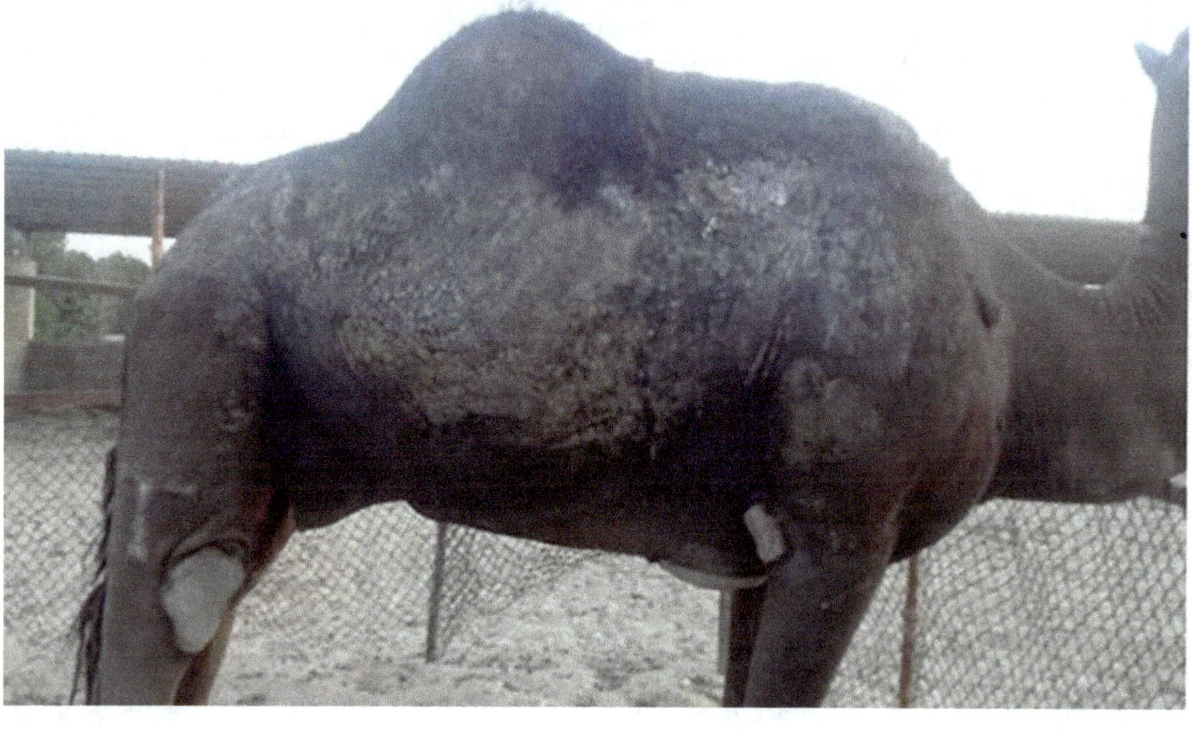

Figure 1. A camel showing some clinical manifestations of sarcoptic mange that includes multiple clinical signs, including thickening and corrugation of the skin, scab formation, pruritic dermatitis and hair loss.

3.2. *Parasitological Examination, Mange Prevalence and Risk Factors*

The parasitological examination revealed the presence of male and female mites, which are shown in Figure 2.

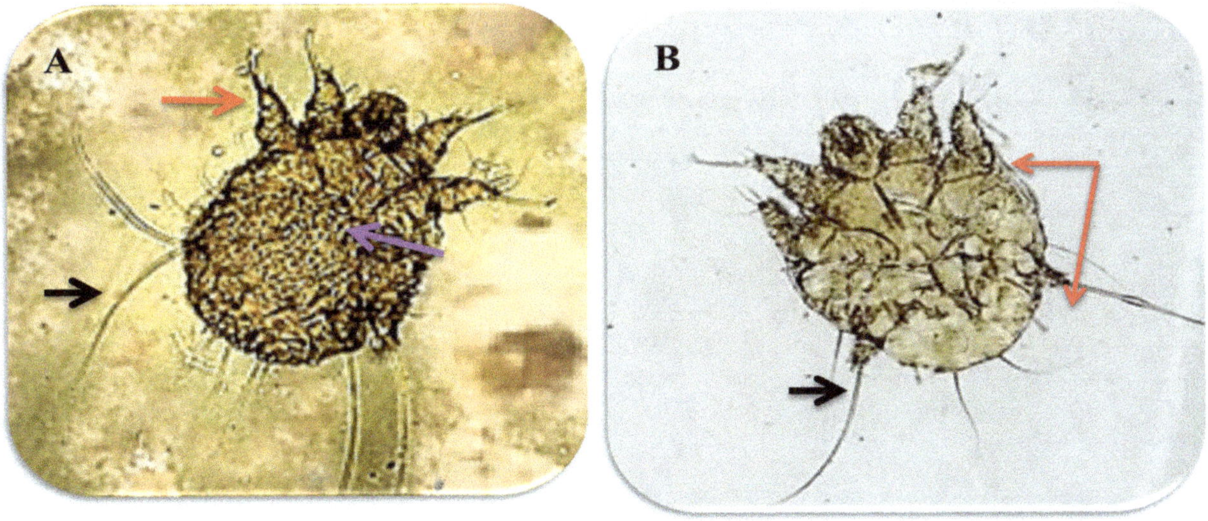

Figure 2. Male and female sarcoptic mange mites under 10× magnification: (**A**) *Sarcoptic scabiei* female, with transverse ridges and triangular scales on the dorsum (pink arrow). The 1st and 2nd pairs of legs ended with cup-shaped suckers (red arrow) while the 3rd and 4th ones ended with bristles (black arrow); (**B**) *Sarcoptic scabiei* male, with the 1st, 2nd and 4th pairs of legs ending with cup-shaped suckers (red arrow) and the 3rd pair ended with bristles (black arrow).

The prevalence of sarcoptic mange in the examined camels was 47.6% (100 out of 210). The mange mite infestation in dromedary camels was significantly affected by the animal's age, sex and season. Camels of age two or older were found to be at higher risk (OR = 2.75; 95% CI, 1.345 to 5.604) than those younger than 2 years (OR = 0.36; 95 CI, 0.1784 to 0.7435). Regarding gender, females were more affected than males with an odds ratio of exposure equal to 2.02 (95% CI, 1.096 to 3.708) and 0.50 (95% CI, 0.2697 to 0.9127), respectively. Moreover, a seasonal variability of the disease was observed and animals were found to be at higher risk in winter than in summer (Table 2).

3.3. *Histopathological Findings*

Interestingly, our present data reveals major histopathological findings that are consistent with sarcoptic mange. The microscopical examination of the affected animals demonstrated histopathological changes in the epidermis and dermis. As previously mentioned, these changes were scored into mild (a score of 1), moderate (a score of 2) and severe (a score of 3). In this regard, the collected samples from animals with severe clinical signs exhibited a score of 3 and were histopathologically represented by thickness in the epidermis, dense hyperkeratosis and acanthosis (Figure 3A,B). Meanwhile, Figure 3C depicts that skin of a camel exposed to the burrowing tunnels of the mites, inflammation and hemorrhage in the dermis, and these samples represent a score of 2 for those animals that showed moderate clinical signs. On the other hand, camels with mild clinical signs showed inflammatory cell infiltration on the dermis near the blood vessels and perifolliculitis that was classified as a score of 1 (Figure 3D). Taken together, the histopathology scoring seems to be consistent with the clinical signs that are shown in Table 1.

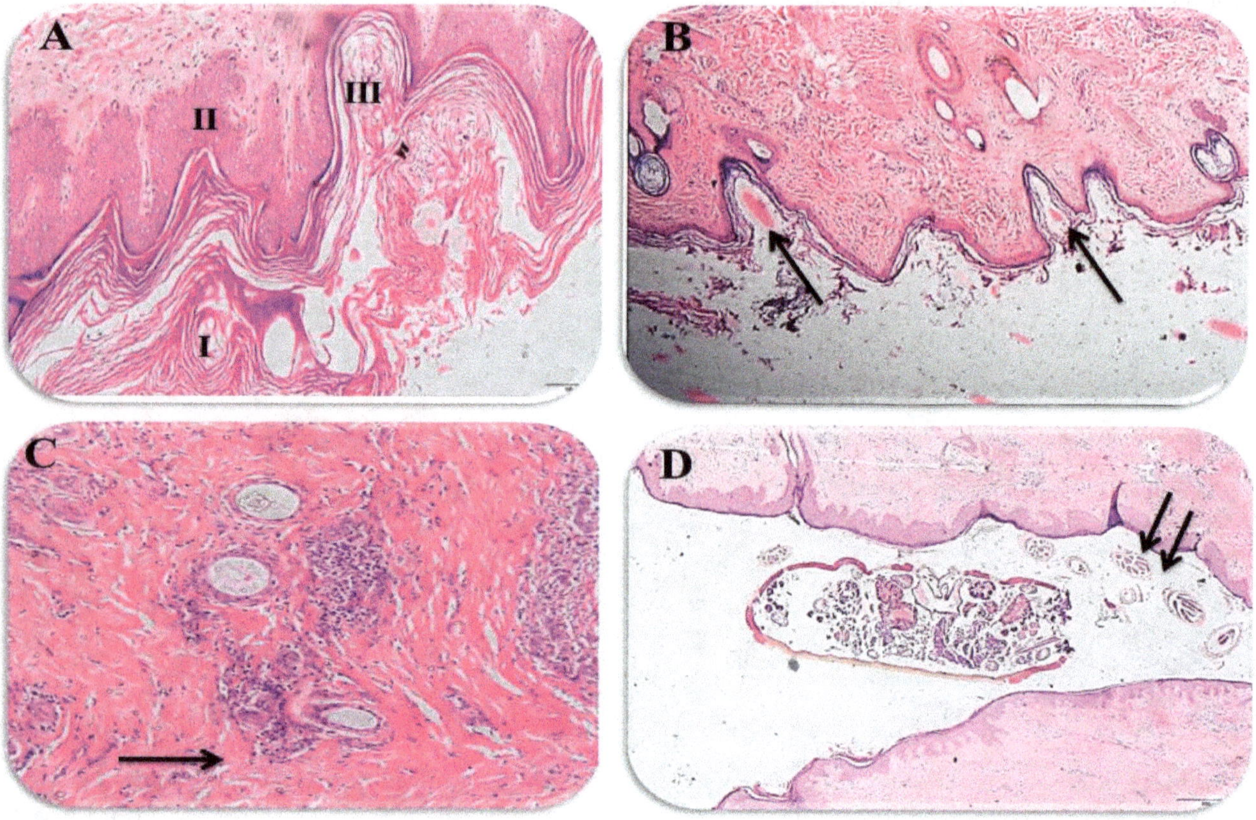

Figure 3. Histopathological findings for the infected camels: (**A**) the epidermis is thickened by compact hyperkeratosis (I) and acanthosis (II), which are in response to both the mite itself and also to the self-trauma caused by intense pruritus, and also shows the burrowing tunnels of the mites (III), ×100 magnification; (**B**) histological section showing *Sarcoptic scabiei* eggs in tunnels in the epidermis of an infested camel (arrow), ×200; (**C**) dermis showing inflammatory cell infiltration around the blood vessels and perifolliculitis (arrow), ×100; and (**D**) adult *Sarcoptic scabiei* and its eggs within the migrating tunnels of the camel skin (arrow), ×200.

4. Discussion

Despite its veterinary and zoonotic burden, camel mange research is minimal at the national and international level. Clearly, there is an obvious scarcity in the available data about the disease in Egypt, with the exception of one previous study in upper Egypt [29], making it difficult to set out the appropriate mange control measures. To the authors' knowledge, camels can be infected by sarcoptic and chorioptic mange mites [24]. However, it should be understood that sarcoptic mange, caused mainly by *Sarcoptes scabiei* var. *cameli*, is considered the most common type of mange in camels while chorioptic mange is relatively rare worldwide [13,14]. Besides being the most common and reported, sarcoptic mange has been considered an extremely contagious and serious zoonosis in camels [15,34]. Our work provides novel interesting data related to the high occurrence of sarcoptic mange in Egypt. Furthermore, our study investigated the major associated risk factors with the occurrence of mange combined with very interesting histopathological changes of the disease among the studied animals. The southernmost Aswan Governorate is considered the primary station of imported camels, which from there are further distributed to the entire country.

As shown in our results, the prevalence of mange mite infestation in the examined camels was 47.6%. Our study reports a higher prevalence than a previous study in Upper Egypt, which reported a mange prevalence of 6.06% among 660 examined one-humped camels [29]. Moreover, a lower prevalence rate of 25% was recorded among camels in Sudan [35]. In Ethiopia, prevalence rates of 16.7% and 35.4% were documented [23,36]. Furthermore, lower prevalence rates of 11.28% and 42.22%

were reported for camel mange in Pakistan [21,37]. On the other hand, our results are slightly lower than a previous study in Sudan where a prevalence rate of 55.2% was recorded for mange among camels [38]. The variation in the prevalence rate of our present study versus previous studies seems to be multifactorial in origin. The potential factors that could be attributed to the contagiousness of mange, besides other factors, are bad management practices in animal premises, inadequate veterinary care, and a lack of awareness among camel owners, which might also have contributed to the high infestation rate among the examined camels [7,39]. Tracking of the precise origin of the disease remains difficult due to the long incubation period of camel mange (2–3 weeks), and the imported Sudanese camels are quarantined in the Abu Simbel or Shelateen facilities only for 10–15 days before release to markets and slaughterhouses [40].

Among the analyzed variables in this study, age was found to be a significant factor affecting mange infestation in camels. Animals of more two years of age had a greater odds ratio of exposure than those of younger age. Similarly, older camels were found more susceptible to infection compared to younger ones in previous studies [21,36]. A previous study in sheep reported a higher prevalence of mange infestation in adult sheep compared to young ones [41]. However, a previous study reported an opposite conclusion related to the higher occurrence of the disease in younger camels than older ones [29,36]. Furthermore, our present results are not consistent with previous reports in domestic animals, such as cattle, and wild animals, such as Iberian wolves and cheetahs, that reported a higher prevalence in young animals [42]. Meanwhile, another previous study has stated that both very young and aged camels are mostly liable [43]. It is noteworthy to state the fact that young camels are usually kept indoors under intensive rearing while older ones participate in work and grazing that might justify the higher susceptibility of older animals than younger ones [35].

Gender was another significant risk factor in our present investigation, whereas females were at higher risk of being infested by mange compared to males. Our finding is consistent with a previous study in Pakistan [37]. Furthermore, the present results are similar to previous studies carried out in domestic and wild animals from Kenya [42]. It seems that the higher level of prolactin and progesterone hormones enhances the vulnerability of the females to any infection. Furthermore, pregnancy, lactation and the breeding behavior of mange-infected males may aggravate the problem and could be an additional risk factor [37]. In stark contrast, other previous reports recorded a higher prevalence of sarcoptic mange in males than females, as was reported in Egypt, Ethiopia and Sudan [29,35,36]. However, a previously published report detected a similar infestation rate of mange in male and female sheep [41]. Several studies documented the impact of seasonality on camel mange [12,23,24,29,37,43]. Among others, one study demonstrated that camel mange is more prevalent in summer than winter [43], while the remaining studies reported the opposite, a higher prevalence of mange in winter than summer, which is consistent with our present findings [21,23,29,37]. The explanation behind the seasonal variability was reported in the latter studies, where low temperatures combined with the overcrowding during the winter months were reported to provide favorable conditions for rapid propagation of the mite life cycle as well as easy spread between susceptible animals [44,45].

To the authors' knowledge, a histopathological examination of tissue biopsies is an important diagnostic tool for detection of various infectious agents in situ [46,47]. In our study, infection by camel mange was associated with certain histopathological changes that were scored into mild, moderate and severe degrees. Importantly, those histopathological changes were in the form of dermal hyperkeratosis (orthokeratosis and parakeratosis), epidermal hyperplasia, epidermal tunnels, creation of a crust and dermatitis, which is consistent with several previous reports [48]. Furthermore, the reported histopathological features in the current study are in agreement with previous studies regarding mange in various animal species [49,50]. Despite this consistency, discrepancies in severity and dispersal of the skin lesions were encountered even with animals of the same species, possibly due to the variation in immune responses between different animals [33]. It should be stressed that the histopathological changes triggered by mange mites in the examined camels are largely due to the parasite's burrowing behavior as well as the defensive response from the affected hosts [51]. Sarcoptic mange is widely known as burrowing mites that make tunnels in the skin of the infested host where they lay eggs and continue their lifecycle [52,53]. Along this course, an enormous aggregate of antigenic material is released in the skin, including dead mites, sloughed skin of the living adult and immature mites, and eggshells, leading to an increase the hypersensitivity to the mites [53,54]. Moreover, excavations on the skin, particularly those made by mature females, resulted in induction of thickening of the epidermis and crust formation [55], and these observations are consistent with our present findings. It is noteworthy to mention that the histopathologic findings in the present study were consistent with the macroscopic lesions, which is in agreement with a previously published report [33].

5. Conclusions

Given the above information, the present study demonstrates a high occurrence of sarcoptic mange infestation among camels in Aswan, Egypt, which is supported by the interesting histopathological data. Though underestimated, this could be associated with loss of productivity among the affected individuals and a zoonotic risk for camel traders, camel breeders and slaughterhouse workers. Clearly, it is of utmost importance to undergo periodical studies to track its prevalence in camels and contact people. The role of veterinary services is also important to advise farmers about the zoonotic importance of disease and to maintain their animals free from ectoparasites by keeping the animals under hygienic conditions. Further future investigation and a wide surveillance strategy seems warranted to explore this parasitic zoonosis in the entire country, which is crucial for combating this disease of public health concern.

Author Contributions: M.A.A., E.K.E., A.G., A.E.A., F.A.E.-G., N.M.E., E.E., A.K.D. and M.F.N.A. were involved in the conception of the research idea and methodology design, and performed the data analysis and interpretation; M.A.A., E.K.E., A.G., F.A.E.-G., N.M.E., E.E., A.K.D. and M.F.N.A. participated in the methodology, sampling, the laboratory work and data analysis, and prepared the manuscript for publication; E.K.E., A.G., M.F.N.A. and S.M.M. contributed their scientific advice, and prepared the manuscript for publication and revision. All authors have read and agreed to the published version of the manuscript.

Acknowledgments: The authors thank the veterinarians and farm owners for their support and help in providing data and samples collection throughout the study. Also, we would like to express our thanks to Jeffrey Adamovicz, University of Missouri-Columbia, USA, for his input and critical review of the manuscript.

References

1. Rabana, J.L.; Kumshe, H.A.; Kamani, J.; Hafsat, G.; Turaki, U.A.; Dilli, H.K. Effects of parasitic infections on erythrocyte indices of camels in Nigeria. *Vet. Res. Forum* **2011**, *2*, 59–63.
2. Momenah, M.A. Some blood parameters of one humped she-camels (Camelus 261 dromedaries) in response to parasitic infection. *Life Sci. J.* **2014**, *11*, 118–123.
3. Hoter, A.; Rizk, S.; Naim, H.Y. Cellular and molecular adaptation of arabian camel to heat stress. *Front. Genet.* **2019**, *10*, 588. [CrossRef] [PubMed]
4. Held, C. *Middle East Patterns, Student Economy Edition: Places, People, and Politics (Inglés)*, 6th ed.; Routledge: London, UK, 2015.
5. Ali, M.A.; Shehata, M.M.; Gomaa, M.R.; Kandeil, A.; El-Shesheny, R.; Kayed, A.S.; El-Taweel, A.N.; Atea, M.; Hassan, N.; Bagato, O.; et al. Systematic, active surveillance for Middle East respiratory syndrome coronavirus in camels in Egypt. *Emerg. Microbes Infect.* **2017**, *6*, e1. [CrossRef]
6. Megersa, B. *An Epidemiological Study of Major Camel Diseases in the Borana Lowland, Southern Ethiopia*; The Drylands Coordination Group: Oslo, Norway, 2010.
7. Lamuka, P.O.; Njeruh, F.M.; Gitao, G.C.; Abey, K.A. Camel health management and pastoralists' knowledge and information on zoonoses and food safety risks in Isiolo County, Kenya. *Pastoralism* **2017**, *7*, 20. [CrossRef]
8. Mochabo, K.O.; Kitala, P.M.; Gathura, P.B.; Ogara, W.O.; Catley, A.; Eregae, E.M.; Kaitho, T.D. Community perceptions of important camel diseases in Lapur Division of Turkana District, Kenya. *Trop. Anim. Health Prod.* **2005**, *37*, 187–204. [CrossRef]

9. Sazmand, A.; Joachim, A.; Otranto, D. Zoonotic parasites of dromedary camels: So important, so ignored. *Parasit Vectors* **2019**, *12*, 610. [CrossRef]
10. Tadjbakhsh, H. Traditional methods used for controlling animal diseases in Iran. *Rev. Sci Tech.* **1994**, *13*, 599–614. [CrossRef]
11. Muthusami, P.; Thangapandian, M.; Gopinath, P. Therapeutic management of sarcoptic mange in a camel (Camelus Dromedarius). *J. Wildl. Res.* **2015**, *3*, 5–7.
12. Feyera, T.; Admasu, P.; Abdilahi, Z.; Mummed, B. Epidemiological and therapeutic studies of camel mange in Fafan zone, Eastern Ethiopia. *Parasit Vectors* **2015**, *8*, 612. [CrossRef]
13. Parsani, H.R.; Momin, R.R. Common parasitic diseases of camel. *Vet. World* **2008**, *1*, 317–318. [CrossRef]
14. Higgins, A.J. Common ectoparasites of the camel and their control. *Br. Vet. J.* **1985**, *141*, 197–216. [CrossRef]
15. Timoney, P. Infectious diseases in camelids. *Vet. J.* **2002**, *164*, 300–301. [CrossRef]
16. Longstaffe, J. Helminths, arthropods and protozoa of domesticated animals EJL Soulsby, 1982. London: Baillière Tindall, 809 pp., illus. ISBN 0-7020-0820-6. *R. Soc. Trop. Med. Hyg.* **1984**. [CrossRef]
17. Higgins, A.J.; Al Mezaini, S.A.; Abukhamseen, A.M. Observations on the incidence and control of Sarcoptes scabiei var cameli in the Arabian camel. *Vet. Rec.* **1984**, *115*, 15–16. [CrossRef] [PubMed]
18. Bornstein, S. Important ectoparasites of Alpaca (Vicugna pacos). *Acta Vet. Scand.* **2010**, *52*, S17. [CrossRef]
19. Parmar, A.J.; Singh, V. Pathomorphological studies on sarcoptic mange in Camelus dromedarius in Banaskantha district. *J. Vet. Parasitol.* **2008**, *22*, 29–31.
20. Schillinger, D. Mange in camels-an important zoonosis. *Rec. Sci. Tech. Off. Int. Epiz.* **1987**, *6*, 479–480. [CrossRef]
21. Qamar, M.; Ayaz, M.; Nazir, M. Isolation and identification of ectoparasites in single humped camels (Camelus dromedarius) of Cholistan area, Pakistan. *Iraqi J. Vet. Sci.* **2019**, *32*, 291–297. [CrossRef]
22. Bandi, K.M.; Saikumar, C. Sarcoptic mange: A zoonotic ectoparasitic skin disease. *J. Clin. Diagn. Res.* **2013**, *7*, 156–157. [CrossRef]
23. Awol, N.; Kiros, S.; Tsegaye, Y.; Ali, M.; Hadush, B. Study on mange mite of camel in Raya-Azebo district, northern Ethiopia. *Vet. Res. Forum* **2014**, *5*, 61–64. [PubMed]
24. Zewdie, W.; Debano, J.; Sibhat, B. Review on Epidemiology of Camel Mange Mites. *Biomed. J. Sci. Tech. Res. (BJSTR)* **2018**, *8*, 6313–6316.
25. Abu-Samra, M.T.; Imbabi, S.E.; Mahgoub, E.S. Mange in domestic animals in the Sudan. *Ann. Trop. Med. Parasitol.* **1981**, *75*, 627–637. [CrossRef] [PubMed]
26. Fassi-Fehri, M. Diseases of camels. *Rev. Sci. Tech. Off. Int. Epiz* **1987**, *6*, 337–354.
27. Saleh, M.A.; Mahran, O.M.; Al-Salahy, M.B. Circulating oxidative stress status in dromedary camels infested with sarcoptic mange. *Vet. Res. Commun.* **2011**, *35*, 35–45. [CrossRef]
28. Rendle, D.; Cottle, H.; Love, S.; Hughes, K. Comparative study of doramectin and fipronil in the treatment of equine chorioptic mange. *Vet. Rec.* **2007**, *161*, 335–338. [CrossRef]
29. Kotb, S.; Abdel-Rady, A. Sarcoptic mange of camel in upper Egypt: Prevalence, risk assessment, and control measures. *J. Adv. Vet. Anim. Res.* **2015**, *2*, 410–417. [CrossRef]
30. Köhler-Rollefson, I.; Mundy, P.; Mathias, E. *A Field Manual of Camel Diseases; Traditional and Modern Health Care for the Dromedary*; Practical Action: Rugby, UK, 2001, p. 272.
31. Espinosa, J.; Raez-Bravo, A.; Lopez-Olvera, J.R.; Perez, J.M.; Lavin, S.; Tvarijonaviciute, A.; Cano-Manuel, F.J.; Fandos, P.; Soriguer, R.C.; Granados, J.E.; et al. Histopathology, microbiology and the inflammatory process associated with Sarcoptes scabiei infection in the Iberian ibex, Capra pyrenaica. *Parasit Vectors* **2017**, *10*, 596. [CrossRef]
32. Bancroft, J.D.; Gamble, M. *Theory and Practice of Histological Techniques*, 6th ed.; Elsevier; Churchill Livingstone: London, UK, 2008.
33. Nimmervoll, H.; Hoby, S.; Robert, N.; Lommano, E.; Welle, M.; Ryser-Degiorgis, M.-P. Pathology of sarcoptic mange in red foxes (vulpes vulpes): Macroscopic and histologic characterization of three disease stages. *J. Wildl. Dis.* **2013**, *49*, 91–102. [CrossRef]
34. Pegram, R.; Higgins, A. Camel ectoparasites: A review. In Proceedings of the first international camel conference, Dubai, UAE, 2–6 February 1992; Newmarket Press: London, UK, 1992.
35. Hakem, M.K.A.; Abu-Samra, M.T. Prevalence and Risk Factors Associated with Mange, Ringworm and Dermatophilus Infection in the One-Humped Camel (Camelus Dromedarius) in Al-Butana Area, El-Gazira

State. Master's Thesis, Sudan University of Science and Technology, Khartoum, Sudan, 2019. Available online: http://repository.sustech.edu/handle/123456789/23312 (accessed on 14 June 2020).

36. Regassa, A.; Awol, N.; Birhanu, H.; Redda, Y.; Teshale, S. Internal and external parasites of camels (Camelusdromedarius) slaughtered at Addis Ababa Abattoir, Ethiopia. *J. Vet. Med. Anim. Health* **2014**, *7*. [CrossRef]
37. Zahid, M.I.; Maqbool, A.; Anjum, S.; Ashraf, K.; Khan, M.; Ahmad, N. Prevalence of sarcoptic mange in camels in Punjab, Pakistan. *J. Anim. Plant. Sci.* **2015**, *25*, 1259–1263.
38. Nayel, N.M.; Abu-Samra, M.T. Sarcoptic mange in the one-humped camel (Camelus dromedarius): A clinico-pathological and epizootiological study of the disease and its treatment. *J. Arid Environ.* **1986**, *10*, 199–211. [CrossRef]
39. Farah, K.; Nyariki, D.; Ngugi, K.; Noor, I.M.; Guliye, A.Y. The somali and the camel: Ecology, management and economics. *Anthropologist* **2004**, *6*, 45–55. [CrossRef]
40. Kaufmann, J. *Parasitic Infections of Domestic Animals: A Diagnostic Manual*; Birkhäuser: Basel, Switzerland, 2013.
41. Geresu, M.; Deferes, D. Sheep mange mites and lice: Prevalence and risk factors in asella and its surroundings, South Eastern Ethiopia. *J. Vet. Sci. Technol.* **2016**, *7*, 1–6. [CrossRef]
42. Gakuya, F.; Ombui, J.; Maingi, N.; Muchemi, G.; Ogara, W.; Soriguer, R.C.; Alasaad, S. Sarcoptic mange and cheetah conservation in Masai Mara (Kenya): Epidemiological study in a wildlife/livestock system. *Parasitology* **2012**, *139*, 1587–1595. [CrossRef]
43. Khan, S.; Rashid Chaudhry, H.; Chaudhry, M.; Iqbal, Z.; Ali, M.; Jamil, T.; Sial, N.; Shahzad, M.i.; Basheer, F.; Akhtar, S.; et al. Prevalence of common diseases in camels of Cholistan Desert, Pakistan. *J. Infect. Mol. Biol.* **2014**, *2*, 49–52. [CrossRef]
44. Delano, M.L.; Mischler, S.A.; Underwood, W.J. Biology and diseases of ruminants: Sheep, goats, and cattle. *Lab. Anim. Med.* **2002**, 519–614. [CrossRef]
45. D'Amato, G.; Holgate, S.T.; Pawankar, R.; Ledford, D.K.; Cecchi, L.; Al-Ahmad, M.; Al-Enezi, F.; Al-Muhsen, S.; Ansotegui, I.; Baena-Cagnani, C.E.; et al. Meteorological conditions, climate change, new emerging factors, and asthma and related allergic disorders. A statement of the World Allergy Organization. *World Allergy Organ. J.* **2015**, *8*, 25. [CrossRef]
46. Gupta, E.; Bhalla, P.; Khurana, N.; Singh, T. Histopathology for the diagnosis of infectious diseases. *Indian J. Med. Microbiol.* **2009**, *27*, 100–106. [CrossRef]
47. Shieh, W.-J. Advanced pathology techniques for detecting emerging infectious disease pathogens. In *Advanced Techniques in Diagnostic Microbiology*; Springer: Berlin/Heidelberg, Germany, 2018; pp. 543–561.
48. Al-Salihi, K.; AbdHatem, A.; Ekman, E. Pathological studies on mixed dermatomycosis and mange infection in camels accompanied with chronic granulomatous hidradenitis. *J. Camel Pract. Res.* **2013**, *20*, 309–315.
49. Deem, S.L.; Noss, A.J.; Cuellar, R.L.; Villarroel, R.; Linn, M.J.; Forrester, D.J. Sarcoptic mange in free-ranging pampas foxes in the Gran Chaco, Bolivia. *J. Wildl. Dis.* **2002**, *38*, 625–628. [CrossRef] [PubMed]
50. Pence, D.; Ueckermann, E. Sarcoptic mange in wildlife. *Rev. Sci. Tech. Off. Int. Epizoot.* **2002**, *21*, 385–398. [CrossRef]
51. Arlian, L.G.; Morgan, M.S. A review of Sarcoptes scabiei: Past, present and future. *Parasites Vectors* **2017**, *10*, 297. [CrossRef] [PubMed]
52. Jimenez, M.D.; Bangs, E.E.; Sime, C.; Asher, V.J. Sarcoptic mange found in wolves in the Rocky Mountains in western United States. *J. Wildl. Dis.* **2010**, *46*, 1120–1125. [CrossRef] [PubMed]
53. Niedringhaus, K.D.; Brown, J.D.; Sweeley, K.M.; Yabsley, M.J. A review of sarcoptic mange in North American wildlife. *Int. J. Parasitol. Parasites Wildl.* **2019**, *9*, 285–297. [CrossRef]
54. Morgan, M.S.; Arlian, L.G.; Rider, S.D., Jr.; Grunwald, W.C., Jr.; Cool, D.R. A proteomic analysis of Sarcoptes scabiei (Acari: Sarcoptidae). *J. Med. Entomol.* **2016**, *53*, 553–561. [CrossRef]
55. Teodoro, T.G.W.; Lima, P.A.; Stehling, P.C.; Oliveira Junior, I.M.; Varaschin, M.S.; Wouters, F.; Wouters, A.T.B. Sarcoptic mange (Sarcoptes scabiei) in wild canids (Cerdocyon thous). *Pesqui. Veterinária Bras.* **2018**, *38*, 1444–1448. [CrossRef]

3

Zoonotic Viruses in Three Species of Voles

Maciej Grzybek [1,*,†], Katarzyna Tołkacz [2,3,†], Tarja Sironen [4], Sanna Mäki [4], Mohammed Alsarraf [2], Jolanta Behnke-Borowczyk [5], Beata Biernat [1], Joanna Nowicka [1], Antti Vaheri [4], Heikki Henttonen [6], Jerzy M. Behnke [7,‡] and Anna Bajer [2,‡]

1 Department of Tropical Parasitology, Institute of Maritime and Tropical Medicine, Medical University of Gdansk, Powstania Styczniowego 9B, 81-519 Gdynia, Poland; beata.biernat@gumed.edu.pl (B.B.); joanna.nowicka@gumed.edu.pl (J.N.)

2 Department of Eco-Epidemiology for Parasitic Diseases, Faculty of Biology, University of Warsaw, 1 Miecznikowa Str, 02-096 Warsaw, Poland; k.tolkacz@ibb.waw.pl (K.T.); muha@biol.uw.edu.pl (M.A.); anabena@biol.uw.edu.pl (A.B.)

3 Department of Antarctic Biology, Institute of Biochemistry and Biophysics, Polish Academy of Sciences, 5A Pawińskiego Str, 02-106 Warsaw, Poland

4 Department of Virology, University of Helsinki, Haartmaninkatu 3, 00014 Helsinki, Finland; tarja.sironen@helsinki.fi (T.S.); sanna.z.maki@helsinki.fi (S.M.); antti.vaheri@helsinki.fi (A.V.)

5 Department of Forest Pathology, Poznan University of Life Sciences, Wojska Polskiego 71c, 60-625 Poznan, Poland; jbehnke@up.poznan.pl

6 Natural Resources Institute Finland, Latokartanonkaari 9, 00790 Helsinki, Finland; ext.Heikki.Henttonen@luke.fi

7 School of Life Sciences, University of Nottingham, University Park, Nottingham NG7 2RD, UK; jerzy.behnke@nottingham.ac.uk

* Correspondence: maciej.grzybek@gumed.edu.pl.

† These authors contributed equally to this work.

‡ These authors contributed equally to this work.

Simple Summary: Wild rodents constitute a significant threat to public health. We tested 77 voles from northeastern Poland for the presence of antibodies to hantaviruses, arenaviruses and cowpox viruses. We report 18.2% overall seroprevalence of zoonotic viruses. Our results contribute to knowledge about the role of Polish voles as possible reservoirs of viral infections.

Abstract: Rodents are known to be reservoir hosts for a plethora of zoonotic viruses and therefore play a significant role in the dissemination of these pathogens. We trapped three vole species (*Microtus arvalis, Alexandromys oeconomus* and *Microtus agrestis*) in northeastern Poland, all of which are widely distributed species in Europe. Using immunofluorescence assays, we assessed serum samples for the presence of antibodies to hantaviruses, arenaviruses and cowpox viruses (CPXV). We detected antibodies against CPXV and Puumala hantavirus (PUUV), the overall seroprevalence of combined viral infections being 18.2% [10.5–29.3] and mostly attributed to CPXV. We detected only one PUUV/TULV cross-reaction in *Microtus arvalis* (1.3% [0.1–7.9]), but found similar levels of antibodies against CPXV in all three vole species. There were no significant differences in seroprevalence of CPXV among host species and age categories, nor between the sexes. These results contribute to our understanding of the distribution and abundance of CPXV in voles in Europe, and confirm that CPXV circulates also in *Microtus* and *Alexandromys* voles in northeastern Poland.

Keywords: arenavirus; hantavirus; LCMV; CPXV; PUUV; TULV; microtus; Alexandromys; vole; seroprevalence; Poland

1. Introduction

The identification of possible hosts, and the study of transmission dynamics in their populations, are both crucial steps in controlling zoonotic diseases [1,2]. Rodents, the most widespread and abundant mammals, are considered to be a significant source of zoonotic pathogens [1,3]. Studies of the population dynamics of wild rodents have demonstrated that European rodent populations experience multiannual and cyclic density fluctuations [4,5]. This has been linked with variation in the incidence of zoonoses spread by rodents [4,5].

Rodent-borne hanta-, mammarena- and orthopox viral pathogens are maintained in nature by direct intraspecies, or, as probably is the case with cowpox virus (CPXV), interspecies transmission from rodent to rodent without the participation of arthropod vectors. Transmission among rodents occurs by contact with body fluids or excretions [6–9].

The most prevalent rodent-borne viruses carried by European rodents include hantaviruses, the Mammarena lymphocytic choriomeningitis virus (LCMV), and the Orthopox CPXV [10–15]. The Puumala hantavirus (PUUV) is widely prevalent in bank vole (*Myodes glareolus*) populations [7,16]. Hantavirus infections in bank voles are chronic and therefore viral replication and shedding are persistent [9,17]. As a consequence, after being infected, the rodent host may be infectious for the rest of its lifespan [18].

CPXV is the only known wildlife-borne orthopox virus (OPV) in Europe [11]. Field voles (*Microtus agrestis)*, among other rodent species (i.e., *Apodemus sylvaticus* and *Myodes glareolus*), are known to act as reservoir hosts for CPXV [11,19,20]. LCMV, the only arenavirus in Europe, was thought to be prevalent in the house mouse (*Mus musculus*) [21]. However, further studies have revealed that the virus is present also in other murine and vole species [21–24]. Ledesma et al. [25] identified an independent genetic lineage of LCMV in wood mice and this led to the suggestion of spillover and the circulation of multiple related and cross-reactive Mammarena viruses.

In 2018, 29 European countries reported 1826 cases of hantavirus disease, mainly caused by Puumala virus [26]. The first outbreak of hantavirus infections in Poland was reported in 2007 when nine human cases were diagnosed, and was followed by a further 93 cases in the period 2014–2018 [26]. One human cowpox infection was reported in Poland in 2015 [27].

Voles (*Microtus* spp., *Myodes* spp. and *Alexandromys* spp.) are the most abundant rodents in European grasslands and forests [28]. This study aimed to evaluate zoonotic and potentially zoonotic viruses in populations of Microtus and Alexandromys spp. in northeastern Poland. Our results contribute to the understanding of the role of vole populations in the maintenance and dissemination of viral pathogens in this geographical region.

2. Materials and Methods

2.1. Ethical Approval

This study was carried out with due regard for the principles required by the European Union and the Polish Law on Animal Protection. Formal permits were obtained, allowing trapping in the field and subsequent laboratory analysis of sampled materials. Our project was approved by the First Warsaw Local Ethics Committee for Animal Experimentation (ethical license numbers: 148/2011 and 406/2013).

2.2. Collection of Voles

The study site was located in the Mazury Lake District region in the northeastern corner of Poland (Urwitałt, near Mikołajki; 53°48′50.25″N, 21°39′7.17″E) and previously described [29,30]. Voles were collected in August 2013 during the late summer season, when rodent population density is at its highest in the annual cycle. Voles were live-trapped using mixed bait comprising fruit (apple), vegetables (carrot and cucumber), and grain. Two traps were set every 10 m along the trap lines at dusk. The following morning traps were checked and closed to prevent animals from entering during daytime and to avoid losses from excessive heat from exposure of traps to direct sunlight. Traps were then re-baited and reset on the following afternoon. All traps were also closed during periods of intensive rainfall. All captured voles were transported in their traps to the laboratory for inspection.

The autopsies were carried out under terminal isoflurane anaesthesia. Animals were weighed to the nearest gram, total body length, and tail length were measured in millimetres. Animals were allocated to three age classes (juveniles, subadult, and adults), based on body weight and nose-to-anus length together with a reproductive condition (scrotal, semi-scrotal, or non-scrotal for males; lactating, pregnant or receptive for females) [29–32]. Recent reports suggest taxonomic changes within vole species [33]. Here, we refer to *Alexandromys oeconomus* (=*Microtus eoconomus*) following Lissovsky et al. [34] and Zorentko et al. [35]. We confirmed species identity by examination of the lower molars M_1 and M_2 and the second upper molar M^2, especially to distinguish between juvenile individuals of *A. oeconomus* and *M. agrestis* [36].

Blood samples were collected directly from the heart using a sterile 1.5 mL syringe immediately after death from over-exposure to Isoflurane (Baxter, Deerfield, IL, USA) anaesthetic. Samples were centrifuged at 5000 rpm for 10 min. Serum was collected and stored at −80 °C until the samples could be analyzed on completion of the fieldwork.

2.3. Serological Screening ofAnti-Virus Antibodies

Serum samples were analyzed using an immunofluorescence assay (IFA). The serum samples were diluted 1:10 in PBS and the reactivity of the samples to hantaviruses was tested with PUUV-(Puumala virus)-IFA, to cowpox viruses with CPXV (Cowpox virus)-IFA and arenaviruses with LCMV (Lymphocytic choriomeningitis virus)-IFA. PUUV (Sotkamo strain), CPXV, and LCMV (Armstrong strain)-infected Vero E6 cells were detached with trypsin, mixed with uninfected Vero E6 cells (in a ratio of 1:3), washed with PBS, spotted on IFA slides, air-dried, and fixed with acetone as described earlier [37]. The slides were stored at −70 °C until use. TULA orthohantavirus (TULV), specific for *Microtus* voles, is known to cross-react strongly with PUUV antibodies (and vice versa). Thus, we report it as PUUV/TULV seroprevalence.

IFAs were carried out as previously described [38] with seropositive human serum as a positive control for the PUUV- and CPXV-IFA; and LCMV mouse monoclonal antibody (Progen, Heidelberg, Germany) for the LCMV-IFA. The slides were read under a fluorescence microscope and photographs were taken with a ZOE™ fluorescent cell imager (BioRad, Hercules, CA, USA).

2.4. Statistical Analysis

Prevalence values (percentage of animals infected) are given with 95% confidence limits in parenthesis (CL_{95}) or error bars on figures, calculated by bespoke software based on the tables of Rohlf and Sokal [39].

The statistical approach has been documented comprehensively in our earlier publications [40–44]. For analysis of prevalence, we used maximum likelihood techniques based on log-linear analysis of contingency tables in the software package IBM SPSS Statistics Version 21 (IBM Corporation, Armonk, NY, USA).

3. Results

We screened a total of 77 *Microtus* and *Alexandromys* spp. serum samples for the presence of mammarena-, orthopox- and hantavirus antibodies. We confirmed the presence of antibodies against CPXV and PUUV/TULV. No individuals were seropositive for LCMV.

The overall seroprevalence of zoonotic viruses was 18.2% (10.5–29.3). Most of the seropositivity was for CPXV (16.9% [9.4–27.9]) with only one individual (*M. arvalis*) showing evidence of the presence of anti-hantaviral antibodies (1.3% [0.1–7.9]). Further analysis is therefore confined to the seroprevalence of CPXV.

CPXV antibodies were present in all three vole species. However, there were no significant differences between vole species (Figure 1A). Female voles had a marginally higher value for CPXV seroprevalence than males (18.2% [8.4–34.8] and 15.2% [7.0–28.7], respectively) (Figure 1B), but the difference between the sexes was not significant. There was no significant effect of host age on CPXV seroprevalence (Figure 1C).

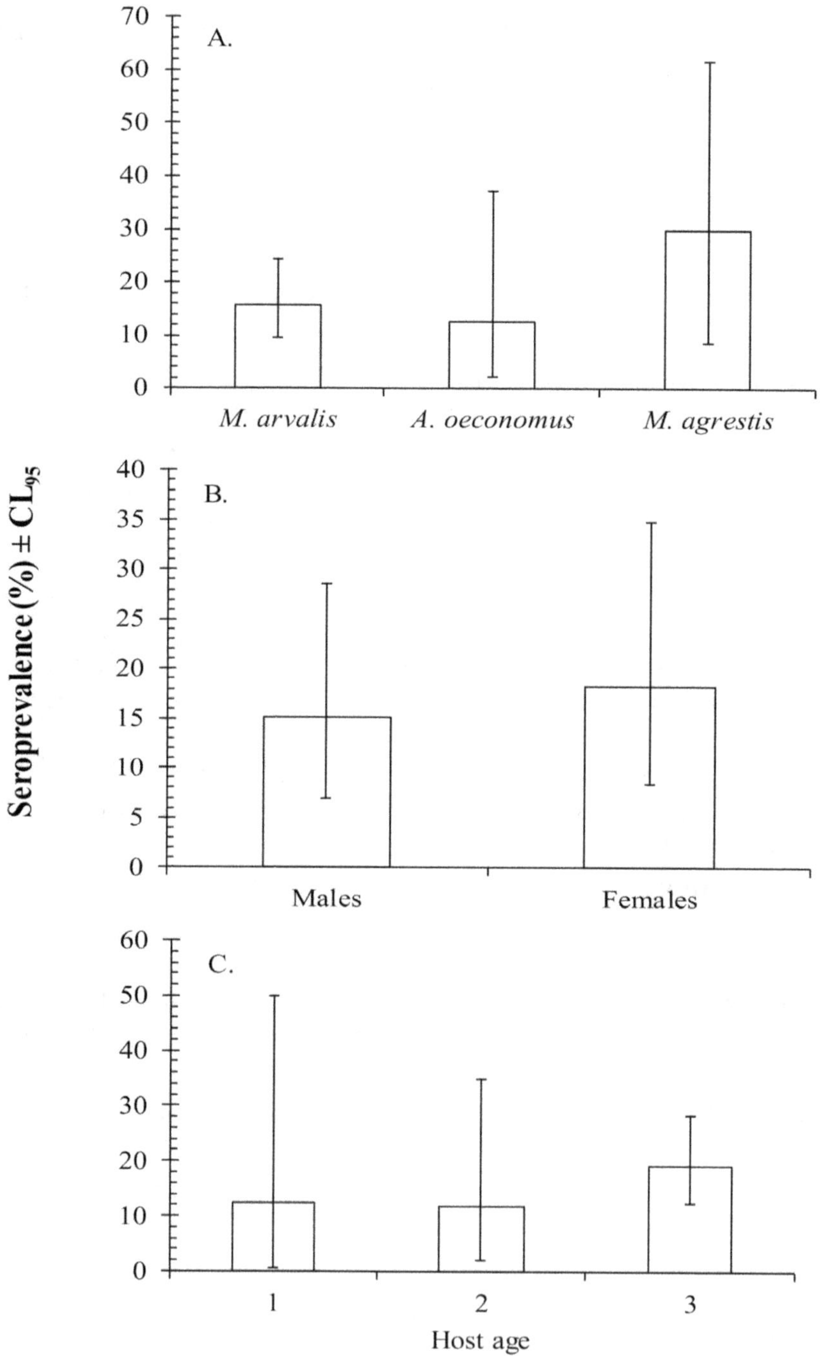

Figure 1. Seroprevalence of cowpox virus within: (**A**) three vole species; (**B**) host sex; (**C**) host age. Number of animals sampled: *Microtus arvalis* (n = 51); *Alexandromys oeconomus* (n = 16); *Microtus agrestis* (n = 10).

4. Discussion

We report a high overall seroprevalence of two common viral infections, mostly CPXV (18.2%) in voles from northeastern Poland. These findings are not only of considerable relevance to public health in the region but by inference are likely to have relevance also for other European regions populated by *Microtus* spp. High seroprevalence of CPXV is consistent with our report on seroprevalence of zoonotic viruses in bank voles (*M. glareolus*) from the same geographical region [14]. It is also in agreement with those obtained in different parts of Europe (e.g., Finland, England, and Turkey) where CPXV, PUUV, and TULV virus species have been detected in voles [22,45–51]. We did not detect any seropositivity to LCMV in the vole species we sampled, although LCMV has been found in other rodent populations (both mice and vole species) in different parts of Europe [21–23,38].

The current work was based on the presence/absence of specific antibody against viruses, and hence positivity in our assay reflected the history of previous infections and not necessarily current infection [41]. Serological tests may provide false positive results due to crossreactivity. This may be caused by the circulation of multiple related and cross-reactive arenaviruses and hantaviruses in rodents [52]. The "gold standard" for detection of zoonotic viruses in rodents should include serological and molecular approaches. Searching for antibodies followed by immunoblotting of spleen/lung tissues, and PCR/RT-PCR for detection of viral DNA/RNA may be applied [53,54]. However, this requires adequate types of samples (host tissues: spleen, lungs, brain), preservation methods (−80 °C), reagents (for RNA preservation), and increased field and laboratory workload [55]. Nevertheless, all these methods may still have limitations because of virus biology. For example, CPXV is a DNA virus with viremia lasting for 2–3 weeks, whereas hantaviruses and arenaviruses cause chronic infection. Therefore, the transmission dynamics of these viruses differ [47]. For the same reason, PCR identification of CPXV-positive individuals can create similar difficulties [11].

Intrinsic factors such as host age, maturity, and host sex may all influence the host's exposure and susceptibility to viral infections [14,40]. On this basis, we would have expected to find a higher seroprevalence among the older animals, which would have had more opportunity for exposure to, and hence experience of infection than juveniles, but the difference between the age classes in the current study was not significant.

In summary, we found serological evidence for the presence of CPXV in three vole species, and PUUV/TULV in a single *M. arvalis* vole, from wild vole populations in northeastern Poland. We believe that identifying rodent species that can serve as reservoirs of zoonotic diseases and predicting regions where new outbreaks are most likely to happen are crucial steps in preventing and minimising the extent of zoonotic diseases in humans [56]. Our results help to consolidate the gap in knowledge about the role of Polish voles as possible candidates for reservoirs of viral infections.

Author Contributions: Conceptualization, M.G., T.S., B.B. and J.M.B.; Data curation, K.T.; Formal analysis, M.G., H.H. and J.M.B.; Investigation, M.G., K.T., S.M., M.A., J.B.-B., J.N., A.V., J.M.B. and A.B.; Methodology, M.G., K.T., T.S., S.M., M.A., H.H., J.M.B. and A.B.; Project administration, K.T.; Supervision, T.S., A.V., J.M.B. and A.B.; Visualization, M.G.; Writing—original draft, M.G. and B.B.; Writing—review and editing, M.G., H.H., J.M.B. and A.B. All authors have read and agreed to the published version of the manuscript.

Acknowledgments: We thank the University of Nottingham, Warsaw University and the Medical University of Gdansk for financial support. M.G. thanks Alicja Rost and Ewa Zieliniewicz for their assistance in the laboratory. Special thanks to Francis S. Gilbert from the University of Nottingham, UK for sharing the statistical software.

References

1. Luis, A.D.; Hayman, D.T.S.; O'Shea, T.J.; Cryan, P.M.; Gilbert, A.T.; Pulliam, J.R.C.; Mills, J.N.; Timonin, M.E.; Willis, C.K.R.; Cunningham, A.A.; et al. A comparison of bats and rodents as reservoirs of zoonotic viruses: Are bats special? *Proc. R. Soc. B Biol. Sci.* **2013**, *280*, 20122753. [CrossRef] [PubMed]
2. Mills, J. Ecologic Studies of Rodent Reservoirs: Their Relevance for Human Health. *Emerg. Infect. Dis.* **1998**, *4*, 529–537. [CrossRef] [PubMed]
3. Bordes, F.; Blasdell, K.; Morand, S. Transmission ecology of rodent-borne diseases: New frontiers. *Integr. Zool.* **2015**, *10*, 424–435. [CrossRef] [PubMed]
4. Kallio, E.R.; Begon, M.; Henttonen, H.; Koskela, E.; Mappes, T.; Vaheri, A.; Vapalahti, O. Cyclic hantavirus epidemics in humans—Predicted by rodent host dynamics. *Epidemics* **2009**, *1*, 101–107. [CrossRef] [PubMed]
5. Olsson, G.E.; Hjertqvist, M.; Lundkvist, Å.; Hörnfeldt, B. Predicting High Risk for Human Hantavirus Infections, Sweden. *Emerg. Infect. Dis.* **2009**, *15*, 104–106. [CrossRef] [PubMed]
6. Carroll, K.; Hobden, J.; Miller, S.; Morse, S.; Mietzner, T.; Detrick, B.; Mitchell, T.; McKerrow, J.; Sakanari, J. Arthropod-Borne and Rodent-Borne Viral Diseases. In *Jawetz Melnick & Adelbergs Medical Microbiology*; McGraw-Hill: New York, NY, USA, 2015; ISBN 0071824987.
7. Vapalahti, O.; Mustonen, J.; Lundkvist, A.; Henttonen, H.; Plyusnin, A.; Vaheri, A. Hantavirus infections in Europe. *Lancet Infect. Dis.* **2003**, *3*, 653–661. [CrossRef]
8. Charrel, R.N.; de Lamballerie, X. Zoonotic aspects of arenavirus infections. *Vet. Microbiol.* **2010**, *140*, 213–220. [CrossRef]
9. Kallio, E.R.; Voutilainen, L.; Vapalahti, O.; Vaheri, A.; Henttonen, H.; Koskela, E.; Mappes, T. Endemic hantavirus infection impairs the winter survival of its rodent host. *Ecology* **2007**, *88*, 1911–1916. [CrossRef]
10. Kallio-Kokko, H.; Uzcategui, N.; Vapalahti, O.; Vaheri, A. Viral zoonoses in Europe. *FEMS Microbiol. Rev.* **2005**, *29*, 1051–1077. [CrossRef]
11. Kinnunen, P.M.; Henttonen, H.; Hoffmann, B.; Kallio, E.R.; Korthase, C.; Laakkonen, J.; Niemimaa, J.; Palva, A.; Schlegel, M.; Ali, H.S.; et al. Orthopox Virus Infections in Eurasian Wild Rodents. *Vector-Borne Zoonotic Dis.* **2011**, *11*, 1133–1140. [CrossRef]
12. Tonteri, E.; Kipar, A.; Voutilainen, L.; Vene, S.; Vaheri, A.; Vapalahti, O.; Lundkvist, Å. The three subtypes of tick-borne encephalitis virus induce encephalitis in a natural host, the bank vole (*Myodes glareolus*). *PLoS ONE* **2013**, *8*, e81214. [CrossRef] [PubMed]
13. Jääskeläinen, A.J.; Kolehmainen, P.; Voutilainen, L.; Hauffe, H.C.; Kallio-Kokko, H.; Lappalainen, M.; Tolf, C.; Lindberg, A.M.; Henttonen, H.; Vaheri, A.; et al. Evidence of Ljungan Virus specific antibodies in humans and rodents, Finland. *J. Med. Virol.* **2013**, *85*, 2001–2008. [CrossRef] [PubMed]
14. Grzybek, M.; Sironen, T.; Mäki, S.; Tołkacz, K.; Alsarraf, M.; Strachecka, A.; Paleolog, J.; Biernat, B.; Szczepaniak, K.; Behnke-Borowczyk, J.; et al. Zoonotic Virus Seroprevalence among Bank Voles, Poland, 2002–2010. *Emerg. Infect. Dis.* **2019**, *25*, 1607–1609. [CrossRef] [PubMed]
15. Goeijenbier, M.; Wagenaar, J.; Goris, M.; Martina, B.; Henttonen, H.; Vaheri, A.; Reusken, C.; Hartskeerl, R.; Osterhaus, A.; Van Gorp, E. Rodent-borne hemorrhagic fevers: Under-recognized, widely spread and preventable—Epidemiology, diagnostics and treatment. *Crit. Rev. Microbiol.* **2013**, *39*, 26–42. [CrossRef] [PubMed]
16. Brummer-Korvenkontio, M.; Henttonen, H.; Vaheri, A. Hemorrhagic fever with renal syndrome in Finland: Ecology and virology of nephropathia epidemica. *Scand. J. Infect. Dis. Suppl.* **1982**, *36*, 88–91.
17. Voutilainen, L.; Sironen, T.; Tonteri, E.; Bäck, A.T.; Razzauti, M.; Karlsson, M.; Wahlström, M.; Niemimaa, J.; Henttonen, H.; Lundkvist, Å. Life-long shedding of Puumala hantavirus in wild bank voles (*Myodes glareolus*). *J. Gen. Virol.* **2015**, *96*, 1238–1247. [CrossRef]
18. Meyer, B.J.; Schmaljohn, C.S. Persistent hantavirus infections: Characteristics and mechanisms. *Trends Microbiol.* **2000**, *8*, 61–67. [CrossRef]
19. Crouch, A.C.; Baxby, D.; Mccracken, C.M.; Gaskell, R.M.; Bennett, M. Serological evidence for the reservoir hosts of cowpox virus in British wildlife. *Epidemiol. Infect.* **1995**, *115*, 185–191. [CrossRef]
20. Chantrey, J.; Meyer, H.; Baxby, D.; Begon, M.; Bown, K.J.; Hazel, S.M.; Jones, T.; Montgomery, W.I.; Bennett, M. Cowpox: Reservoir hosts and geographic range. *Epidemiol. Infect.* **1999**, *122*, 455–460. [CrossRef]
21. Blasdell, K.R.; Becker, S.D.; Hurst, J.; Begon, M.; Bennett, M. Host Range and Genetic Diversity of Arenaviruses in Rodents, United Kingdom. *Emerg. Infect. Dis.* **2008**, *14*, 1455–1458. [CrossRef]

22. Laakkonen, J.; Kallio-Kokko, H.; Öktem, M.A.; Blasdell, K.; Plyusnina, A.; Niemimaa, J.; Karataş, A.; Plyusnin, A.; Vaheri, A.; Henttonen, H. Serological Survey for Viral Pathogens in Turkish Rodents. *J. Wildl. Dis.* **2006**, *42*, 672–676. [CrossRef] [PubMed]
23. Tagliapietra, V.; Rosà, R.; Hauffe, H.C.; Laakkonen, J.; Voutilainen, L.; Vapalahti, O.; Vaheri, A.; Henttonen, H.; Rizzoli, A. Spatial and temporal dynamics of lymphocytic choriomeningitis virus in wild rodents, northern Italy. *Emerg. Infect. Dis.* **2009**, *15*, 1019–1025. [CrossRef] [PubMed]
24. Kallio, E.R.; Klingström, J.; Gustafsson, E.; Manni, T.; Vaheri, A.; Henttonen, H.; Vapalahti, O.; Lundkvist, Å. Prolonged survival of Puumala hantavirus outside the host: Evidence for indirect transmission via the environment. *J. Gen. Virol.* **2006**, *87*, 2127–2134. [CrossRef] [PubMed]
25. Ledesma, J.; Fedele, C.G.; Carro, F.; Lledó, L.; Sánchez-Seco, M.P.; Tenorio, A.; Soriguer, R.C.; Saz, J.V.; Domínguez, G.; Rosas, M.F.; et al. Independent Lineage of Lymphocytic Choriomeningitis Virus in Wood Mice (*Apodemus sylvaticus*), Spain. *Emerg. Infect. Dis.* **2009**, *15*, 1677–1680. [CrossRef] [PubMed]
26. ECDC. Annual Epidemiological Report for 2018. Stockholm, 2020. Available online: https://www.ecdc.europa.eu/sites/default/files/documents/hantavirus-annual-epidemiological-report-2018.pdf (accessed on 7 August 2020).
27. Świtaj, K.; Kajfasz, P.; Kurth, A.; Nitsche, A. Cowpox after a cat scratch—case report from Poland. *Ann. Agric. Environ. Med.* **2015**, *22*, 456–458. [CrossRef]
28. Hanski, I.; Henttonen, H. Predation on Competing Rodent Species: A Simple Explanation of Complex Patterns. *J. Anim. Ecol.* **1996**, *65*, 220–232. [CrossRef]
29. Tołkacz, K.; Alsarraf, M.; Kowalec, M.; Dwużnik, D.; Grzybek, M.; Behnke, J.M.; Bajer, A. Bartonella infections in three species of Microtus: Prevalence and genetic diversity, vertical transmission and the effect of concurrent *Babesia microti* infection on its success. *Parasites Vectors* **2018**, *11*, 491. [CrossRef]
30. Tołkacz, K.; Bednarska, M.; Alsarraf, M.; Dwużnik, D.; Grzybek, M.; Welc-Faleçiak, R.; Behnke, J.M.; Bajer, A. Prevalence, genetic identity and vertical transmission of Babesia microti in three naturally infected species of vole, *Microtus* spp. (Cricetidae). *Parasites Vectors* **2017**, *10*, 1–12. [CrossRef]
31. Pawelczyk, A.; Bajer, A.; Behnke, J.M.; Gilbert, F.S.; Sinski, E. Factors affecting the component community structure of haemoparasites in common voles (*Microtus arvalis*) from the Mazury Lake District region of Poland. *Parasitol. Res.* **2004**, *92*, 270–284. [CrossRef]
32. Haukisalmi, V.; Henttonen, H.; Tenora, F. Population Dynamics of Common and Rare Helminths in Cyclic Vole Populations. *J. Anim. Ecol.* **1988**, *57*, 807–825. [CrossRef]
33. Bannikova, A.A.; Lebedev, V.S.; Lissovsky, A.A.; Matrosova, V.; Abramson, N.I.; Obolenskaya, E.V.; Tesakov, A.S. Molecular phylogeny and evolution of the Asian lineage of vole genus Microtus (Rodentia: Arvicolinae) inferred from mitochondrial cytochrome b sequence. *Biol. J. Linn. Soc.* **2010**, *99*, 595–613. [CrossRef]
34. Lissovsky, A.A.; Petrova, T.V.; Yatsentyuk, S.P.; Golenishchev, F.N.; Putincev, N.I.; Kartavtseva, I.V.; Sheremetyeva, I.N.; Abramson, N.I. Multilocus phylogeny and taxonomy of East Asian voles Alexandromys (Rodentia, Arvicolinae). *Zool. Scr.* **2018**, *47*, 9–20. [CrossRef]
35. Zorenko, T.A.; Atanasov, N.I. Copulatory behavior supports a new insight into taxonomic status of root vole Alexandromys oeconomus (Rodentia, Arvicolinae). *Russ. J. Theriol.* **2018**, *17*, 48–57. [CrossRef]
36. Pucek, Z. *Keys to Vertebrates of Poland. Mammals*; Polish Scientific Publishers: Warsaw, Poland, 1981; ISBN 8301025530 9788301025533.
37. Hedman, K.; Vaheri, A.; Brummer Korvenkontio, M. Rapid diagnosis of hantavirus disease with an IgG-avidity assay. *Lancet* **1991**, *338*, 1353–1356. [CrossRef]
38. Kallio-Kokko, H.; Laakkonen, J.; Rizzoli, A.; Tagliapietra, V.; Cattadori, I.; Perkins, S.E.; Hudson, P.J.; Cristofolini, A.; Versini, W.; Vapalahti, O.; et al. Hantavirus and arenavirus antibody prevalence in rodents and humans in Trentino, Northern Italy. *Epidemiol. Infect.* **2006**, *134*, 830–836. [CrossRef]
39. Sokal, R.R.; Rohlf, F.J. *Biometry: The Principles and Practices of Statistics in Biological Research*; W. H. Freeman: New York, NY, USA, 1994; ISBN 978-0716724117.
40. Grzybek, M.; Bajer, A.; Bednarska, M.M.; Al-Sarraf, M.; Behnke-Borowczyk, J.; Harris, P.D.; Price, S.J.; Brown, G.S.; Osborne, S.-J.; Siński, E.; et al. Long-term spatiotemporal stability and dynamic changes in helminth infracommunities of bank voles (*Myodes glareolus*) in NE Poland. *Parasitology* **2015**, *142*, 1722–1743. [CrossRef]

41. Grzybek, M.; Alsarraf, M.; Tołkacz, K.; Behnke-Borowczyk, J.; Biernat, B.; Stańczak, J.; Strachecka, A.; Guz, L.; Szczepaniak, K.; Paleolog, J.; et al. Seroprevalence of TBEV in bank voles from Poland—A long-term approach. *Emerg. Microbes Infect.* **2018**, *7*, 145. [CrossRef]
42. Behnke, J.M.; Barnard, C.J.; Bajer, A.; Bray, D.; Dinmore, J.; Frake, K.; Osmond, J.; Race, T.; Sinski, E. Variation in the helminth community structure in bank voles (*Clethrionomys glareolus*) from three comparable localities in the mazury lake istrict region of Poland. *Parasitology* **2001**, *123*, 401–414. [CrossRef]
43. Behnke, J.M.; Bajer, A.; Harris, P.D.; Newington, L.; Pidgeon, E.; Rowlands, G.; Sheriff, C.; Kuliś-Malkowska, K.; Siński, E.; Gilbert, F.S.; et al. Temporal and between-site variation in helminth communities of bank voles (*Myodes glareolus*) from N.E. Poland. 1. Regional fauna and component community levels. *Parasitology* **2008**, *135*, 985–997. [CrossRef]
44. Bajer, A.; Behnke, J.M.; Pawełczyk, A.; Kuliś, K.; Sereda, M.J.; Siński, E. Medium-term temporal stability of the helminth component community structure in bank voles (*Clethrionomys glareolus*) from the Mazury Lake District region of Poland. *Parasitology* **2005**, *130*, 213–228. [CrossRef]
45. Razzauti, M.; Plyusnina, A.; Sironen, T.; Henttonen, H.; Plyusnin, A. Analysis of Puumala hantavirus in a bank vole population in northern Finland: Evidence for co-circulation of two genetic lineages and frequent reassortment between strains. *J. Gen. Virol.* **2009**, *90*, 1923–1931. [CrossRef] [PubMed]
46. Thomason, A.G.; Begon, M.; Bradley, J.E.; Paterson, S.; Jackson, J.A. Endemic Hantavirus in Field Voles, Northern England. *Emerg. Infect. Dis.* **2017**, *23*, 1033–1035. [CrossRef] [PubMed]
47. Forbes, K.M.; Voutilainen, L.; Jääskeläinen, A.; Sironen, T.; Kinnunen, P.M.; Stuart, P.; Vapalahti, O.; Henttonen, H.; Huitu, O. Serological Survey of Rodent-Borne Viruses in Finnish Field Voles. *Vector-Borne Zoonotic Dis.* **2014**, *14*, 278–283. [CrossRef] [PubMed]
48. Schmidt-Chanasit, J.; Essbauer, S.; Petraityte, R.; Yoshimatsu, K.; Tackmann, K.; Conraths, F.J.; Sasnauskas, K.; Arikawa, J.; Thomas, A.; Pfeffer, M.; et al. Extensive Host Sharing of Central European Tula Virus. *J. Virol.* **2010**, *84*, 459–474. [CrossRef]
49. Olsson, G.E.; Leirs, H.; Henttonen, H. Hantaviruses and Their Hosts in Europe: Reservoirs Here and There, But Not Everywhere? *Vector-Borne Zoonotic Dis.* **2010**, *10*, 549–561. [CrossRef]
50. Vaheri, A.; Henttonen, H.; Voutilainen, L.; Mustonen, J.; Sironen, T.; Vapalahti, O. Hantavirus infections in Europe and their impact on public health. *Rev. Med. Virol.* **2013**, *23*, 35–49. [CrossRef]
51. Sironen, T.; Plyusnina, A.; Andersen, H.K.; Lodal, J.; Leirs, H.; Niemimaa, J.; Henttonen, H.; Vaheri, A.; Lundkvist, Å.; Plyusnin, A. Distribution of Puumala Hantavirus in Denmark: Analysis of Bank Voles (*Clethrionomys glareolus*) from Fyn and Jutland. *Vector-Borne Zoonotic Dis.* **2002**, *2*, 37–45. [CrossRef]
52. Vaheri, A.; Vapalahti, O.; Plyusnin, A. How to diagnose hantavirus infections and detect them in rodents and insectivores. *Rev. Med. Virol.* **2008**, *18*, 277–288. [CrossRef]
53. Vieth, S.; Drosten, C.; Lenz, O.; Vincent, M.; Omilabu, S.; Hass, M.; Becker-Ziaja, B.; ter Meulen, J.; Nichol, S.T.; Schmitz, H.; et al. RT-PCR assay for detection of Lassa virus and related Old World arenaviruses targeting the L gene. *Trans. R. Soc. Trop. Med. Hyg.* **2007**, *101*, 1253–1264. [CrossRef]
54. Jonsson, C.B.; Figueiredo, L.T.M.; Vapalahti, O. A Global Perspective on Hantavirus Ecology, Epidemiology, and Disease. *Clin. Microbiol. Rev.* **2010**, *23*, 412–441. [CrossRef]
55. Yee, J.; Wortman, I.A.; Nofchissey, R.A.; Goade, D.; Bennett, S.G.; Webb, J.P.; Irwin, W.; Hjelle, B. Rapid and simple method for screening wild rodents for antibodies to Sin Nombre hantavirus. *J. Wildl. Dis.* **2003**, *39*, 271–277. [CrossRef] [PubMed]
56. Han, B.A.; Schmidt, J.P.; Bowden, S.E.; Drake, J.M. Rodent reservoirs of future zoonotic diseases. *Proc. Natl. Acad. Sci. USA* **2015**, *112*, 7039–7044. [CrossRef] [PubMed]

4

High Exposure to *Toxoplasma gondii* and *Neospora* Spp. in Donkeys

Sharon Tirosh-Levy [1,2], Amir Steinman [1], Avital Minderigiu [1], Ori Arieli [1], Igor Savitski [2], Ludmila Fleiderovitz [2], Nir Edery [3], Gili Schvartz [1,4] and Monica Leszkowicz Mazuz [2,*]

1 Koret School of Veterinary Medicine, The Robert H. Smith Faculty of Agriculture, Food and Environment, The Hebrew University of Jerusalem, Rehovot 7610001, Israel; sharontirosh@gmail.com (S.T.-L.); amirst@savion.huji.ac.il (A.S.); avitalmind@gmail.com (A.M.); oriarieli6@gmail.com (O.A.); giliun@gmail.com (G.S.)
2 Division of Parasitology, Kimron Veterinary Institute, Bet Dagan 50250, Israel; igors@moag.gov.il (I.S.); ludaf@moag.gov.il (L.F.)
3 Division of Pathology, Kimron Veterinary Institute, Bet Dagan 50250, Israel; nire@moag.gov.il
4 Division of Virology, Kimron Veterinary Institute, Bet Dagan 50250, Israel
* Correspondence: monical@moag.gov.il.

Simple Summary: *Toxoplasma gondii* and *Neospora* spp. are major pathogenic parasites of animals worldwide, with the first also affecting humans. These parasites have two-host life cycles, with the cat and the dog being the definitive hosts of *T. gondii* and *N. caninum*, respectively. Both parasites can infect various animal species, as intermediate hosts, in which they form tissue cysts and may cause abortions and neurological disease. Both parasites have been reported in wild and domestic animals in Israel. This study aimed to evaluate the serologic exposure of donkeys to these parasites. A total of 98 donkeys were examined. Half of them ($n = 49$) were from animal shelters in Israel, and the rest ($n = 49$) were working donkeys from the Palestinian Authority. Anti-*T. gondii* antibodies and anti-*Neospora* spp. antibodies were found in 94% and in 70% of the donkeys, respectively. In addition, two cases of donkeys presenting *N. caninum* tissue cysts, which were detected during post-mortem examination, were described. This is the first report of the exposure of donkeys to *Toxoplasma gondii* and *Neospora* spp. in the area. The exposure of donkeys to both parasites was considerably higher than the exposure of other species in the area and may be the result of poor husbandry conditions and higher exposure to infection. These results indicate that donkeys may have an important role in the maintenance and transmission of these parasites.

Abstract: *Toxoplasma gondii* and *Neospora* spp. are closely related cyst-forming coccidian parasites, which infect various animal species and have considerable zoonotic and economic implications, respectively. Both parasites are endemic in Israel and have been reported to infect wild and domestic animals. This study was conceived to evaluate the serologic exposure of donkeys to these parasites. Serum samples were collected from 98 donkeys. Half of them ($n = 49$) were from animal shelters in Israel, and the rest ($n = 49$) were working donkeys from the Palestinian Authority. The donkeys were screened for the presence of anti-*Toxoplasma* and anti-*Neospora* antibodies by immunofluorescence antibody tests (IFATs). The seroprevalence of *T. gondii* and *Neospora* spp. was 94% and 70%, respectively, and 69% of the donkeys were exposed to both parasites. In addition, *N. caninum* tissue cysts were documented in two donkeys during post-mortem examination. This is the first report of the exposure of donkeys to *T. gondii* and *Neospora* spp. in the area. The high prevalence found in this study suggests that donkeys may have a role in the maintenance of these parasites in the area, thus serving as a source of infection for the definitive hosts.

Keywords: *Toxoplasma gondii*; *Neospora*; donkey; IFAT; serology

1. Introduction

Cyst-forming coccidian parasites, mainly *Toxoplasma gondii* and *Neospora* spp., are major pathogens of animals with worldwide distribution. These closely related apicomplexan intracellular parasites have heteroxenous life cycles, with felids being the definitive hosts of *T. gondii* and canids of *N. caninum*. Both parasites infect various mammalian species as intermediate hosts in which they form tissue cysts [1].

Toxoplasmosis may cause abortions, fetal damage or neurologic disease in a wide range of animals and humans. It is a prominent cause of abortion in sheep and a common zoonosis [1–4]. The clinical significance of *T. gondii* infection in horses is unclear. Nevertheless, horses may be exposed to or infected by the *T. gondii* parasite with no apparent clinical signs, and may pose a zoonotic risk through the consumption of infective horse or donkey meat [5–7]. In Israel, the seroprevalence of *T. gondii* was evaluated as 20–60% in humans [8], 25% in sheep [9], 36% in dogs [10], 17% in cats [11], 43% in crows, 40% in Griffon vultures [12] and 2.5% in horses [13].

Neosporosis causes abortion and neurologic disease in various animals. *Neospora caninum* is a major cause of abortion and economic loss in the cattle industry, and has been reported in horses [1,14]. *Neospora hughesi* is known to affect only equids and was isolated from cases of neurological disease in horses [14,15]. These two species are indistinguishable when using standard serological methods [16]. Horses may be infected with both parasites, and since most surveys were based on serology, the reported prevalence in horses and donkeys was of *Neospora* spp. In Israel, the seroprevalence of *Neospora* spp. was evaluated as 51% in cattle [17], 1.3–67% in wild animals [18] and 12% in horses [19]. The seroprevalence in aborting mares and cows was significantly higher than in the general population [17,19].

Domestic donkeys (*Equus africanus acinus*) in Israel are used as draught animals, riding animals, as pets and in petting zoos, and therefore are in close contact with humans. In other countries, donkeys are also used for their meat as food, and certain donkey-derived items are also important for traditional Chinese medicinal purposes [20]. Since donkeys are closely related to horses, they may be affected by similar pathogens. Exposure to both parasites has been reported in donkeys worldwide [5,6,21–27]. However, little is known about the role of donkeys in the epidemiology of these parasites. In Israel, data concerning the exposure of donkeys to infectious diseases are scarce. The aim of this study was to assess whether donkeys in Israel are exposed to *T. gondii* and *Neospora* spp. protozoan parasites, and to report two neosporosis cases of affected donkeys.

2. Materials and Methods

2.1. Sample Collection for Serological Survey

The sample size was calculated according to the prevalence of *Neospora* spp. in horses in Israel (12%) [19] using WinPepi 11.43®. A sample size of 77 donkeys met the criteria for an expected prevalence under 30%, with a relative error of ≤20% and 95% confidence level.

Since no data are available for estimating the distribution of donkeys in Israel, it was unfeasible to design a sample that would reliably represent the donkey population in the area. Therefore, donkeys were sampled at two donkey shelters in Israel that receive donkeys from different locations (49 donkeys), and at three locations in the Palestinian Authority (PA) to which working animals were brought to receive veterinary care given through a humanitarian association (49 donkeys).

Blood collections were performed with owners' consent, and the study was approved by the Internal Research Review Committee of the Koret School of Veterinary Medicine—Veterinary Teaching Hospital (KSVM-VTH/23_2014). Blood was collected from the jugular vein of each animal into a sterile vacuum tube without anticoagulant. Sera were obtained from the clotted blood samples by centrifugation (4000× *g* for 10 min) and stored at −20 °C until processing. During sample collection, data for each donkey were recorded including the farm's location, sex, age, and origin of the donkey, when available. At the time of sampling, all donkeys were apparently healthy according to both the owners and the veterinarians who collected the samples.

2.2. Serological Screening Using Immunofluorescence Antibody Test (IFAT)

Serological screening for the presence of anti-*T. gondii* antibodies was conducted on 1:2 serial dilutions of the sera, starting at 1:64 as a cut-off value for screening [28,29], up to a final dilution of 1:16,384.

Serological screening for the presence of anti-*Neospora* spp. antibodies was conducted on 1:2 serial dilutions of the sera, starting at 1:50 as a cut-off value for screening [19,25,29], up to a final dilution of 1:3200.

In-house antigens were prepared as previously described [30]. Briefly, free tachyzoites were obtained from an infected Vero cell culture, separated by centrifugation, diluted in phosphate buffered saline (PBS), dropped onto slides and stored at −80 °C until use. The slides were thawed at 37 °C for 30 min and air dried. The sera were diluted in PBS with 1% bovine serum albumin (BSA). A volume of 35 μL of serum was added to each antigen drop well and incubated in a humid chamber at 37 °C for 30 min. The slides were washed for 10 min in carbonate buffer (pH 9, diluted 1:4 in distilled water) before the application of 35 μL of anti-horse fluorescein isothiocyanate (FITC) secondary antibody (Sigma-Aldrich, St. Louis, MO, USA) diluted 1:80 with PBS–BSA, and incubation at 37 °C for 30 min in a humid chamber. The slides were later washed for 10 min in carbonate buffer, dried, mounted with glycerol/carbonate buffer (50%) and examined under a fluorescence microscope. Positive and negative control serum samples from positive horses were added to each run.

2.3. Statistical Analysis of Serology Results

Risk factors associated with exposure to either parasite or both parasites were assessed separately and included the farm, the geographical area (Israel versus the Palestinian Authority), the donkey's sex and age. Association with nominal independent variables was assessed by using the χ^2 test or Fisher's exact test, as appropriate, and odds ratios were calculated. Association with quantitative parameters was assessed using *t*-tests. Association between potential risk factors and antibody titer was assessed using ANOVA. Statistical significance was set at $p < 0.05$. The analysis was performed using the SPSS 22.0® and Win Pepi 11.43® statistical software.

2.4. Sample Collection, Histopathology and Polymerase Chain Reaction (PCR) of Clinical Samples

Skeletal muscle tissue from the triceps brachi muscle was collected from two donkeys (Donkeys 1 and 2) and was sent to the Kimron Veterinary Institute pathology department for post-mortem examination. Brain tissue was collected from one of these donkeys (Donkey 1), which was reported to have neurological signs prior to euthanasia, and stored at −20 °C until processing. Muscle tissue samples were transferred into 4% formaldehyde solution before the preparation of histological slides with hematoxylin and eosin (H&E) staining.

DNA was extracted from the paraffin-embedded muscle tissue dissolved in xylene and washed with PBS, using the DNeasy blood and tissue kit (QIAGEN, Hilden, Germany) according to the manufacturer's instructions. The presence of coccidian parasites was confirmed using PCR targeting the small-subunit rRNA (COC1 F: AAGTATAAGCTTTTATACGGCT, COC2 R: CACTGCCACGGTAGTCCAATAC), and the classification of the species was achieved by sequence- and species-specific PCRs targeting *Besnoitia besnoiti*, *Hammonidia*, *N. caninum*, *Sarcocystis* spp., *T. gondii* and *Trypanosoma* spp. (the primers and targets are specified in Table 1).

RNA was extracted from brain tissue, and the presence of West Nile virus (WNV) RNA was tested for and confirmed by real-time reverse transcription PCR (qRT-PCR) and further amplified and sequenced, as previously described [31].

Table 1. The PCR primers used to identify the coccidian species of the tissue cysts found in donkeys' muscle tissue.

Organism	Primer	Sequence	Amplicon Size (bp)	Target Gene	Reference
Besnoitia spp.	ITS1-F	TGACATTTAATAACAATCAACCCTT	250	ITS	[32]
	ITS1-R	GGTTTGTATTAACCAATCCGTGA			
	Bes-F	ATTGGGACCGTTTTGTGG		ITS	
	Bes-R	CCTCTCGAGGCTACAAGTCG			
	Bes-F2	CCTCCTCACTCTGCTATCACG	750	(nested)	
	Bes-R2	TTCCACTGGTAACGCCTCT			
Sarcocyst spp.	71-F	CGGATCGCATTATGACCTTT		18S rRNA	
	894-R	GGTGCAGGAGAAGTCAAGGA			
	317-F	ATTGGAATGATGGGAATCCA	300	(nested)	
	548-R	TGCCACCAACACAATGAAGT			
Toxoplasma gondii	Tox4	CGCTGCAGGGAGGAAGACGAAAG	500	Non-coding	[33]
	Tox5	CGCTGCAGACACAGTGCATCTGG			
Hammondia spp.	JS4	CGAAATGGGAAGTTTTGTGAAAC	270	ITS	[34]
	JS5	CAGCAGCTACATACGTAGA			
Neospora spp.	476-F	CTGCTGACGTGTCGTTGT		NC5	[35]
	1014-R	CATCTACCAGGCCGCTCTTC			
	631-F	GCGTCAGGGTGAGGACAGTG	279	(nested)	
	910-R	CTCTCCGTTCGCCAGCAGTG			
	ITS1D-F	TACCGATTGAGTGTTCCGGTG		ITS	[36]
	ITS1D-R	GCAATTCACATTGCGTTTCGC			
	ITS1Di-F	CGTAACAAGGTTTCCGTAGG	480	(nested)	
	ITS1Di-R	TTCATCGTTGCGCGAGCCAAG			
Trypanosoma spp.	ITS1	GATTACGTCCCTGCCATTTG		ITS	
	ITS2	TTGTTCGCTATCGGTCTTCC			
	ITS3	GGAAGCAAAAGTCGTAACAAGG	1200	(nested)	
	ITS4	TGTTTTCTTTTCCTCCGCTG			

All positive PCR products were sent for sequencing by HyLabs (Rehovot, Israel). Sequences were evaluated using the Chromas software (Technelysium Pty Ltd., Tewantin, QLD, Australia, version 2.6) and assembled using the MEGA7 software (http://www.megasoftware.net, version 7.0.18). Consensus sequences were created for each gene from both donkeys and were submitted to GenBank.

3. Results

3.1. Serologic Exposure to T. gondii and Neospora Spp. in Donkeys

The study population comprised donkeys from Israel ($n = 49$) and the Palestinian Authority ($n = 49$). Sixty of the donkeys were males (61%), and 38 were females (39%). Age was available for 70 of the donkeys and ranged between four months and 25 years (mean = 7.6 years, median = 7.0 years, standard deviation = 5.1 years). All donkeys were apparently healthy during blood collection.

Anti-*T. gondii* antibodies were detected in 92 of 98 donkeys (94%). The antibody titers ranged between 1:64 and 1:16,384 (Figure 1a), while high titers (≥1:256) were found in 66% of the animals. No significant risk factors for exposure were identified.

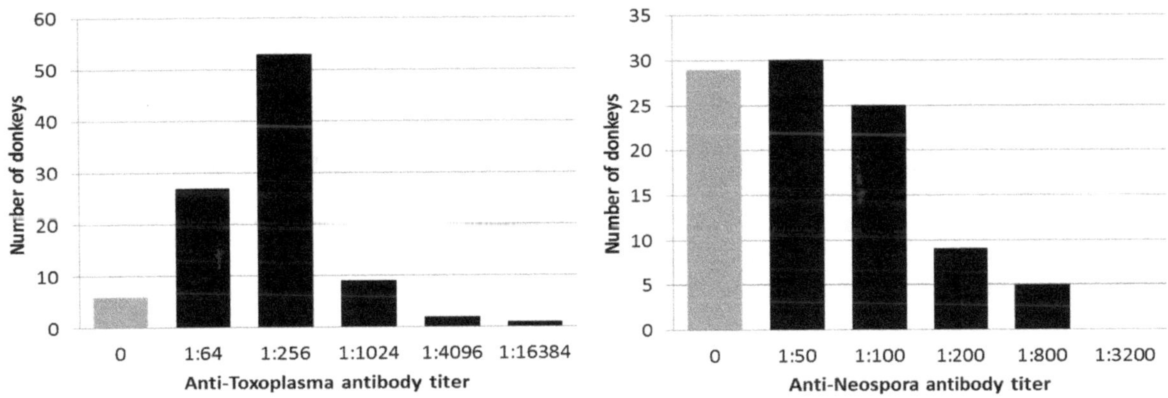

(a) (b)

Figure 1. The distribution of anti-*T. gondii* (**a**) and anti-*Neospora* spp. (**b**) antibody titers in 98 donkeys, as detected by immunofluorescence antibody tests (IFATs).

Anti-*Neospora* spp. antibodies were detected in 69 of 98 donkeys (70%). The antibody titers ranged between 1:50 and 1:800 (Figure 1b), while high titers (≥1:200) were found in 14% of the animals. No significant risk factors for exposure were identified. High antibody titers (≥1:200) were associated with one farm in Israel. In this farm, 10 out of 25 donkeys had high antibody titers, representing 71.4% (10 of 14) of the donkeys with high antibody titers ($p > 0.001$, odds ratio (OR) = 11.5, 95% confidence interval (CI) = 2.76–55.29).

The majority of donkeys (68/98, 69.4%) were exposed to both parasites. An additional 24 donkeys (24.5%) were exposed only to *Toxoplasma gondii*, one donkey (1%) was exposed only to *Neospora* spp., and five donkeys (5.1%) were not exposed to any of these parasites. No significant risk factors for co-exposure were identified.

3.2. Clinical Cases of Neosporosis in Donkeys

Parasitic tissue cysts were identified in the skeletal muscles of two donkeys sent for post-mortem examination (Figure 2). Both donkeys were sent from the same animal shelter. The first donkey (Donkey 1) was over 30 years old and presented with neurological signs and severe weakness before euthanasia. The second donkey (Donkey 2) was over 20 years old, and his left thoracic limb had been amputated several years prior to his death from unrelated causes. After his demise, the right thoracic limb was sent for evaluation for any potential effect of the amputation on the contralateral limb. The donkey that had presented with neurological signs (Donkey 1) was diagnosed as being infected with WNV after viral RNA was isolated and sequenced from its brain tissue (MT828577). In both donkeys, multifocal tissue cysts containing parasites were observed (Figure 2). *Neospora caninum* DNA was identified in the skeletal muscle tissue of both donkeys and was confirmed by the sequencing of two different species-specific target genes (NC5 (MT831977) and ITS1 (MT826198), over 97% homology with species-specific sequences in GenBank). Specific PCRs targeting *Besnoitia* spp., *Hammonidia*, *T. gondii*, *Neospora* spp., *Sarcocystis* spp., *T. gondii* and *Trypanosoma* spp. were negative, and the presence of these related cyst-forming parasites was ruled out.

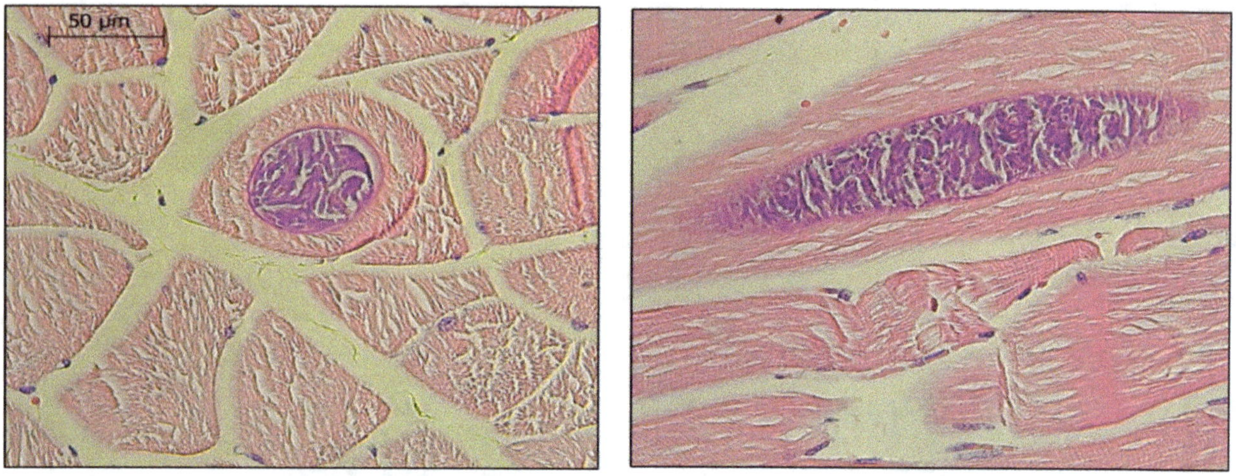

(a) (b)

Figure 2. *Neospora caninum* tissue cysts in the skeletal muscles of the front limb of Donkey 1: (**a**) transverse section; (**b**) longitudinal section. Giemsa, ×1000.

4. Discussion

The seroprevalence of both *T. gondii* and *N. caninum* in donkeys in Israel is high, and higher than the recorded prevalence in any other mammalian species in the area, including horses [13,18]. Donkeys in Israel are sometimes kept as burden animals, being more prevalent in Arab and Bedouin villages and often receiving little veterinary care, in comparison to horses. Half of the donkeys in this survey were sampled in animal shelters that receive neglected donkeys from various locations, while the other half were sampled in Arab villages in the Palestinian authority, by a veterinarian giving free veterinary care through a humanitarian organization. The high exposure to both parasites may be the result of the poor sanitation associated with low-income populations, which may increase the chance of exposure to oocysts in water sources or the environment. The association between low income and higher exposure to *T. gondii* has been previously described in humans and in horses [7,37,38]. In addition, in poor sanitary conditions, stray dogs and cats may have access to and feed on donkey carcasses, thus enhancing the maintenance and transmission of Neosporosis and Toxoplasmosis in these areas.

The seroprevalence of *T. gondii* in horses varies between countries and ranges between 1.2% in Sweden [39] and 71.2% in Iran [40]. The differences in prevalence may be associated with housing, stable hygiene and feeding practices [7,41]. The prevalence of *T. gondii* was higher in donkeys (72.7%) than in horses (27.7%) in a recent study from Brazil [42], as well as in other studies from Spain [23] and Pakistan [43]. However, since there are fewer studies evaluating both horses and donkeys in similar cohorts, it is difficult to determine whether these differences reflect a higher susceptibility of donkeys, or merely reflect differences in sanitation or management practices between these species. Since horses are considered to be naturally resistant to *T. gondii* infection [42], it is possible that they develop lower antibody titers that are not detected by serological tests.

In Israel, *T. gondii* seroprevalence was significantly higher in the Arab population (60.4%) than in Bedouins (27.5%) or Jews (19.9%) [8], and similar to the reported prevalence in Lebanon (62.2%) [44]. The seroprevalence was age-dependent and reached 96% in Arabs over 60 years of age [8].

The differences within ethnic groups in Israel may be attributable to a combination of economic status, exposure to animals and climate [8]. Since donkeys in Israel are more abundant in Arab settlements, the high seroprevalence may reflect similar conditions for exposure.

Although the consumption of donkey or horse meat is not common in this area, infection from contaminated meat is still a potential source for zoonotic transmission. Viable *T. gondii* parasites have been isolated from horse and donkey meat intended for human consumption worldwide [5,6,45–47], with a possible link to human disease [46].

In a recent study [48], an association between *T. gondii* seropositivity and the prevalence of impaired cognitive function was demonstrated in humans. Researchers theorize that behavior manipulation increases the parasite's likelihood of transmission by manipulating the host to engage in risky behaviors so that the host is likely to be preyed upon, particularly by a feline [48]. This was demonstrated in rats [49]. In this study, behavioral changes were not observed in any of the animals. To the best of our knowledge, behavioral changes have never been reported in equids in regard to *T. gondii* infection.

Neosporosis is not considered zoonotic, and its main impact is economic, mostly due to its effect on the reproduction of cattle and small ruminants, which are considered as the main intermediate hosts [14,50]. Therefore, fewer data are available regarding its prevalence in equines. In Israel, the prevalence in horses (12%) [19] was considerably lower than our findings in donkeys (70%). In neighboring Jordan, the reported seroprevalence in horses was 32% [51], and that in small ruminants was 63% [52]. Both dogs and donkeys often accompany small ruminant flocks in the Middle East, which may increase the chance of infection of both the primary and secondary hosts. In 1998, a new species of *Neospora*, *N. hughesi*, was identified in a horse from California [15]. Since then, *N. hughesi* has been reported only in horses and mostly from North America; however, since the two *Neospora* species are indistinguishable serologically, the global distribution of *N. hughesi* is unclear [14]. In the two cases of tissue cysts described here, parasites were classified as *N. caninum* based on two loci. In addition, *N. caninum* was identified in several cases of *Neospora*-induced abortion in mares in Israel (Mazuz et al., unpublished data), while *N. hughesi* has never been described in the area.

In horses, both toxoplasmosis and neosporosis had been associated with neurological disease, while neosporosis had also been described as a cause of abortions and neonatal disease [53,54]. However, reports of equine clinical cases are rare, and the majority of seropositive horses are asymptomatic. The clinical significance of high exposure to these parasites in donkeys is unclear. All donkeys in this study were apparently healthy, and to the best of our knowledge, clinical toxoplasmosis or neosporosis in donkeys has never been reported in Israel or elsewhere. Although one of the clinical cases in this report (Donkey 1) exhibited marked neurological signs, the cause of the neurological disease was determined as WNV, which is the most common cause of neurological disease in horses in the area [55]. Nevertheless, the identification of *N. caninum* tissue cysts in muscle specimens from two donkeys suggests that donkeys may be susceptible to clinical infection.

5. Conclusions

This is the first epidemiological survey investigating the exposure of donkeys to *T. gondii* and *N. caninum* in Israel. The high seroprevalence of both parasites in donkeys may reflect a high susceptibility of this species or high exposure due to poor husbandry conditions. The pathological findings of *N. caninum* tissue cysts in two donkeys suggest that donkeys may also be clinically infected and highlight the potential of donkeys to be a source of infection to other animal species. The higher exposure of donkeys in relation to other animal species in these areas suggests that donkeys could be used as sentinels to monitor exposure to these important, and potentially zoonotic, parasites.

Author Contributions: Conceptualization, A.S., M.L.M. and S.T.-L.; formal analysis, S.T.-L.; investigation, A.M., G.S., L.F., N.E. and I.S.; resources, S.T.-L., M.L.M., A.S. and O.A.; writing—original draft preparation, S.T.-L.; writing—review and editing, A.S. and M.L.M.; supervision, M.L.M. All authors have read and agreed to the published version of the manuscript.

Acknowledgments: The authors wish to thank the workers of the donkey shelters and the workers in the veterinary clinics in the Palestinian Authority for their assistance and collaboration.

References

1. Dubey, J.P.; Lindsay, D.S. Neosporosis, toxoplasmosis, and sarcocystosis in ruminants. *Vet. Clin. North. Am. Food Anim. Pract.* **2006**, *22*, 645–671. [CrossRef] [PubMed]
2. Benavides, J.; Fernandez, M.; Castano, P.; Ferreras, M.C.; Ortega-Mora, L.; Perez, V. Ovine toxoplasmosis: A new look at its pathogenesis. *J. Comp. Pathol.* **2017**, *157*, 34–38. [CrossRef] [PubMed]
3. Dubey, J.P. Toxoplasmosis in sheep-The last 20 years. *Vet. Parasitol.* **2009**, *163*, 1–14. [CrossRef]
4. Dubey, J.P. *Toxoplasmosis of Animals and Humans*; CRC Press: Boca Raton, FL, USA, 2016.
5. Alvarado-Esquivel, C.; Alvarado-Esquivel, D.; Dubey, J.P. Prevalence of *Toxoplasma gondii* antibodies in domestic donkeys (*Equus asinus*) in Durango, Mexico slaughtered for human consumption. *BMC Vet. Res.* **2015**, *11*, 6. [CrossRef]
6. Cong, W.; Chen, L.; Shan, X.F.; Qian, A.D.; Meng, Q.F. First genetic characterization of *Toxoplasma gondii* infection in donkey meat slaughtered for human consumption in Shandong province, eastern China. *Infect. Genet. Evol.* **2018**, *61*, 1–3. [CrossRef] [PubMed]
7. Li, X.; Ni, H.B.; Ren, W.X.; Jiang, J.; Gong, Q.L.; Zhang, X.X. Seroprevalence of *Toxoplasma gondii* in horses: A global systematic review and meta-analysis. *Acta Trop.* **2020**, *201*, 105222. [CrossRef] [PubMed]
8. Markovich, M.P.; Shohat, T.; Riklis, I.; Avni, R.; Yujelevski-Rozenblit, D.; Bassal, R.; Cohen, D.; Rorman, E. Seroepidemiology of *Toxoplasma gondii* infection in the Israeli population. *Epidemiol. Infect.* **2014**, *142*, 149–155. [CrossRef] [PubMed]
9. Shkap, V.; Pipano, E.; Marcus, S.; Rapoport, E. The prevalence of *Toxoplasma gondii* antibodies in sheep and cattle in Israel. *Isr. J. Vet. Med.* **1992**, *47*, 100.
10. Baneth, G.; Shkap, V.; Savitsky, I.; Pipano, E. The prevalence of antibodies to *Toxoplasma gondii* in dogs in Israel. *Isr. J. Vet. Med.* **1996**, *51*, 31–34.
11. Salant, H.; Spira, D.T. A cross-sectional survey of anti-*Toxoplasma gondii* antibodies in Jerusalem cats. *Vet. Parasitol.* **2004**, *124*, 167–177. [CrossRef]
12. Salant, H.; Hamburger, J.; King, R.; Baneth, G. *Toxoplasma gondii* prevalence in Israeli crows and Griffon vultures. *Vet. Parasitol.* **2013**, *191*, 23–28. [CrossRef]
13. Aharonson-Raz, K.; Baneth, G.; Lopes, A.P.; Brancal, H.; Schallig, H.; Cardoso, L.; Steinman, A. Low Seroprevalence of *Leishmania infantum* and *Toxoplasma gondii* in the Horse Population in Israel. *Vector Borne Zoonotic Dis.* **2015**, *15*, 726–731. [CrossRef]
14. Dubey, J.; Hemphill, A.; Calero-Bernal, R.; Schares, G. *Neosporosis in Animals*; CRC Press: Boca Raton, FL, USA, 2017.
15. Marsh, A.E.; Barr, B.C.; Packham, A.E.; Conrad, P.A. Description of a new *Neospora* species (Protozoa: Apicomplexa: Sarcocystidae). *J. Parasitol.* **1998**, *84*, 983–991. [CrossRef] [PubMed]
16. Marsh, A.E.; Howe, D.K.; Wang, G.; Barr, B.C.; Cannon, N.; Conrad, P.A. Differentiation of *Neospora hughesi* from *Neospora caninum* based on their immunodominant surface antigen, SAG1 and SRS2. *Int. J. Parasitol.* **1999**, *29*, 1575–1582. [CrossRef]
17. Mazuz, L.M.; Fish, L.; Molad, T.; Savitsky, I.; Wolkomirsky, R.; Leibovitz, B.; Shkap, V. *Neospora Caninum* as Causative-Pathogen of Abortion in Cattle. *Isr. J. Vet. Med.* **2011**, *66*, 14–18.
18. Mazuz, M.L.; Alvarez-Garcia, G.; King, R.; Savisky, I.; Shkap, V.; Ortega-Mora, L.M.; Gutierrez-Exposito, D. Exposure to *Neospora* spp. and *Besnoitia* spp. in wildlife from Israel. *Int. J. Parasitol. Parasites Wildl.* **2018**, *7*, 317–321. [CrossRef] [PubMed]
19. Kligler, E.B.; Shkap, V.; Baneth, G.; Mildenberg, Z.; Steinman, A. Seroprevalence of *Neospora* spp. among asymptomatic horses, aborted mares and horses demonstrating neurological signs in Israel. *Vet. Parasitol.* **2007**, *148*, 109–113. [CrossRef] [PubMed]
20. Bennett, R.; Pfuderer, S. The Potential for New Donkey Farming Systems to Supply the Growing Demand for Hides. *Animals* **2020**, *10*, 718. [CrossRef]
21. Cong, W.; Nie, L.B.; Qin, S.Y.; Wang, W.L.; Qian, A.D.; Meng, Q.F. Prevalence of *Neospora* spp. in donkeys in China. *Parasite* **2018**, *25*. [CrossRef]

22. Galvao, C.M.M.D.; Rezende-Gondim, M.M.; Chaves, A.C.R.; Schares, G.; Ribas, J.R.L.; Gondim, L.F.P. Brazilian donkeys (*Equus asinus*) have a low exposure to *Neospora* spp. *Rev. Bras. Parasitol.* **2015**, *24*, 340–344. [CrossRef] [PubMed]
23. Garcia-Bocanegra, I.; Cabezon, O.; Arenas-Montes, A.; Carbonero, A.; Dubey, J.P.; Perea, A.; Almeria, S. Seroprevalence of *Toxoplasma gondii* in equids from Southern Spain. *Parasitol. Int.* **2012**, *61*, 421–424. [CrossRef]
24. Gennari, S.M.; Esmerini, P.D.; Lopes, M.G.; Soares, H.S.; Vitaliano, S.N.; Cabral, A.D.; Pena, H.F.J.; Horta, M.C.; Cavalcante, P.H.; Fortes, K.P.; et al. Occurrence of antibodies against *Toxoplasma gondii* and its isolation and genotyping in donkeys, mules, and horses in Brazil. *Vet. Parasitol.* **2015**, *209*, 129–132. [CrossRef] [PubMed]
25. Gennari, S.M.; Pena, H.F.D.; Lindsay, D.S.; Lopes, M.G.; Soares, H.S.; Cabral, A.D.; Vitaliano, S.N.; Amaku, M. Prevalence of antibodies against *Neospora* spp. and *Sarcocystis neurona* in donkeys from northeastern Brazil. *Rev. Bras. Parasitol.* **2016**, *25*, 109–111. [CrossRef] [PubMed]
26. Machacova, T.; Bartova, E.; Di Loria, A.; Sedlak, K.; Guccione, J.; Fulgione, D.; Veneziano, V. Seroprevalence and risk factors of *Neospora* spp. in donkeys from Southern Italy. *Vet. Parasitol.* **2013**, *198*, 201–204. [CrossRef] [PubMed]
27. Nazir, M.M.; Ayaz, M.M.; Ahmed, A.N.; Rasheed, I.; Faraz, A.; Akram, Q.; Althtar, S.; Maqbool, A.; Tabassum, S.; Zheng, Y.D.; et al. Prevalence and risk factors for IgG antibodies to *Neospora* spp. in three types of equids from Southern Punjab, Pakistan. *Acta Trop.* **2018**, *188*, 240–243. [CrossRef] [PubMed]
28. Dubey, J.P.; Murata, F.H.A.; Cerqueira-Cezar, C.K.; Kwok, O.C.H. *Toxoplasma gondii* infections in horses, donkeys, and other equids: The last decade. *Res. Vet. Sci.* **2020**, *132*, 492–499. [CrossRef]
29. Moreira, T.R.; Sarturi, C.; Stelmachtchuk, F.N.; Andersson, E.; Norlander, E.; de Oliveira, F.L.C.; Machado Portela, J.; Marcili, A.; Emanuelson, U.; Gennari, S.M.; et al. Prevalence of antibodies against *Toxoplasma gondii* and *Neospora* spp. in equids of Western Para, Brazil. *Acta Trop.* **2019**, *189*, 39–45. [CrossRef]
30. Shkap, V.; Reske, A.; Pipano, E.; Fish, L.; Baszler, T. Immunological relationship *between Neospora caninum* and *Besnoitia besnoiti*. *Vet. Parasitol.* **2002**, *106*, 35–43. [CrossRef]
31. Schvartz, G.; Farnoushi, Y.; Berkowitz, A.; Edery, N.; Hann, S.; Steinman, A.; Lublin, A.; Erster, O. Molecular characterization of the re-emerging *West Nile Virus* in avian species and equids in Israel, and pathological description of the disease. *Parasit. Vectors* **2018**, in press.
32. Cortes, H.C.; Reis, Y.; Gottstein, B.; Hemphill, A.; Leitao, A.; Muller, N. Application of conventional and real-time fluorescent ITS1 rDNA PCR for detection of *Besnoitia besnoiti* infections in bovine skin biopsies. *Vet. Parasitol.* **2007**, *146*, 352–356. [CrossRef]
33. Homan, W.L.; Vercammen, M.; De Braekeleer, J.; Verschueren, H. Identification of a 200- to 300-fold repetitive 529 bp DNA fragment in *Toxoplasma gondii*, and its use for diagnostic and quantitative PCR. *Int. J. Parasitol.* **2000**, *30*, 69–75. [CrossRef]
34. Slapeta, J.R.; Koudela, B.; Votypka, J.; Modry, D.; Horejs, R.; Lukes, J. Coprodiagnosis of *Hammondia heydorni* in dogs by PCR based amplification of ITS 1 rRNA: Differentiation from morphologically indistinguishable oocysts of *Neospora caninum*. *Vet. J.* **2002**, *163*, 147–154. [CrossRef] [PubMed]
35. Fish, L.; Mazuz, M.; Molad, T.; Savitsky, I.; Shkap, V. Isolation of *Neospora caninum* from dairy zero grazing cattle in Israel. *Vet. Parasitol.* **2007**, *149*, 167–171. [CrossRef] [PubMed]
36. Wobeser, B.K.; Godson, D.L.; Rejmanek, D.; Dowling, P. Equine protozoal myeloencephalitis caused by *Neospora hughesi* in an adult horse in Saskatchewan. *Can. Vet. J.* **2009**, *50*, 851–853. [PubMed]
37. Rostami, A.; Riahi, S.M.; Contopoulos-Ioannidis, D.G.; Gamble, H.R.; Fakhri, Y.; Shiadeh, M.N.; Foroutan, M.; Behniafar, H.; Taghipour, A.; Maldonado, Y.A.; et al. Acute *Toxoplasma* infection in pregnant women worldwide: A systematic review and meta-analysis. *PLoS Negl. Trop. Dis.* **2019**, *13*, e0007807. [CrossRef] [PubMed]
38. Rostami, A.; Riahi, S.M.; Gamble, H.R.; Fakhri, Y.; Nourollahpour Shiadeh, M.; Danesh, M.; Behniafar, H.; Paktinat, S.; Foroutan, M.; Mokdad, A.H.; et al. Global prevalence of latent toxoplasmosis in pregnant women: A systematic review and meta-analysis. *Clin. Microbiol. Infect.* **2020**, *26*, 673–683. [CrossRef] [PubMed]
39. Jakubek, E.B.; Lunden, A.; Uggla, A. Seroprevalences of *Toxoplasma gondii* and *Neospora* sp. infections in Swedish horses. *Vet. Parasitol.* **2006**, *138*, 194–199. [CrossRef] [PubMed]
40. Hajialilo, E.; Ziaali, N.; Harandi, M.F.; Saraei, M.; Hajialilo, M. Prevalence of anti-*Toxoplasma gondii* antibodies in sport horses from Qazvin, Iran. *Trop. Anim. Health Prod.* **2010**, *42*, 1321–1322. [CrossRef]

41. Tenter, A.M.; Heckeroth, A.R.; Weiss, L.M. *Toxoplasma gondii*: From animals to humans. *Int. J. Parasitol.* **2000**, *30*, 1217–1258. [CrossRef]
42. Munhoz, A.D.; Souza, M.A.; Costa, S.C.L.; Freitas, J.S.; Silva, A.N.D.; Lacerda, L.C.; Cruz, R.D.S.; Albuquerque, G.R.; Pereira, M.J.S. Factors associated with the distribution of natural *Toxoplasma gondii* infection among equids in Northeastern Brazil. *Rev. Bras. Parasitol. Vet.* **2019**, *28*, 283–290. [CrossRef]
43. Saqib, M.; Hussain, M.H.; Sajid, M.S.; Mansoor, M.K.; Asi, M.N.; Fadya, A.A.; Zohaib, A.; Sial, A.U.; Muhammad, G.; Ullah, I. Sero-epidemiology of equine toxoplasmosis using a latex agglutination test in the three metropolises of Punjab, Pakistan. *Trop. Biomed.* **2015**, *32*, 276–285. [PubMed]
44. Bouhamdan, S.F.; Bitar, L.K.; Saghir, H.J.; Bayan, A.; Araj, G.F. Seroprevalence of *Toxoplasma* antibodies among individuals tested at hospitals and private laboratories in Beirut. *J. Med. Liban* **2010**, *58*, 8–11.
45. Shaapan, R.M.; Ghazy, A.A. Isolation of *Toxoplasma gondii* from horse meat in Egypt. *Pak. J. Biol. Sci.* **2007**, *10*, 174–177. [CrossRef]
46. Pomares, C.; Ajzenberg, D.; Bornard, L.; Bernardin, G.; Hasseine, L.; Darde, M.L.; Marty, P. Toxoplasmosis and horse meat, France. *Emerg. Infect. Dis.* **2011**, *17*, 1327–1328. [CrossRef] [PubMed]
47. Pastiu, A.I.; Gyorke, A.; Kalmar, Z.; Bolfa, P.; Rosenthal, B.M.; Oltean, M.; Villena, I.; Spinu, M.; Cozma, V. *Toxoplasma gondii* in horse meat intended for human consumption in Romania. *Vet. Parasitol.* **2015**, *212*, 393–395. [CrossRef]
48. Wiener, R.C.; Waters, C.; Bhandari, R. The association of *Toxoplasma gondii* IgG and cognitive function scores: NHANES 2013-2014. *Parasitol. Int.* **2020**, *78*, 102123. [CrossRef] [PubMed]
49. da Silva, R.C.; Langoni, H. *Toxoplasma gondii*: Host-parasite interaction and behavior manipulation. *Parasitol. Res.* **2009**, *105*, 893–898. [CrossRef]
50. Reichel, M.P.; Ayanegui-Alcérreca, M.A.; Gondim, L.F.; Ellis, J.T. What is the global economic impact of *Neospora caninum* in cattle—the billion dollar question. *Int. J. Parasitol.* **2013**, *43*, 133–142. [CrossRef] [PubMed]
51. Talafha, A.Q.; Abutarbush, S.M.; Rutley, D.L. Seroprevalence and Potential Risk Factors Associated with *Neospora* spp. Infection among Asymptomatic Horses in Jordan. *Korean J. Parasitol.* **2015**, *53*, 163–167. [CrossRef]
52. Abo-Shehada, M.N.; Abu-Halaweh, M.M. Flock-level seroprevalence of, and risk factors for, *Neospora caninum* among sheep and goats in northern Jordan. *Prev. Vet. Med.* **2010**, *93*, 25–32. [CrossRef]
53. James, K.E.; Smith, W.A.; Packham, A.E.; Conrad, P.A.; Pusterla, N. *Toxoplasma gondii* seroprevalence and association with equine protozoal myeloencephalitis: A case-control study of Californian horses. *Vet. J.* **2017**, *224*, 38–43. [CrossRef] [PubMed]
54. Lindsay, D.S. Neosporosis: An emerging protozoal disease of horses. *Equine Vet. J.* **2001**, *33*, 116–118. [CrossRef] [PubMed]
55. Aharonson-Raz, K.; Lichter-Peled, A.; Tal, S.; Gelman, B.; Cohen, D.; Klement, E.; Steinman, A. Spatial and temporal distribution of *West Nile virus* in horses in Israel (1997–2013)—from endemic to epidemics. *PLoS ONE* **2014**, *9*, e113149. [CrossRef] [PubMed]

5

Broad Range Screening of Vector-Borne Pathogens in Arctic Foxes (*Vulpes lagopus*)

Sándor Hornok [1,*], Kristin Mühldorfer [2], Nóra Takács [1], Regina Hofmann-Lehmann [3], Marina L. Meli [3], Miklós Gyuranecz [4], Ester R. Unnsteinsdóttir [5], Alex D. Greenwood [2,6] and Gábor Á. Czirják [2,*]

1 Department of Parasitology and Zoology, University of Veterinary Medicine, 1078 Budapest, Hungary; takacs.nora@univet.hu
2 Department of Wildlife Diseases, Leibniz Institute for Zoo and Wildlife Research, 10315 Berlin, Germany; muehldorfer@izw-berlin.de (K.M.); greenwood@izw-berlin.de (A.D.G.)
3 Clinical Laboratory, Department of Clinical Diagnostics and Services, and Center for Clinical Studies, Vetsuisse Faculty, University of Zurich, 8057 Zurich, Switzerland; rhofmann@vetclinics.uzh.ch (R.H.-L.); mmeli@vetclinics.uzh.ch (M.L.M.)
4 Institute for Veterinary Medical Research, Centre for Agricultural Research, 1143 Budapest, Hungary; m.gyuranecz@gmail.com
5 Ecology and Consultancy Department, Icelandic Institute of Natural History, 210 Garðabær, Iceland; Ester.R.Unnsteinsdottir@ni.is
6 Department of Veterinary Medicine, Freie Universität Berlin, 14163 Berlin, Germany
* Correspondence: hornok.sandor@univet.hu (S.H.); czirjak@izw-berlin.de (G.Á.C.)

Simple Summary: The arctic fox is the only native terrestrial mammal in Iceland. The population comprises both "coastal" and "inland" fox ecotypes, with regard to food resources. Because of the relatively low biodiversity within arctic ecosystems and the involvement of the species in both marine and terrestrial ecosystems, the Icelandic arctic fox population could serve as sentinels for the overall ecosystem health of Iceland. After screening the samples from 60 foxes for tick-/vector-borne pathogens, this study reports the near-absence (very low prevalence) of these pathogens in Icelandic arctic foxes in 2011–2012. Taking into account the broad range of target microorganisms analyzed here, as well as the warming climate and increasing presence of the vector *Ixodes ricinus* in Iceland, our results will be very useful as baseline data for comparison in future monitoring of the emergence of ticks and tick-borne diseases in this country.

Abstract: The arctic fox (*Vulpes lagopus*) is the only native terrestrial mammal in Iceland. While red foxes (*V. vulpes*) are known to be epidemiologically important carriers of several vector-borne pathogens in Europe, arctic foxes have never been evaluated in a similar context on this continent. This has become especially relevant in the last decade, considering the establishing populations of the tick species *Ixodes ricinus* in Iceland. In this study, liver DNA extracts of 60 arctic foxes, hunted between 2011–2012, were molecularly screened for vector-borne protozoan parasites (*Trypanosomatidae, Babesia, Theileria, Hepatozoon*) and bacteria (*Anaplasma, Ehrlichia, Rickettsia, Borrelia*, hemotropic *Mycoplasma*). One sample was real-time qPCR positive for *Anaplasma phagocytophilum*, though this positivity could not be confirmed with sequencing. Samples were negative for all other tested vector-borne pathogens. Results of this study indicate that, except for *A. phagocytophilum*, Icelandic arctic foxes were apparently "not yet infected" with vector-borne pathogens in 2011–2012, or their infections were "below the detection limit" of applied methods. Taking into account the broad range of target microorganisms analyzed here, as well as the warming climate and increasing presence of the vector *I. ricinus* in Iceland, our results will be very useful as baseline data for comparison in future monitoring of the emergence of ticks and tick-borne diseases in this country.

Keywords: arctic fox; Iceland; vector-borne bacteria; vector-borne protozoan parasites; climate change

1. Introduction

The arctic fox (*Vulpes lagopus*) is a small size (ca. 3–5 kg) generalist predator species with circumpolar distribution, associated primarily with arctic and tundra habitats. In Iceland, the arctic fox is the only native terrestrial mammal, divided into coastal and inland ecotypes [1]. While coastal ecotype foxes mainly feed on sea birds and eggs, invertebrates, and marine mammal carcasses, the inland foxes feed on ptarmigans, migrating waterfowl, eggs, reindeer and livestock carcasses, and wood mice [2].

The closest relative of the arctic fox in the Palearctic region is the red fox (*V. vulpes*), and in northern countries, these two species show partly overlapping geographical range and niche [3]. The red fox is widespread in Europe and is known to harbor a broad range of pathogens transmitted by hard ticks (Acari: *Ixodidae*) and other blood-sucking arthropod vectors [4–6]. This implies that red foxes participate in the natural transmission cycle of vector-borne pathogens but may also be used as sentinels for epidemiological surveillance of associated disease risks. On the other hand, a similar epidemiological role has not been postulated for the arctic fox, most likely because they were not found to be tick-infested in early studies [7]. However, this scenario may change with the warming climate, as increasing tick abundance has recently been experienced in Iceland [8].

Eight hard tick species have been reported in Iceland [9], among which *Ixodes ricinus* has the highest veterinary-medical importance in Europe [10]. Since the first record of *I. ricinus* in Iceland, dating back to 1967, its growing significance has been reported [8,9]. Apart from the import of this tick species by migratory birds, its host-questing activity on the vegetation is a likely indicator of established populations [8]. Importantly, arctic foxes are among the possible wildlife reproduction hosts of *I. ricinus* (i.e., feeding adults), while rodents, such as wood mice (*Apodemus sylvaticus*), can support larvae and nymphs.

Between 2012–2013, vector-borne pathogens were examined in 28 arctic foxes in Canada, and *Bartonella henselae*, *Mycoplasma haemocanis*, and *Ehrlichia canis* were detected [11]. However, despite the emergence of *I. ricinus* in Iceland, arctic foxes have not been screened for vector-borne pathogens in this country. Thus, the aim of the present study was to screen liver samples of 60 arctic foxes from Iceland for DNA of vector-borne protozoa (Euglenozoa: *Trypanosomatidae*; Apicomplexa: *Babesia*, *Theileria*, *Hepatozoon*) and bacteria (Proteobacteria: *Anaplasma*, *Ehrlichia*, *Rickettsia*, *Bartonella*; *Spirochaetes*: *Borrelia*; Tenericutes: hemotropic *Mycoplasma*), with emphasis on tick-borne pathogens.

2. Materials and Methods

All experimental procedures described in the materials and methods section were approved by the Internal Committee for Ethics and Animal Welfare of the Leibniz Institute for Zoo and Wildlife Research (permit #2010-01-03). All experiments were carried out in compliance with the approved guidelines of the Leibniz Institute for Zoo and Wildlife Research and the laws of Germany, Hungary, and Iceland.

Liver samples of 60 arctic foxes hunted between 2011 and 2012 in various inland and coastal regions of Iceland were used in this study. Hunting was covered by the government and managed by The Environmental Agency, under the wildlife act (64/1994) and animal welfare act (55/2013). Scientific use of the harvest was organized by the Icelandic Institute of Natural History, courtesy of The Icelandic Ministry for the Environment and Natural Resources. The animals included 40 adults (23 males, 17 females) and 20 juveniles (11 males, 9 females). Age determination of the arctic foxes was performed by X-ray measurements based on dental pulp cavity volume and cementum analysis. Juveniles were defined as younger than 1 year and adults as older than 1 year of age [12]. Carcasses were stored at −20 °C until necropsy was performed.

During necropsy, approximately 10 g of liver tissue was sampled and then stored at −80 °C until further analysis. The liver was chosen as the target organ, because it contains blood from both the portal and systemic circulation and is rich in cells of the reticuloendothelial system, i.e., components that are the most likely to contain the DNA of hemotropic, vector-borne microorganisms. Ectoparasites were not seen on the foxes post-mortem at the time of sample collection.

DNA was extracted from liver samples, using the NucleoSpin Tissue kit (Macherey-Nagel GmbH, Düren, Germany), individually from each fox. A total of 100 μL of homogenized tissue was digested with Proteinase-K overnight at 56 °C and prepared as described in the user manual. Quality and quantity of extracted DNA were assessed by ND-1000 UV-Vis Spectrophotometer (Nanodrop Technologies, Wilmington, DE, USA) measurements.

All 60 DNA extracts were screened for a broad range of tick-/vector-borne pathogens with PCRs summarized in the Supplementary Material (Table S1). For *Anaplasma phagocytophilum*, the assay consisted of 40 cycles and the results were regarded as positive if the threshold cycle (Ct) value was below 39. The detection limit of this qPCR was a 0.125 ratio (one-eighths) of an *A. phagocytophilum* infected cell [13]. For Sanger sequencing of *A. phagocytophilum* from the real-time qPCR-positive sample, two conventional PCRs were attempted, the first by using the msp2 primers and annealing temperature, as in method "A" (Supplementary Materials, Table S1), and the second to amplify part of the heat shock chaperonin GroEL gene [14]. The latter PCR was repeated, but no sequenceable product was obtained.

3. Results and Discussion

Out of 60 samples, one adult female arctic fox from the costal ecotype was positive for *A. phagocytophilum*-specific real-time qPCR (Ct = 36.71; sequencing was repeatedly not successful). In line with this finding, red foxes have been reported to carry *A. phagocytophilum* DNA in at least 10 European countries [4,5]. *Anaplasma phygocytophilum* (Rickettsiales: Anaplasmataceae) is the causative agent of granulocytic anaplasmosis in multiple hosts (including humans) and tick-borne fever in ruminants [15]. In Europe, *A. phagocytophilum* is transmitted by *I. ricinus*, the tick-species increasingly recognized to affect animals in Iceland [8]. Nevertheless, to the best of our knowledge, this is the first molecular evidence of *A. phagocytophilum* in arctic foxes and the first autochthonous occurrence of this tick-borne species in Iceland. However, since this real-time qPCR positivity for *A. phagocytophilum* could not be confirmed with sequencing, probably because of the low amount of DNA, as reflected by the high Ct value in the more sensitive real-time qPCR, further studies are needed to verify the presence of this species in arctic foxes in Iceland. Although seropositivity to *A. phagocytophilum* has already been reported in humans in Iceland, in the absence of published data on the autochthonous occurrence of its vector in the country, this finding was explained by exposure during travel abroad [16].

All 60 samples were negative or contained DNA below the PCR detection limit for other tested vector-borne pathogens. Taking into account that red foxes are known to harbor a broad range of the vector-borne protozoa and bacteria targeted here (e.g., in northern Europe [5]; in southern Europe [4,6]), PCR-negativity of most samples implies that the warming climate of Iceland has not entailed changes of similar magnitude in the distribution of tick-borne pathogens in 2011–2012, as reported in the same period from Scandinavia [17]. This is further confirmed by the absence of any ticks on the 60 foxes analyzed here, as well as on 315 arctic foxes examined in 2015–2016 [8].

Unlike what is shown here, arctic foxes were reported to harbor *Bartonella* spp., *M. haemocanis*, and *E. canis* in northern Canada [11,18]. However, in the latter case, the majority of positive samples were flea-borne bartonellae and not tick-borne pathogens. At least three rodent species are known to occur in Iceland [19], but their mite and flea species are usually not shared with foxes [20]. Despite this, during prey consumption, the role of temporary infestation of arctic foxes with these non-host specific ectoparasites, in the transmission of vector-borne pathogens, should not be discounted [18].

Nevertheless, results of the present study suggest that different spectra of vector-borne bacteria might emerge in arctic foxes in Iceland compared to Canada.

4. Conclusions

The above results provide baseline data on the near-absence (very low prevalence) of tick-/vector-borne pathogens in Icelandic arctic foxes in 2011–2012. Already observed and foreseeable climate changes in Iceland (milder winter, warmer spring and autumn [8]) will most likely promote multi-focal establishment of *I. ricinus* and possibly other tick species in this country, with increased risks of autochthonous transmission of tick-borne pathogens [8]. This warrants continuous monitoring of emerging vector-borne pathogens in Iceland, similar to all arctic ecosystems. Taking into account the broad range of target microorganisms analyzed here (for which red foxes are known to be susceptible), as well as the warming climate and increasing presence of *I. ricinus* in Iceland, our results will be very useful as baseline data for comparison in future monitoring of the emergence of ticks and tick-borne diseases in this country.

Author Contributions: S.H., K.M., and G.Á.C. designed the study; M.G., E.R.U., A.D.G., and G.Á.C. coordinated different parts of the study; E.R.U. collected the samples; S.H., K.M., N.T., R.H.-L., and M.L.M. performed laboratory analysis; S.H. wrote the manuscript with the contributions of all the co-authors. All authors have read and agreed to the published version of the manuscript.

Acknowledgments: We would like to thank Katja Pohle and Nadine Jahn for their help with curating the samples and conducting the laboratory analyses. The laboratory work was partly performed using the logistics of the Center for Clinical Studies at the Vetsuisse Faculty of the University of Zurich. This manuscript benefited from comments of six anonymous referees.

References

1. Carbonell Ellgutter, J.A.; Ehrich, D.; Killengreen, S.T.; Ims, R.A.; Unnsteinsdóttir, E.R. Dietary variation in Icelandic arctic fox (*Vulpes lagopus*) over a period of 30 years assessed through stable isotopes. *Oecologia* **2020**, *192*, 403–414. [PubMed]
2. Bocharova, N.; Treu, G.; Czirják, G.Á.; Krone, O.; Stefanski, V.; Wibbelt, G.; Unnsteinsdóttir, E.R.; Hersteinsson, P.; Schares, G.; Doronina, L.; et al. Correlates between feeding ecology and mercury levels in historical and modern arctic foxes (*Vulpes lagopus*). *PLoS ONE* **2013**, *8*, e60879. [CrossRef] [PubMed]
3. Elmhagen, B.; Tannerfeldt, M.; Angerbjorn, A. Food-niche overlap between arctic and red foxes. *Can. J. Zool.* **2002**, *80*, 1274–1285. [CrossRef]
4. Hodžić, A.; Alić, A.; Fuehrer, H.P.; Harl, J.; Wille-Piazzai, W.; Duscher, G.G. A molecular survey of vector-borne pathogens in red foxes (*Vulpes vulpes*) from Bosnia and Herzegovina. *Parasites Vectors* **2015**, *8*, 88. [CrossRef] [PubMed]
5. Sakalauskas, P.; Lipatova, I.; Radzijevskaja, J.; Paulauskas, A. Pathogen screening in the red fox (*Vulpes vulpes*) from Lithuania. *Biologija* **2019**, *65*, 283–295. [CrossRef]
6. Sukara, R.; Juwaid, S.; Ćirović, D.; Penezić, A.; Mihaljica, D.; Veinović, G.; Radojičić, S.; Hodžić, A.; Duscher, G.G.; Tomanović, S. *Candidatus Neoehrlichia* sp. (FU98) and *Borrelia burgdorferi sensu lato* in red foxes (*Vulpes vulpes*) from Serbia. *Acta Vet-Beogr.* **2019**, *69*, 312–324. [CrossRef]
7. Hersteinsson, P. (Ed.) *Íslensk Spendýr [Icelandic Mammals]*; Vaka-Helgafell: Reykjavík, Iceland, 2004; p. 344. (In Icelandic)
8. Alfredsson, M.; Olafsson, E.; Eydal, M.; Unnsteinsdóttir, E.R.; Hansford, K.; Wint, W.; Alexander, N.; Medlock, J.M. Surveillance of *Ixodes ricinus* ticks (Acari: Ixodidae) in Iceland. *Parasites Vectors* **2017**, *10*, 466. [CrossRef] [PubMed]
9. Richter, S.H.; Eydal, M.; Skírnisson, K.; Ólafsson, E. Tick species (Ixodida) identified in Iceland. *Icel. Agric. Sci.* **2013**, *26*, 3–10.

10. Gray, J.S. The development and seasonal activity of the tick *Ixodes ricinus*: A vector of Lyme borreliosis. *Rev. Med. Vet. Entomol.* **1991**, *79*, 323–333.
11. Mascarelli, P.E.; Elmore, S.A.; Jenkins, E.J.; Alisauskas, R.T.; Walsh, M.; Breitschwerdt, E.B.; Maggi, R.G. Vector-borne pathogens in arctic foxes, *Vulpes lagopus*, from Canada. *Res. Vet. Sci.* **2015**, *99*, 58–59. [CrossRef]
12. Treu, G.; Krone, O.; Unnsteinsdóttir, E.R.; Greenwood, A.D.; Czirják, G.Á. Correlations between hair and tissue mercury concentrations in Icelandic arctic foxes (*Vulpes lagopus*). *Sci. Total Environ.* **2018**, *619–620*, 1589–1598. [CrossRef]
13. Courtney, J.W.; Kostelnik, L.M.; Zeidner, N.S.; Massung, R.F. Multiplex real-time PCR for detection of *Anaplasma phagocytophilum* and *Borrelia burgdorferi*. *J. Clin. Microbiol.* **2004**, *42*, 3164–3168. [CrossRef] [PubMed]
14. Alberti, A.; Zobba, R.; Chessa, B.; Addis, M.F.; Sparagano, O.; Pinna Parpaglia, M.L.; Cubeddu, T.; Pintori, G.; Pittau, M. Equine and canine *Anaplasma phagocytophilum* strains isolated on the island of Sardinia (Italy) are phylogenetically related to pathogenic strains from the United States. *Appl. Environ. Microbiol.* **2005**, *71*, 6418–6422. [CrossRef]
15. Woldehiwet, Z. The natural history of *Anaplasma phagocytophilum*. *Vet. Parasitol.* **2010**, *167*, 108–122. [CrossRef]
16. Skarpheðinsson, S.; Søgaard, P.; Pedersen, C. Seroprevalence of human granulocytic ehrlichiosis in high-risk groups in Denmark. *Scand. J. Inf. Dis.* **2001**, *33*, 206–210.
17. Jaenson, T.G.; Jaenson, D.G.; Eisen, L.; Petersson, E.; Lindgren, E. Changes in the geographical distribution and abundance of the tick *Ixodes ricinus* during the past 30 years in Sweden. *Parasites Vectors* **2012**, *5*, 8. [CrossRef] [PubMed]
18. Buhler, K.J.; Maggi, R.G.; Gailius, J.; Galloway, T.D.; Chilton, N.B.; Alisauskas, R.T.; Samelius, G.; Bouchard, É.; Jenkins, E.J. Hopping species and borders: Detection of *Bartonella* spp. in avian nest fleas and arctic foxes from Nunavut, Canada. *Parasites Vectors* **2020**, *13*, 469. [CrossRef]
19. Bengtson, S.A.; Brinck-Lindroth, G.; Lundqvist, L.; Nilsson, A.; Rundgren, S. Ectoparasites on small mammals in Iceland: Origin and population characteristics of a species-poor insular community. *Holarct. Ecol.* **1986**, *9*, 143–148. [CrossRef]
20. Brinck-Lindroth, G.; Smit, F.G.A.M. *The Fleas (Siphonaptera) of Fennoscandia and Denmark*; Brill Academic Publishers: Leiden, The Netherlands, 2007.

6

Fatal Pulmonary Hypertension and Right-Sided Congestive Heart Failure in a Kitten Infected with *Aelurostrongylus abstrusus*

Tommaso Vezzosi [1], Stefania Perrucci [1], Francesca Parisi [1], Simone Morelli [2], Michela Maestrini [1], Giulia Mennuni [3], Donato Traversa [2] and Alessandro Poli [1,*]

[1] Department of Veterinary Sciences, University of Pisa, Viale delle Piagge n. 2, 56124 Pisa, Italy; tommaso.vezzosi86@gmail.com (T.V.); stefania.perrucci@unipi.it (S.P.); francesca.parisi@vet.unipi.it (F.P.); michela.maestrini@phd.unipi.it (M.M.)

[2] Faculty of Veterinary Medicine, University of Teramo, Piano d'Accio, 64100 Teramo, Italy; smorelli@unite.it (S.M.); dtraversa@unite.it (D.T.)

[3] Studio Associato Veterinario Razzauti Daolio Anguillesi, 57100 Livorno, Italy; giulia_mennuni@yahoo.it

* Correspondence: alessandro.poli@unipi.it

Simple Summary: Infections caused by lungworms are an emerging issue in feline medicine. Clinical features in cats may vary from subclinical infections to a severe disease, occasionally including fatal pneumonia, depending on different factors, e.g., lungworm species, parasitic burden, and age of the animal. A case of infection caused by *Aelurostrongylus abstrusus* in a domestic kitten presenting acute dyspnoea and ascites is presented here. Clinical, radiological, echocardiographic, parasitological, molecular, and pathological data are described. This is the first report of life-threatening pulmonary hypertension inducing congestive heart failure caused by *A. abstrusus* infection in a domestic kitten.

Abstract: *Aelurostrongylus abstrusus* is considered the most important respiratory nematode of domestic cats worldwide. This parasite inhabits the alveoli, alveolar ducts, and bronchioles and causes a subacute to chronic respiratory clinical disease. Clinical signs may occur in domestic cats of any age, though they are more often described in young animals. Physical examination, echocardiography, thoracic radiography, pulmonary and cardiac pathological findings, classical, and molecular parasitological analysis of a six-month-old kitten referred at the Veterinary Teaching Hospital of the University of Pisa (Italy) led to a diagnosis of parasitic bronchopneumonia caused by *A. abstrusus*, which was complicated by severe pulmonary hypertension (PH) and right-sided congestive heart failure (R-CHF) that caused the death of the animal. Cases of reversible PH associated with *A. abstrusus* infection have been seldom reported in cats. This is the first report of fatal PH and R-CHF in a kitten with clinical aelurostrongylosis.

Keywords: *Aelurostrongylus abstrusus*; ascites; cardiology; congestive heart failure; domestic cat; echocardiography; parasitic bronchopneumonia; pulmonary hypertension

---

1. Introduction

The cosmopolitan metastrongylid *Aelurostrongylus abstrusus*, known as the "cat lungworm", is the most prevalent respiratory nematode of the domestic cat [1,2]. This respiratory nematode infects cats of all ages, regardless of their habitat, lifestyle, breed, or gender [2,3]. In Europe, *A. abstrusus* is distributed throughout countries, and in Italy, especially in central-southern regions [4,5]. In Europe, infection rates vary widely from 1.2% in owned to 50% in free roaming cats [2]. In the Americas,

A. abstrusus has been recorded with rates from 0.08% in client-owned to 5.1% in shelter cats in North America [6,7], and from 0.21% to 39.2% in different domestic cat populations of South America [8].

The life cycle of *A. abstrusus* involves gastropod intermediate hosts, though cats most often become infected preying on small vertebrates, such as mice, birds, reptiles, and amphibians, serving as paratenic hosts [1,2]. The continuous availability of paratenic hosts is the most important reason why cats are at risk of being infected throughout the year [1,3]. Furthermore, kittens may acquire the infection through the ingestion of tissues of preys offered or regurgitated by the queen during the weaning period [1,9].

Adults of *A. abstrusus* infect alveoli, alveolar ducts, and bronchioles of the cat, and cause subacute, acute, or chronic respiratory diseases in cats of any age, although clinical signs are usually more frequent and severe in young subjects [1,2,10,11]. Cough, tachypnoea, and dyspnoea of varying severity, but rarely with a fatal outcome, are the most frequent findings in *A. abstrusus*-infected cats [1–3]. In more severe cases, pneumothorax, pleural effusions, and asthma-like clinical signs can be observed [3,11].

The main pathological findings associated with cat aelurostrongylosis are caused by nematode adults, larvae, and eggs, and are represented by multifocal granulomatous and inflammatory cell infiltrates in the pulmonary parenchyma and in the alveoli of peribronchial areas, alveolar wall thickening, and musculature hypertrophy [12,13]. Cell infiltrates in the bronchial walls, presence of mucus and inflammatory cells in the bronchial lumen, and smooth muscle hypertrophy have also been reported [13].

Pulmonary hypertension (PH) in cats has been described in association with congenital heart diseases [14–16], pulmonary thromboembolism [17], pulmonary fibrosis [18], chronic upper airway obstruction [19], and left-sided congestive heart failure [20]. PH has been occasionally diagnosed in infected cats, i.e., a single case of irreversible PH in a cat infected by *Troglostrongylus brevior* in Italy [21] and reversible PH in one kitten with aelurostrongylosis in the Netherlands [22]. This study describes the first report of severe and life-threatening PH inducing R-CHF caused by *A. abstrusus* in a domestic kitten.

2. Materials and Methods

2.1. Clinical Case

A 6-month-old female shorthair kitten, 1 kg in weight, was referred to the Veterinary Teaching Hospital of the University of Pisa, central Italy, for progressive cough, worsening dyspnoea, and dysorexia in the last 5 days. The kitten had mainly an outdoor lifestyle in a countryside environment. Physical examination revealed pink-pale mucous membranes, cachexia, and tachypnoea (55 breaths per minute) with a restrictive breathing pattern. Lung auscultation revealed diffuse pulmonary crackles. Weak femoral pulse was present bilaterally. Heart rate was 180 beats per minute with regular rhythm, and the cardiac auscultation revealed a grade 4/6 right basilar holosystolic murmur. The kitten was mildly hypothermic (rectal temperature, 37.3 °C) and had an abdominal distention. The animal was immediately hospitalized in critical clinical condition. The main differential diagnosis based on history and physical examination included: congestive heart failure, pneumonia, feline infectious peritonitis. Thoracic radiology and echocardiography were performed, and faeces (about 3 g) were collected for parasitological examinations. Based on diagnostic findings (see results section), the cat was diagnosed with parasitic bronchopneumonia with secondary PH and R-CHF. Oxygen therapy was administered through an oxygen cage. The kitten was treated with methylprednisolone 0.5 mg/kg IV q24h, furosemide 1 mg/kg IV q12h, and sildenafil 1 mg/kg PO q12h. Nevertheless, a few hours after hospitalization, the clinical conditions progressively worsened until a sudden cardiorespiratory arrest. Written informed consent was obtained from the owners to perform the necropsy.

2.2. Thoracic Radiology and Echocardiography

Chest radiographs were performed using a digital system (FPD 4343A GOS/CSI, Isomedic srl, Lodi, Italy). The respiratory distress of the patient allowed for only lateral views.

Standard echocardiography was performed in a standing position due to the patient's critical condition. The echocardiographic examination was performed using an ultrasonographic unit (Aplio 300, Canon Medical Systems Europe, Zoetermeer, The Netherlands) equipped with an electronic phased-array transducer (4–9 Mhz). Left chamber dimensions, wall thicknesses, and ventricular function were assessed as previously described [20]. Right-heart dimension and function were subjectively and objectively assessed [20,23,24]. The presence of interventricular septal flattening was subjectively assessed. The dimension of the pulmonary artery was calculated as the ratio between the pulmonary trunk and the aorta, and the pulmonary systolic flow profile was assessed using pulsed wave Doppler [20]. The tricuspid regurgitation was evaluated using colour and continuous wave Doppler. Pulmonary hypertension was defined as a peak tricuspid regurgitation velocity > 2.7 m/s [20].

2.3. Parasitological and Molecular Analysis

Faecal samples were microscopically analysed by a conventional flotation assay using a saturated NaCl solution (specific gravity 1.2), and by the Baermann migration test [25]. First stage larvae (L1) recovered at the Baermann test were counted and then identified based on their morphologic and morphometric features [25]. After the post mortem examination (Section 3.2), a portion of a lung was opened, and pulmonary tissue smears were examined for nematode eggs and larvae. Then, the lung piece was washed in saline solution in a conic beaker for 12 h at 4 °C. Then, the pulmonary lavage liquid was microscopically analysed under an inverted and an optical microscope, for the detection and identification of larval nematodes [26]. An aliquot of faeces, Baermann's sediment, and the lung lavage liquid found positive for larvae in the microscopic examinations were subjected to a previously described molecular test specific for the most common feline metastrongyloids [27]. Briefly, a multiplex PCR method able to simultaneously identify *A. abstrusus*, *T. brevior*, and *Angiostrongylus chabaudi*, and consisting of a first step with universal primers NC1 and NC2 and a second step using diagnostic primers in combination with NC2 to achieve specific amplifications for the three nematodes, was used [27].

2.4. Histopathological Methods

Representative tissue samples of stomach, intestine, lymph nodes (peripheral, mesenteric, and mediastinal), spleen, liver, kidney, adrenal glands, ovary, uterus, lung, heart, thymus, encephalon (telencephalon, diencephalon, mesencephalon, pons, cerebellum, and medulla), and spinal cord were fixed in 10% neutral buffered formalin and routinely embedded in paraffin wax. Four micron thick sections were stained with Haematoxylin and Eosin, Goldner's Trichrome, and Periodic Acid Schiff, Perls, and Toluidine Blue stains.

3. Results

3.1. Clinical Evaluation

Thoracic radiographs showed a diffuse interstitial and alveolar pattern, with mild pleural effusion (Figure 1). The increased sternal contact of the cardiac silhouette suggested right-side cardiomegaly.

Echocardiography showed severe right atrial and ventricular dilation (Figure 2a,b) associated with right ventricular hypokinesia. Flattening of the interventricular septum was present and the internal dimension of the left ventricle was reduced. Moderate to severe tricuspid regurgitation was evident (Figure 2c) with normal morphology of the valvular leaflets. The peak velocity of the tricuspid regurgitation was 2.9 m/s. The pulmonary artery was dilated, with a pulmonary trunk to aorta ratio of 1.42. The pulmonary artery systolic flow had a proto-systolic peak (Figure 2d). Mild pericardial and pleural effusion and moderate abdominal effusion were evident. The analysis of the abdominal effusion indicated a modified transudate. All these findings were consistent with severe pre-capillary PH and R-CHF. The presence of congenital heart diseases was verified and excluded by two-dimensional and Doppler echocardiography.

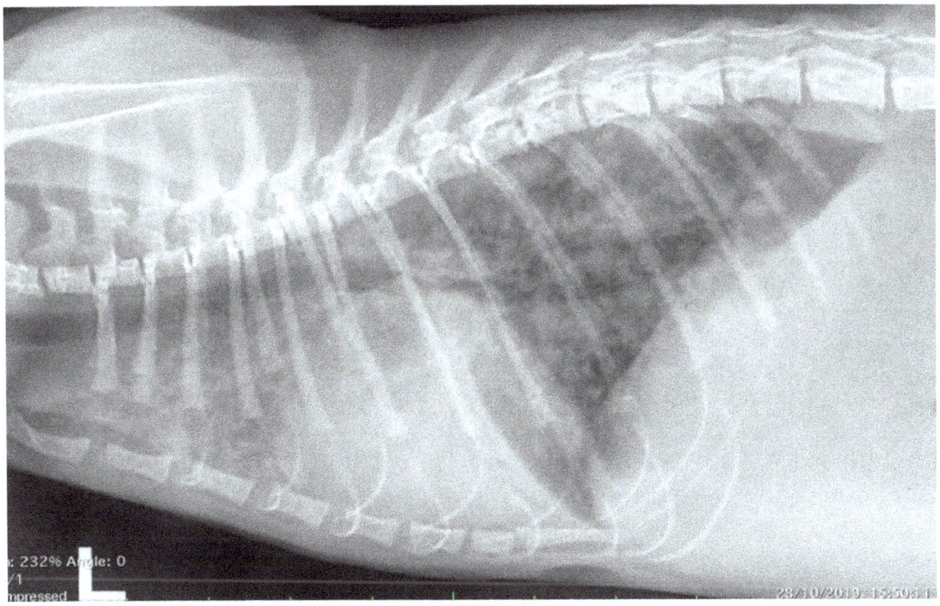

Figure 1. Thoracic radiograph (lateral view) from a 6-month-old domestic kitten with progressive dyspnoea. Diffuse interstitial and alveolar pattern, with mild pleural effusion, was evident. The increased sternal contact of the cardiac silhouette suggested right-side cardiomegaly.

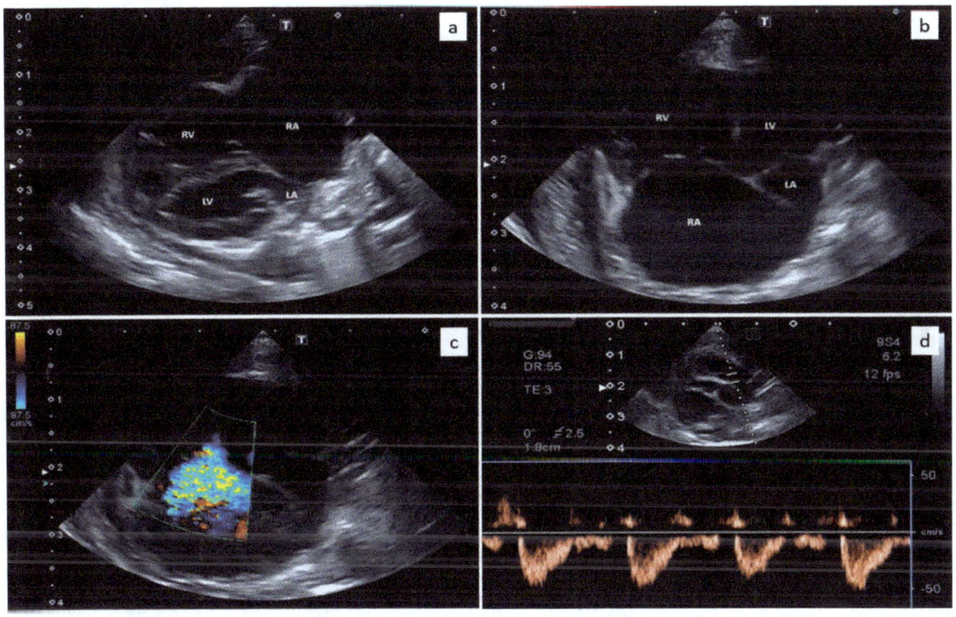

Figure 2. Echocardiography from the domestic kitten showing severe right atrial (RA) and right ventricular (RV) dilation, with reduced dimensions of the left atrium (LA) and the left ventricle (LV) (**a**,**b**). Moderate to severe tricuspid regurgitation was evident (**c**) with normal morphology of the valvular leaflets. The pulmonary artery systolic flow had a proto-systolic peak (**d**).

Several nematode L1s were found in the sediment of the Baermann test (about 20 L1/microscopic field at 40x, and about 4260 L1 per gram of faeces, LPG). In the microscopic examination, L1s were 360–415 μm in length and about 18–19 μm in width, showed a rounded head with a terminal opening (Figure 3a), and an S-shaped tail with distinct knob-like or small finger-like projections at the tip of cuticular spines (Figure 3b). For all these features, they were identified as *A. abstrusus* L1 [26].

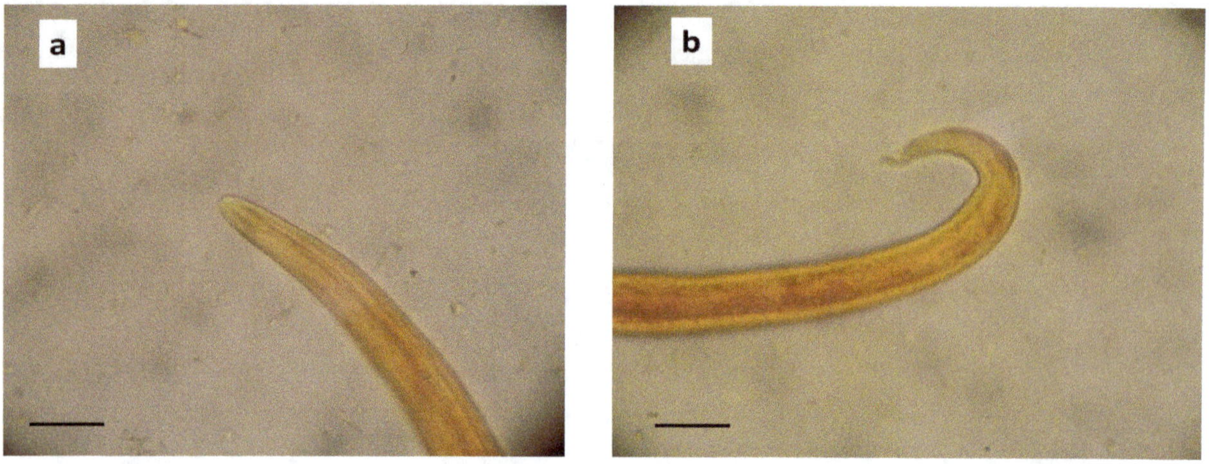

Figure 3. *Aelurostrongylus abstrusus* first stage larva (L1) in the Baermann examination of the kitten faecal sample. (**a**) Anterior end, (**b**) posterior end showing the S-shaped tail. 400x, (scale bar = 20 μm).

Based on the clinical, parasitological, and molecular results, a parasitic bronchopneumonia caused by *A. abstrusus* infection, with secondary severe PH and R-CHF, was diagnosed.

3.2. Post-Mortem Examination

At necropsy, 50 mL of blood-tinged serous transudate was collected from the peritoneal cavity, and the liver surface was markedly covered with thin fibrin deposits. Other organs in the abdominal cavity were normal at gross examination. A total of 20 ml of blood-tinged transudate fluid was collected from the thoracic cavity and both lungs showed lobar areas of reddish consolidation, as well as sparse subpleural soft to firm greyish/whitish slightly raised nodules (Figure 4a). Pulmonary oedema and multifocal emphysema were present at the periphery of these lesions. On the cut surface of lung parenchyma, marked oedema, thickening of bronchiolar walls, and the presence of catarrhal exudate in the bronchial lumen were observed. No adult nematodes were macroscopically visible in the trachea, bronchi, and bronchioles lumen. Tracheobronchial lymph nodes were moderately enlarged. A small amount of transudate fluid was detected in the pericardial sac. The heart weighted 12 g and marked enlargement of the right atrial and ventricular cavities was evident (Figure 4b). Macroscopic examination of encephalon revealed congestion of blood vessels in the meninges.

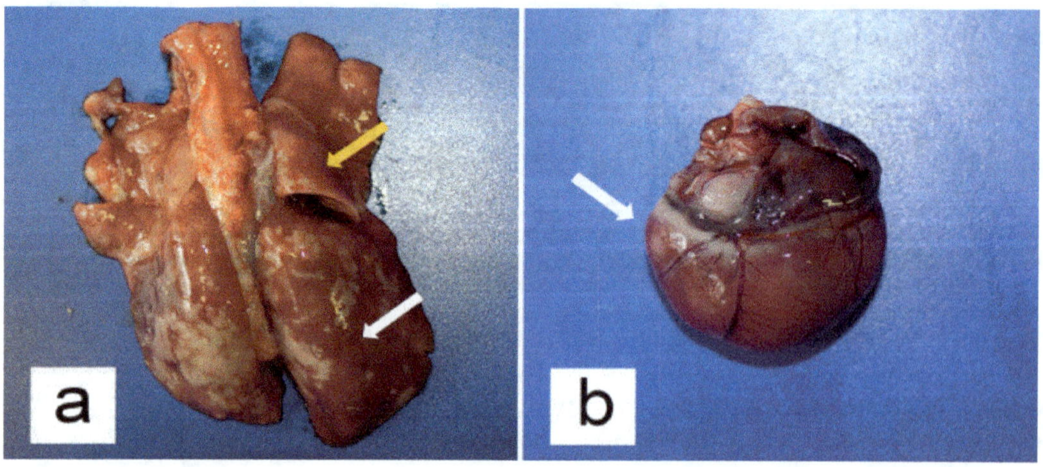

Figure 4. Gross pathological findings from the examined kitten. (**a**) Lungs showed diffuse hyperaemia (orange arrow) with lobular areas of consolidation (white arrow) and sparse whitish, slightly raised nodules. (**b**) Marked right-sided cardiac enlargement was evident (white arrow).

At the examination of the post mortem lung lavage fluid, a countless number of L1 were evidenced. Molecular analysis of all biological samples taken from the kitten, i.e., lung lavage liquid, the Baermann sediment, and the faecal sample, confirmed the microscopic identification of the parasite as *A. abstrusus*.

Histopathologic examination revealed marked liver congestion with the accumulation of red blood cells in the centrilobular areas without acute swelling or necrosis of hepatocytes. Fibrin deposits were evident on the liver capsule in the absence of inflammatory infiltrates. In large areas of pulmonary parenchyma, alveolar lumen was filled by thin-walled morulated eggs and larvae accompanied by a diffuse thickening of the alveolar walls due to the presence of mixed inflammatory cell infiltrates constituted by eosinophils, neutrophils, and macrophages (Figure 5a), whereas granulomatous inflammation was rarely observed. Inflammatory lesions were mostly located in the peribronchial area. Alveolar capillary congestion and alveolar lumen dilatation were detected at the periphery of peribronchial areas. Cross-sections of adult nematodes (from 55 to 75 μm in diameter) were detected within the inflammatory infiltrates (Figure 5b). Inflammatory infiltrates were detected in the wall of larger and smaller bronchi and bronchioles, including lymphocytes and plasma cells. A mild hyperplasia of the bronchial-associated lymphoid tissue and the peribronchial glands was evident, in association with mucus and inflammatory cells in the bronchial lumina. The smooth muscles of bronchiolar walls and alveolar ducts were slightly hypertrophied. Pulmonary artery changes included the presence of mild inflammatory cell infiltrates located in the subintimal areas, aggregated into a cluster of periarteriolar areas (Figure 5c). Thickening of the smooth muscle of the arterial wall was not evident. Reactive lymphoid hyperplasia was detected in the tracheobronchial lymph nodes. Histopathologic examination of the heart samples revealed myocardial oedema with myocardiocyte spacing and arteriolar changes, characterized by the presence of mild inflammatory infiltrates located in the periarteriolar areas and constituted by mononuclear cells (Figure 5d). Significant histopathologic changes were not detected in the other examined tissues.

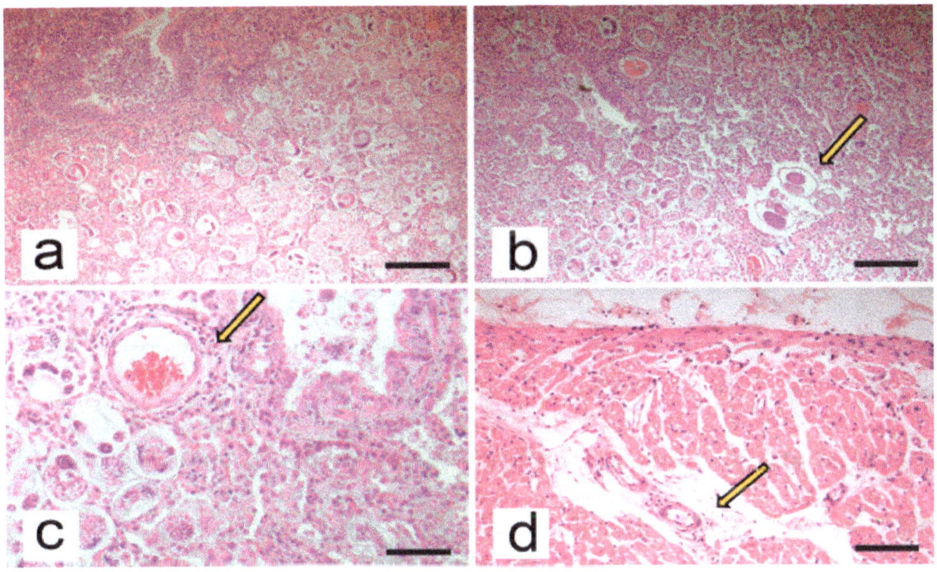

Figure 5. Histopathological findings from the examined kitten. (**a**) Lung. Alveolar lumen filled with eggs and larvae (Haematoxylin-Eosin stain, bar = 100 μm). (**b**) Lung. Scattered adult *Aelurostrongylus abstrusus* (arrow) were present within the inflammatory tissue, where the alveoli were filled by morulated eggs (Haematoxylin-Eosin stain, bar = 100 μm). (**c**) Lung. Absence of smooth muscle hypertrophy of arteriolar wall and presence of mild inflammatory cell infiltrate in the periarteriolar area (arrow; Haematoxylin-Eosin stain, bar = 50 μm). (**d**) Heart. Myocardial oedema with myocardiocyte spacing and presence of mild inflammatory infiltrates located in the periarteriolar areas (Haematoxylin-Eosin stain, bar = 100 μm).

4. Discussion

Cat aelurostrongylosis may be subclinical, acute, or chronic, but it causes fatal pneumonia very rarely [1,10,28]. Most *A. abstrusus*-infected cats are subclinical or show a chronic cough with gradually increasing tachypnoea and respiratory distress, or other respiratory signs, as wheezing, sneezing, nasal discharge, frequently associated to apathy, anorexia, and fever [10,11,29,30]. Some kittens may develop more severe clinical forms than adult cats, probably due to a quicker occlusion of the airways by *A. abstrusus* due to the smaller diameter of the bronchi and the concomitant inflammation [31]. This happens more frequently in troglostrongylosis of kittens due to the size of *T. brevior* adults [1], as *A. abstrusus* is a tiny nematode, thus only highly parasitic burdens may occlude the airways of cats. In fact, lung damages in aelurostrongylosis are rather caused by the egg deposition with consequent pulmonary inflammation [12].

The present kitten presented PH. Based on the veterinary literature, the main differential diagnosis for PH in young cats includes congenital heart diseases (patent ductus arteriosus, supravalvular mitral stenosis, cor triatriatum sinister, atrioventricular septal defect) [14–16,20], lungworm diseases [21,22], and upper airway obstruction [19]. Differently from dogs, cats affected by heartworm or lungworm disease rarely develop PH, even if presenting significant pulmonary parenchymal and arterial damage [32,33]. Nevertheless, reversible PH with right ventricular enlargement and large systolic tricuspid regurgitation associated with *A. abstrusus* infection have been previously recorded in one ten-week-old kitten [22]. In this latter case, only moderate right atrial enlargement was described, with no evidence of right-sided congestive heart failure. Conversely, in the clinical case here in described, severe right atrial enlargement was present, and pericardial, pleural, and abdominal effusions were compatible with right-sided congestive heart failure.

No echocardiographic evidence of PH was reported in a study on cats infected by *A. abstrusus* [32]. However, the median age of the included population was 24 months, with the youngest cat ageing 8 months. It can be thus argued that age is a critical factor in triggering the onset of PH, in consideration of the age of the kitten with PH which was described in the Netherlands [22] and of the kitten presented here. Nevertheless, reversible PH with right ventricular enlargement and large systolic tricuspid regurgitation associated with *A. abstrusus* infection have been previously recorded in one ten-week-old kitten [19]. In this latter case, only moderate right atrial enlargement was described, with no evidence of R-CHF. Conversely, in the present clinical case, the evidence of severe right atrial and ventricular dilation, the flattening of the interventricular septum, the reduced left ventricular dimension, and the pulmonary artery enlargement were consistent with severe PH [14–17,20]. Additional Doppler signs of PH were the increased velocity of the tricuspid regurgitation and the proto-systolic peak of the pulmonic flow [14–17,20]. The pericardial, pleural, and abdominal effusions were compatible with R-CHF. A possible higher tricuspid regurgitation peak velocity could have been expected in a case of PH causing R-CHF. However, the presence of right ventricular systolic disfunction, the high right atrial pressure, and possible technical factors such as high frequency transducers and suboptimal alignment, could have produced a lower peak velocity. Differential diagnosis for R-CHF in domestic cats include congenital heart diseases (mainly tricuspid valve dysplasia, tetralogy of Fallot, endocardial cushion defect, patent ductus arteriosus, double chambered right ventricle) [34–36] and acquired cardiomyopathies (mainly restrictive cardiomyopathy and arrhythmogenic right ventricular cardiomyopathy) [37,38]. To the authors' knowledge, this the first report of severe PH and R-CHF of parasitic origin in a kitten.

Other than age, parasite load and other unknown risk factors may play a central role in the development of clinical signs, including PH, in cats naturally infected with *A. abstrusus* [2]. Indeed, in addition to the direct damages caused by adult nematodes to the lung parenchyma, eggs, larvae, and inflammatory exudate induce bronchiolar muscular hypertrophy and hyperplasia of the smooth muscle of the pulmonary arteries, which may gradually obstruct the bronchiolar system and cause PH [12,39,40]. Pulmonary vasoconstriction elicited by mast cells and histamine release, promoting pulmonary vascular resistance, was also hypothesized [2,22].

The LPG found in the kitten faeces in the Baermann test, i.e., about 4260 LPG, can be considered a high value. In fact, a mean number of 1198 LPG was counted in the majority of symptomatic cats showing severe radiographic changes in a previous study [41], although cats experimentally infected with a high dose of *A. abstrusus* L3 and showing severe lung lesions may shed a variable number of L1s, down to 687 [10]. Although the LPG number counted in the Baermann test in the kitten herein examined may be considered consistent with the very high number of L1 found in the lung, in general there is no a constant concordance between number of L1 shed by infected animals and the degree of lung damages and severity of clinical signs. Additionally, the period elapsed between the death of the kitten and the parasitological analysis of the lungs could have allowed the eggs present in the examined lung tissue to hatch, resulting in the detection of an extremely high L1 number.

Interestingly, *A. abstrusus* infection is a frequent finding in cats deceased during anaesthesia [42]. Sedation or anaesthesia may reduce a cat's ability to compensate for diminished gas exchange surface area, compromising lung perfusion and ventilation, which can lead to hypoxia, systemic hypotension, and cardiovascular arrest. For these reasons, pre-anaesthesia parasitological screening for lungworms is strongly suggested [42]. This is particularly true for kittens, given that age could play a role in the onset of PH impacting on cardiorespiratory functions.

Pathologic findings in the clinical case showed in this study are in line with previous studies [10,13,22]. Regarding changes in the pulmonary arteries, hyperplasia, and hypertrophy of the smooth muscle cells of the media and intimal proliferation are commonly reported, resulting in narrowing of the lumen of pulmonary vasculature [12]. However, in the herein described case, no significant changes in the media and intima were noted. Based on the severe pulmonary parenchymal lesions, it is possible that PH occurred secondarily to lung damages and hypoxemia. Similar findings were already reported in a kitten with severe pulmonary parenchymal disease [22]. Diffuse alveolar disease can lead to impaired oxygen exchange in the lungs [43]. In addition, *A. abstrusus* may cause prolonged vasoconstriction mediated by mast cells and histamine release, triggering increased pulmonary vascular resistance and PH [44].

Irreversible pulmonary hypertension was recently reported in a cat infected with the lungworm *T. brevior* [21]. Importantly, this nematode is more pathogenic than *A. abstrusus* and it is known that kittens often develop severe or fatal infections by *T. brevior* rather than cats harbouring *A. abstrusus* [9,45]. Thus, a reliable parasitological diagnostic work-up is important to differentiate these lungworms towards appropriate and efficacious anthelmintic treatments [11]. The detection of L1 in the Baermann test and a thorough microscopic analysis are crucial. It has been recently claimed that the length of *A. abstrusus* and *T. brevior* L1s is distinctively different, i.e., ~360–415 and ~300–357 μm, respectively [26]. Nonetheless, L1s of both species with length outside of these ranges have also been described [1,4]. Therefore, other features should be examined to achieve a definitive identification. In particular, *A. abstrusus* L1s have a rounded head with a terminal oral opening and an S-shaped tail with a distinct knob-like or small finger-like projections at the tip of cuticular spines, while *T. brevior* L1s have a pointed head and a subterminal oral opening, with a tail tapering to the extremity and showing a deep dorsal notch and a shallower ventral one near their tip [26]. DNA based approaches are advisable in doubtful cases [27].

5. Conclusions

This is the first report of fatal severe PH and right-sided congestive heart failure in a kitten infected with *A. abstrusus*. Thus, other than in clinical cases of respiratory distress, *A. abstrusus* should be included in the differentials in the case of PH and right-sided congestive heart failure, especially in kittens and young cats. This is of importance, as cases of PH in association with *A. abstrusus* infection up to now have been reported only sporadically.

Author Contributions: Conceptualization, T.V., G.M. and A.P.; methodology, T.V., S.P., M.M., S.M., D.T. and A.P.; investigation, T.V., S.P., F.P., M.M., S.M., G.M., D.T. and A.P.; resources, S.P., D.T. and A.P.; data curation, T.V., S.P., F.P., M.M., G.M. and A.P.; writing—original draft preparation, T.V., S.P. and F.P.; writing—review and editing, T.V., S.P., D.T. and A.P. All authors have read and agreed to the published version of the manuscript.

Acknowledgments: The authors acknowledge Oscar Daolio for referring the clinical cases, and Luigi Venco for his contribution in the interpretation of clinical findings.

References

1. Traversa, D.; Di Cesare, A. Feline lungworms: What a dilemma. *Trends Parasitol.* **2013**, *29*, 423–430. [CrossRef] [PubMed]
2. Elsheikha, H.M.; Schnyder, M.; Traversa, D.; Di Cesare, A.; Wright, I.; Lacher, D.W. Updates on feline aelurostrongylosis and research priorities for the next decade. *Parasites Vectors* **2016**, *9*, 389. [CrossRef] [PubMed]
3. Traversa, D.; Di Cesare, A. Diagnosis and management of lungworm infections in cats: Cornerstones, dilemmas and new avenues. *J. Feline Med. Surg.* **2016**, *18*, 7–20. [CrossRef] [PubMed]
4. Giannelli, A.; Capelli, G.; Joachim, A.; Hinney, B.; Losson, B.; Kirkova, Z.; René-Martellet, M.; Papadopoulos, E.; Farkas, R.; Napoli, E.; et al. Lungworms and gastrointestinal parasites of domestic cats: A European perspective. *Int. J. Parasitol.* **2017**, *47*, 517–528. [CrossRef]
5. Traversa, D.; Morelli, S.; Cassini, R.; Crisi, P.E.; Russi, I.; Grillotti, E.; Manzocchi, S.; Simonato, G.; Beraldo, P.; Viglietti, A.; et al. Occurrence of canine and feline extra-intestinal nematodes in key endemic regions of Italy. *Acta Trop.* **2019**, *193*, 227–235. [CrossRef]
6. Hoggard, K.R.; Jarriel, D.M.; Bevelock, T.J.; Verocai, G.G. Prevalence survey of gastrointestinal and respiratory parasites of shelter cats in northeastern Georgia, USA. *Vet. Parasitol. Reg. Stud. Rep.* **2019**, *16*, 100270. [CrossRef]
7. Nagamori, Y.; Payton, M.E.; Looper, E.; Apple, H.; Johnson, E.M. Retrospective survey of parasitism identified in feces of client-owned cats in North America from 2007 through 2018. *Vet. Parasitol.* **2020**, *277*, 109008. [CrossRef]
8. Penagos-Tabares, F.; Lange, M.K.; Chaparro-Gutiérrez, J.J.; Taubert, A.; Hermosilla, C. *Angiostrongylus vasorum* and *Aelurostrongylus abstrusus*: Neglected and underestimated parasites in South America. *Parasites Vectors* **2018**, *11*, 208. [CrossRef]
9. Di Cesare, A.; Frangipane di Regalbono, A.; Tessarin, C.; Seghetti, M.; Iorio, R.; Simonato, G.; Traversa, D. Mixed infection by *Aelurostrongylus abstrusus* and *Troglostrongylus brevior* in kittens from the same litter in Italy. *Parasitol. Res.* **2014**, *113*, 613–618. [CrossRef]
10. Schnyder, M.; Di Cesare, A.; Basso, W.; Guscetti, F.; Riond, B.; Glaus, T.; Crisi, P.; Deplazes, P. Clinical, laboratory and pathological findings in cats experimentally infected with *Aelurostrongylus abstrusus*. *Parasitol. Res.* **2014**, *113*, 1425–1433. [CrossRef]
11. Crisi, P.E.; Aste, G.; Traversa, D.; Di Cesare, A.; Febo, E.; Vignoli, M.; Santori, D.; Luciani, A.; Boari, A. Single and mixed feline lungworm infections: Clinical, radiographic and therapeutic features of 26 cases (2013–2015). *J. Feline Med. Surg.* **2017**, *19*, 1017–1029. [CrossRef] [PubMed]
12. Naylor, J.R.; Hamilton, J.M.; Weatherley, A.J. Changes in the ultrastructure of feline pulmonary arteries following infection with the lungworm *Aelurostrongylus abstrusus*. *Br. Vet. J.* **1984**, *140*, 181–190. [CrossRef]
13. Dennler, M.; Bass, D.A.; Gutierrez-Crespo, B.; Schnyder, M.; Guscetti, F.; Di Cesare, A.; Deplazes, P.; Kircher, P.R.; Glaus, T.M. Thoracic computed tomography, angiographic computed tomography, and pathology findings in six cats experimentally infected with *Aelurostrongylus abstrusus*. *Vet. Radiol. Ultrasound* **2013**, *54*, 459–469. [CrossRef] [PubMed]
14. Connolly, D.J.; Lamb, C.R.; Boswood, A. Right-to-left shunting patent ductus arteriosus with pulmonary hypertension in a cat. *J. Small Anim. Pract.* **2003**, *44*, 184–188. [CrossRef]
15. Campbell, F.E.; Thomas, W.P. Congenital supravalvular mitral stenosis in 14 cats. *J. Vet. Cardiol.* **2012**, *14*, 281–292. [CrossRef]

16. Aoki, T.; Sugimoto, K.; Sunahara, H.; Fujii, Y. Patent ductus arteriosus ligation in two young cats with pulmonary hypertension. *J. Vet. Med. Sci.* **2013**, *75*, 199–202. [CrossRef]
17. Toaldo, M.B.; Guglielmini, C.; Diana, A.; Giunti, M.; Dondi, F.; Cipone, M. Reversible pulmonary hypertension in a cat. *J. Small Anim. Pract.* **2011**, *52*, 271–277. [CrossRef]
18. Evola, M.G.; Edmondson, E.F.; Reichle, J.K.; Biller, D.S.; Mitchell, C.W.; Valdés-Martínez, A. Radiographic and histopathologic characteristics of pulmonary fibrosis in nine cats. *Vet. Radiol. Ultrasound* **2014**, *55*, 133–140. [CrossRef]
19. MacPhail, C.M.; Innocenti, C.M.; Kudnig, S.T.; Veir, J.K.; Lappin, M.R. Atypical manifestations of feline inflammatory polyps in three cats. *J. Feline Med. Surg.* **2007**, *9*, 219–225. [CrossRef]
20. Vezzosi, T.; Schober, K.E. Doppler-derived echocardiographic evidence of pulmonary hypertension in cats with left-sided congestive heart failure. *J. Vet. Cardiol.* **2019**, *23*, 58–68. [CrossRef]
21. Crisi, P.E.; Traversa, D.; Di Cesare, A.; Luciani, A.; Civitella, C.; Santori, D.; Boari, A. Irreversible pulmonary hypertension associated with *Troglostrongylus brevior* infection in a kitten. *Res. Vet. Sci.* **2015**, *102*, 223–227. [CrossRef] [PubMed]
22. Dirven, M.; Szatmári, V.; van den Ingh, T.; Nijsse, R. Reversible pulmonary hypertension associated with lungworm infection in a young cat. *J. Vet. Cardiol.* **2012**, *14*, 465–474. [CrossRef] [PubMed]
23. Vezzosi, T.; Domenech, O.; Iacona, M.; Marchesotti, F.; Zini, E.; Venco, L.; Tognetti, R. Echocardiographic evaluation of the right atrial area index in dogs with pulmonary hypertension. *J. Vet. Intern. Med.* **2018**, *32*, 42–47. [CrossRef] [PubMed]
24. Vezzosi, T.; Domenech, O.; Costa, G.; Marchesotti, F.; Venco, L.; Zini, E.; Del Palacio, M.; Tognetti, R. Echocardiographic evaluation of the right ventricular dimension and systolic function in dogs with pulmonary hypertension. *J. Vet. Intern. Med.* **2018**, *32*, 1541–1548. [CrossRef] [PubMed]
25. Sloss, M.W.; Kemp, R.L.; Zajac, A.M. Fecal examination: Dogs and cats. In *Veterinary Clinical Parasitology*, 6th ed.; Iowa State University Press: Ames, IA, USA, 1994; p. 198.
26. Brianti, E.; Giannetto, S.; Dantas-Torres, F.; Otranto, D. Lungworms of the genus *Troglostrongylus* (Strongylida: Crenosomatidae): Neglected parasites for domestic cats. *Vet. Parasitol.* **2014**, *202*, 104–112. [CrossRef] [PubMed]
27. Di Cesare, A.; Veronesi, F.; di Regalbono, A.F.; Iorio, R.; Traversa, D. Novel Molecular Assay for Simultaneous Identification of Neglected Lungworms and Heartworms Affecting Cats. *J. Clin. Microbiol.* **2015**, *53*, 3009–3013. [CrossRef] [PubMed]
28. Philbey, A.W.; Krause, S.; Jeffries, R. Verminous pneumonia and enteritis due to hyperinfection with *Aelurostrongylusabstrusus* in a kitten. *J. Comp. Pathol.* **2014**, *150*, 357–360. [CrossRef]
29. Traversa, D.; Lia, R.P.; Iorio, R.; Boari, A.; Paradies, P.; Capelli, G.; Avolio, S.; Otranto, D. Diagnosis and risk factors of *Aelurostrongylus abstrusus* (Nematoda, Strongylida) infection in cats from Italy. *Vet. Parasitol.* **2008**, *153*, 182–186. [CrossRef]
30. Traversa, D.; Di Cesare, A.; Milillo, P.; Iorio, R.; Otranto, D. *Aelurostrongylus abstrusus* in a feline colony from central Italy: Clinical features, diagnostic procedures and molecular characterization. *Parasitol. Res.* **2008**, *103*, 1191–1196. [CrossRef]
31. Hawley, M.M.; Johnson, L.R.; Traversa, D.; Bucy, D.; Vernau, K.M.; Vernau, W. Respiratory distress associated with lungworm infection in a kitten. *J. Feline Med. Surg. Open Rep.* **2016**, *2*, 2055116916675801. [CrossRef]
32. Lacava, G.; Zini, E.; Marchesotti, F.; Domenech, O.; Romano, F.; Manzocchi, S.; Venco, L.; Auriemma, E. Computed tomography, radiology and echocardiography in cats naturally infected with *Aelurostrongylus abstrusus*. *J. Feline Med. Surg.* **2017**, *19*, 446–453. [CrossRef]
33. Winter, R.L.; Dillon, A.R.; Cattley, R.C.; Blagburn, B.L.; Tillson, D.M.; Johnson, C.M.; Brawner, W.R.; Welles, E.G.; Barney, S. Effect of heartworm disease and heartworm-associated respiratory disease (HARD) on the right ventricle of cats. *Parasites Vectors* **2017**, *10*, 492. [CrossRef] [PubMed]
34. Fossum, T.W.; Miller, M.W.; Rogers, K.S.; Bonagura, J.D.; Meurs, K.M. Chylothorax associated with right-sided heart failure in five cats. *J. Am. Vet. Med. Assoc.* **1994**, *204*, 84–89. [PubMed]
35. Koffas, H.; Fuentes, V.L.; Boswood, A.; Connolly, D.J.; Brockman, D.J.; Bonagura, J.D.; Meurs, K.M.; Koplitz, S.; Baumwart, R. Double chambered right ventricle in 9 cats. *J. Vet. Intern. Med.* **2007**, *21*, 76–80. [CrossRef] [PubMed]

36. Novo-Matos, J.; Hurter, K.; Bektas, R.; Grest, P.; Glaus, T. Patent ductus arteriosus in an adult cat with pulmonary hypertension and right-sided congestive heart failure: Hemodynamic evaluation and clinical outcome following ductal closure. *J. Vet. Cardiol.* **2014**, *16*, 197–203. [CrossRef]
37. Harvey, A.M.; Battersby, I.A.; Faena, M.; Fews, D.; Darke, P.G.; Ferasin, L. Arrhythmogenic right ventricular cardiomyopathy in two cats. *J. Small Anim. Pract.* **2005**, *46*, 151–156. [CrossRef]
38. Chetboul, V.; Passavin, P.; Trehiou-Sechi, E.; Gouni, V.; Poissonnier, C.; Pouchelon, J.L.; Desquilbet, L. Clinical, epidemiological and echocardiographic features and prognostic factors in cats with restrictive cardiomyopathy: A retrospective study of 92 cases (2001–2015). *J. Vet. Intern. Med.* **2019**, *33*, 1222–1231. [CrossRef]
39. Hamilton, J.M. The influence of infestation by *Aelurostrongylus abstrusus* on the pulmonary vasculature of the cat. *Br. Vet. J.* **1970**, *126*, 202–209. [CrossRef]
40. Losonsky, J.M.; Thrall, D.E.; Prestwood, A.K. Radiographic evaluation of pulmonary abnormalities after *Aelurostrogylus abstrusus* inoculation in cats. *Am. J. Vet. Res.* **1983**, *44*, 478–482.
41. Genchi, M.; Ferrari, N.; Fonti, P.; De Francesco, I.; Piazza, C.; Viglietti, A. Relation between *Aelurostrongylus abstrusus* larvae excretion, respiratory and radiographic signs in naturally infected cats. *Vet. Parasitol.* **2014**, *206*, 182–187. [CrossRef]
42. Gerdin, J.A.; Slater, M.R.; Makolinski, K.V.; Looney, A.L.; Appel, L.D.; Martin, N.M.; McDonough, S.P. Post-mortem findings in 54 cases of anesthetic associated death in cats from two spay-neuter programs in New York State. *J. Feline Med. Surg.* **2011**, *13*, 959–966. [CrossRef] [PubMed]
43. Mahaffey, M.B. Radiographic-pathologic findings in experimental *Aelurostrongylus abstrusus* infection in cats. *J. Am. Vet. Rad. Soc.* **1979**, *20*, 81. [CrossRef]
44. Rawlings, C.A.; Losonsky, J.M.; Lewis, R.E.; Hubble, J.J.; Prestwood, A.K. Response of the feline heart to *Aelurostrongylus abstrusus*. *J. Am. Anim. Hosp. Assoc.* **1980**, *16*, 573–578.
45. Di Cesare, A.; Veronesi, F.; Traversa, D. Felid Lungworms and Heartworms in Italy: More Questions than Answers? *Trends Parasitol.* **2015**, *31*, 665–675. [CrossRef]

7

Descriptive Pathological Study of Avian Schistosomes Infection in Whooper Swans (*Cygnus cygnus*)

Mohamed S. Ahmed [1,2], Reda E. Khalafalla [3], Ashraf Al-Brakati [4], Tokuma Yanai [5] and Ehab Kotb Elmahallawy [6,*]

1 Department of Pathology, Faculty of Veterinary Medicine, Kafrelsheikh University, Kafrelsheikh 33516, Egypt; aosayedahmed@yahoo.com
2 Department of Veterinary Pathology, Gifu University, 1-1 Yanagido, Gifu 501-1193, Japan
3 Department of Parasitology, Faculty of Veterinary Medicine, Kafrelsheikh University, Kafrelsheikh 33516, Egypt; redabast@hotmail.de
4 Department of Human Anatomy, College of Medicine, Taif University, P.O. Box 11099, Taif 21944, Saudi Arabia; a.albrakati@tu.edu.sa
5 Laboratory of Wildlife and Forensic Pathology, Biomedical Science Examination and Research Center, Department of Veterinary Medicine, Faculty of Veterinary Medicine, Okayama University of Science, Okayama 700-0005, Japan; tokumayanai@gmail.com
6 Department of Zoonoses, Faculty of Veterinary Medicine, Sohag University, Sohag 82524, Egypt
* Correspondence: eehaa@unileon.es

Simple Summary: Avian schistosomes are a group of parasites responsible for most of the reported cases of cercarial dermatitis outbreaks. Among others, *Trichobilharzia* is considered the largest genus of avian Schistosomatidae, and it infects more than 40 avian species. The present study involves a descriptive pathological study of avian schistosome in 54 whooper swans (*Cygnus cygnus*) from various rescue/rehabilitation centers in Honshu, Japan. Interestingly, adult schistosomes were detected in the lumen of mesenteric, serosal, portal, and testicular veins, in the capillaries of the intestinal lamina propria, and in the sinusoids of the adrenal gland, spleen, and liver of 23 (42.59%) swans. Schistosomes were assumed to be *Allobilharzia visceralis* based on the morphological characteristics of the worm and eggs found at histopathological examination of internal organs, along with suggestive pathological findings as well as the pathological findings. Collectively, the present study provides novel descriptive pathological data about schistosome infection in whooper swans with new insights on their role in the transmission and spreading of avian schistosomes in Japan.

Abstract: Cercarial dermatitis, or Swimmer's itch, is one of the emerging diseases caused by the cercariae of water-borne schistosomes, mainly *Trichobilharzia* spp. Since the zoonotic potential of *Allobilharzia visceralis* is still unknown, studies on this schistosome would be helpful to add knowledge on its possible role in causing human infections. In the present study, 54 whooper swans (*Cygnus cygnus*) from rescue/rehabilitation centers in Honshu, Japan, were necropsied to identify the cause of death. Grossly, 33 (61.11%) swans were severely emaciated and 23 (42.59%) had multiple reddened areas throughout the length of the intestine with no worms detected in the internal organs. Microscopically, adult schistosomes were found in the lumen of the mesenteric, serosal, portal, and testicular veins, in the capillaries of the intestinal lamina propria, and in the sinusoids of the adrenal gland, spleen, and liver of 23 (42.59%) swans. Hypertrophy of veins containing adult worms was identified in 15 (27.77%) swans, and vascular lumen obliteration was observed in 8 (14.81%) swans. Mild to severe villous atrophy and superficial enteritis were observed in 8 birds (14.81%), whereas bile pigments and hemosiderin were detected in the livers of 14 (25.92%) and 18 (33.33%) swans, respectively. In three swans (5.55%), schistosome parasites were found in the subcapsular veins of the testes. The schistosomes in the present study were assumed to be *A. visceralis* based on the microscopical and histological evidence of adult schistosomes found in the lumen of veins as well as the infection pathology, which was very similar to the schistosome-induced pathology previously reported in swans infected by *A. visceralis* in Europe and Australia. The swans examined herein most likely died from obstructive phlebitis associated with *A. visceralis*, but further molecular confirmation is required for identification of this species. However, the present study does not provide new data on the zoonotic potential, but only on the pathogenic potential of this schistosome in swans. Furthermore, our study provides a novel contribution to the description of the pathological effects of avian schistosomes infection in whooper swans in Japan.

Keywords: schistosome; *Allobilharzia visceralis*; whooper swans; obstructive phlebitis

---

1. Introduction

Avian schistosomes are a specialized group of parasites and have a particular importance due to their zoonotic potential [1–3]. These schistosomes inhabit the circulatory system of the definitive avian hosts and are commonly known as "blood flukes." Various species of birds can be infected with schistosomes, but infection is most prevalent in waterfowl [1,4–7]. Among others, *Trichobilharzia* is the largest genus of avian Schistosomatidae, covering more than 40 avian species [8], and they can be divided into visceral and nasal species based on their predilection sites. Visceral species migrate through the viscera and are typically found in mesenteric, renal, cloacal, and portal blood vessels [9,10].

Most of these digenean trematodes have an indirect lifecycle involving a gastropod intermediate host. Fresh-water snails are required for the development of schistosomes belonging to the genera *Bilharziella, Ornithobilharzia, Jilinobilharzia, Macrobilhazia,* and *Trichobilharzia* and salt or brackish mollusks are instead required for genera *Dendritobilharzia, Gigantobilharzia,* and *Austrobilharzia* [3,8,10,11]. Infected aquatic bird excrete schistosome eggs, that hatch and release miracidia that penetrate inside the intermediate hosts where they develop to cercaria [11,12]. Thereafter, cercaria is released from the snail intermediate hosts and invade the warm-blooded vertebrate host via skin penetration, in whose circulatory system they develop to adults [1,4,7].

Avian schistosomiasis is characterized by lesions similar to those present in mammals infected with schistosomes, e.g., obliterative endophlebitis, venous hypertrophy, necrosis, granulomatous reaction combined with a mixed inflammatory response, thrombosis of mesenteric veins, fibrinohemorrhagic colitis, and portal fibroplasia, due to the presence of adults and/or eggs in blood vessels [5,9,13–21]. However, extensive anatomopathological studies on avian schistosomiasis are lacking. In humans, the repeated penetration of the skin causes the human cercarial dermatitis (HCD), an allergic reaction also known as "swimmer's itch" [1,15,22]. Cercarial dermatitis can be caused by several species of avian schistosomes, e.g., those belonging to the genera *Trichobilharzia, Gigantobilharzia,* and *Austrobilharzia* [3,8,10,11,23]. The zoonotic potential of other species, such as the swan schistosome *Allobilharzia visceralis* remains unknown [6,24,25], despite it cannot be excluded that it can produce HCD. Human cercarial dermatitis is considered endemic in Japan and rice farmers are among the occupational groups at high risk of infection [1,15,26]. In many cases, an etiological diagnosis of HCD at species level can be difficult to achieve, and it cannot be excluded that some cases could be due to *A. visceralis*. Swans are present in Japan and can transport their schistosomes during their migrations [15,23,27]. Indeed, *A. visceralis* has been already reported in swans either in Japan other than in North America and Iceland [13,28–30]. Therefore, in the light of the scarce knowledge on the pathology of avian schistosomiasis and of the potential zoonotic implications of blood flukes infecting swans [1,15,31,32], this study evaluated the occurrence of blood flukes in swans from Japan, discussing anatomopathological findings.

2. Materials and Methods

2.1. Ethical Statement

This study was approved by the Animal Care and Use Committee of Gifu University (approval I: EA07-05) and the Department of Veterinary Pathology, Kafrelsheikh University. Appropriate Institutional Animal Care Guidelines were followed during all handling and procedures.

2.2. Animals and Sample Collection

Fifty-four swans were received from rescue/rehabilitation centers in Honshu, Japan, between May 2005 and June 2007. Of these 54 birds, 38 were found dead, 12 swans died shortly after their arrival, whereas 4 swans were severely or moderately emaciated and dehydrated and were euthanized to avoid them unnecessary suffering. To determine the cause of death, the swans were submitted to the veterinary pathology department of the Gifu University for postmortem examination. Thirty-one swans were young (24–36 months), and the remaining were adults (48–72 months). Birds were categorized as immature if they still had brown feathers in their plumage, a pink-gray beak, and gray feet, whereas birds with fully white plumage, an orange beak, and black feet were categorized as mature [19,33]. This study followed the guidelines and measures of the Department of Veterinary Pathology, Gifu University, Japan, for the care and use of animals. In addition, before proceeding with euthanasia, appropriate veterinary care consistent with international, national, and institutional guidelines was guaranteed to the swans.

2.3. Gross and Histopathological Examination

Necropsies were performed on all swans in accordance with a standardized protocol. This procedure began with a review of the relevant history followed a full examination to detect anatomopathological alterations. To identify small foreign fragments or any lesions, the contents of the gizzard and intestine were carefully washed. Tissue samples were collected from all organs and from any noticeable lesions. The specimens were fixed in 10% phosphate-buffered formalin, embedded in paraffin, sectioned at a thickness of 4 μm, and then stained with hematoxylin and eosin [34]. Liver sections were also stained with Hall's bilirubin stain for bile pigment, and specimens of the liver and spleen were stained with Berlin blue stain for iron [34,35].

2.4. Parasitological Examination

It is difficult to describe the morphological features of the worms in this study, because the adult worms were very small and typically present only in the lumen of the affected veins. The different stages of the parasites observed in the various histopathological sections were incidentally reported during the measurement of lead (Pb) content in the soft tissues (liver and kidney). The morphology of the different stages of the adult worm in the blood vessels of different damaged internal organs and the effect of eggs in the intestinal mucosa of the affected birds were used for localization of the parasite during histopathological examination, as reported elsewhere [36].

3. Results

3.1. Gross Examination

Thirty-three out of 54 necropsied whooper swans were severely emaciated and lean, with atrophied pectoral muscles, serious atrophy of pericardial fat, and an absence of fat depots. Twenty-three birds showed multiple reddened areas throughout the entire length of the intestine, which were most prominent in the ileum, cecum, and colon. The main histological lesions were found in the intestinal tract, liver, adrenal gland, spleen, and testis; these lesions were caused by both worms and eggs (Table 1).

Table 1. Summary of histopathological lesions and worm findings in 23 infected whooper swans.

No. of Swans	1	2	3	4	5	6	7	8	9	10	11	12	13	14	15	16	17	18	19	20	21	22	23
Sex/Age	F/A	F/A	F/A	M/Y	M/Y	M/Y	M/Y	F/A	F/A	F/Y	M/A	M/Y	M/Y	F/A	M/Y	F/Y	ND/Y	F/A	F/Y	F/ND	M/Y	F/A	M/Y
Emaciation	++	+++	+	+	+	++	+	+++	+	+	++	+	+	+	++	+	+	++	+++	++	+	+	+
Parasites in serosal vein	+	++	+	++	+	++	+	++	+	+	++	+	+	++	+	+	+	++	+	+	+	++	++
Parasites in mesenteric V	++	++	+	+	++	++	++	+	+	+	+	+	++	+	+	+	+	+	+	+	+	+	+
Parasites in portal vein	+	+	+	-	-	+	+	++	-	-	+	-	-	-	+	-	+	+	+	+	-	+	+
Parasites in hepatic sinusoids	+	+	-	+	-	+	+	+	-	-	++	-	-	-	++	-	+	+	+	+	-	+	+
Parasites in adrenal sinusoids	+	+++	+	-	-	-	++	-	-	+	-	-	+	-	-	+	-	++	+++	-	-	++	-
Parasites *in splenic veins*	-	-	+	+	-	-	+	+	+++	-	+	+	-	-	-	-	+	+	-	-	+	-	-
Parasites *in subcapsular veins*	+++	++	-	-	-	-	-	++	-	-	-	-	-	-	-	-	-	-	-	-	-	-	-
Bile pigment deposition	++	++	-	+	-	+++	-	+++	+	-	++	-	+	-	++	-	-	+	+	+	-	+	+
Hemosiderin pigment	+++	++	-	++	+	++	-	+++	++	-	++	-	+	-	++	+	+	++	++	+	+	+	+
Venous hypertrophy	++	++	-	-	++	-	++	++	-	-	++	-	+	-	++	-	+	++	++	-	-	++	-
Obliterative endophlebitis	+	+	-	-	+	-	-	+	-	-	+	-	-	-	++	-	-	++	+	-	-	-	-
Villous atrophy		+	-	-	+	+	-	+	++	-	+	-	-	+	-	-	-	++	-	-	-	-	-

F: female M: male A: adult Y: young NA: not analyzed ND: not determined N: negative + mild ++ moderate +++ severe.

3.2. *Histopathological Examination*

Adult schistosomes were found in 43% (23/54) of the swans. In these cases, one or more adult worms were detected in the veins but not in the arteries. Adult worms were found in the lumen of the mesenteric veins, serosal veins, portal veins, testicular veins, capillaries of the intestinal lamina propria, and sinusoids of the adrenal gland, spleen and liver. Macrophages containing brownish pigment were occasionally seen in the parenchyma surrounding the worms, most commonly in the splenic veins and the hepatic sinusoids. Some affected veins, mainly the serosal and mesenteric veins, showed endophlebitis, irregular intimal thickening due to the infiltration of inflammatory cells, and hypertrophy of the muscular fibers in the tunica media.

3.2.1. Intestine

Numerous sections of adult schistosomes were found in the mesenteric and serosal veins throughout the intestine in all 23 infected birds, being the ileum, caecum, and colon the most affected areas. Vessels containing adult schistosomes showed endophlebitis characterized by myointimal hyperplasia, with infiltration of plasma cells, heterophils, and eosinophils in the surrounding tissues (Figure 1A,B). In 12 swans, the mesenteric and serosal veins, along with the veins between the muscular layers of the intestine, exhibited nodular hypertrophy of the tunica media. Eight swans suffered from obliterative endophlebitis with complete occlusion of the venous lumen (Figure 1C). Superficial enteritis was present in eight birds, and mild to severe villous atrophy was observed in association with numerous parasitic eggs in the lamina propria (in both the small and large intestine) have been observed by microscopical or histological evidence. The eggs were surrounded by venous congestion and diffuse infiltration of the lamina propria, with a variable number of lymphocytes and a few plasma cells, heterophils, and eosinophils (Figure 1D).

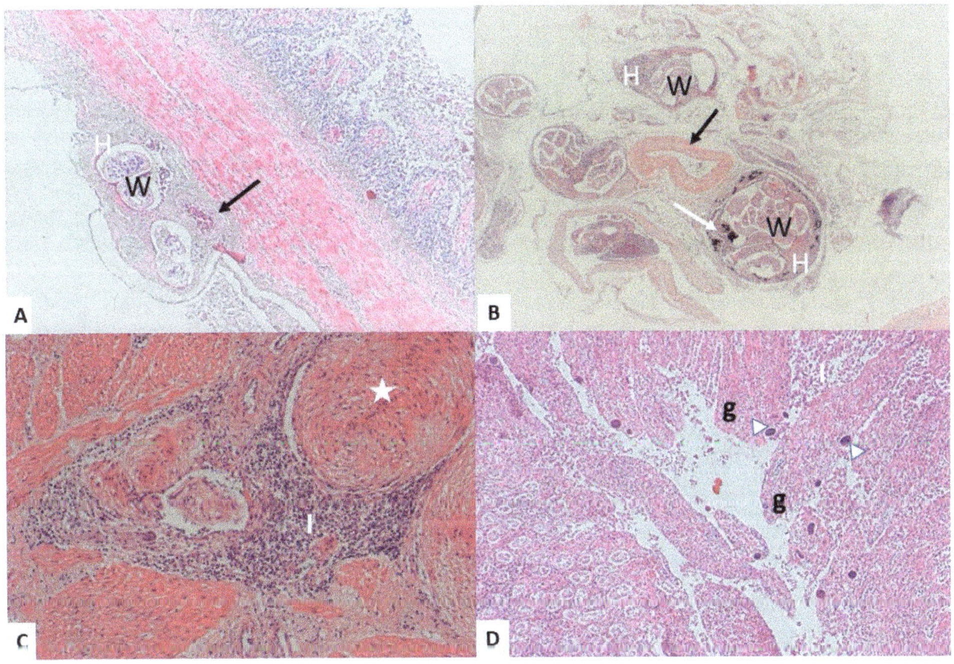

Figure 1. Effect of the parasite in the intestine. (**A**) Adult worms (W) are seen in the thickened walls of the serosal vein (H). Note the normal thickness of the artery (black arrow). (**B**) Brownish pigment–laden macrophages (white arrow) around the worm (W) in the thickened wall of the mesenteric veins (H). (**C**) The vein lumen was almost occluded due to marked myointimal hyperplasia in the veins of the muscular layer of the intestine (white star), with perivascular inflammatory reaction (I). (**D**) Several schistosome eggs (white arrowheads) present in the intestinal lamina propria and surrounded by an inflammatory reaction of lymphocytes and plasma cells (I); the intestinal villi are markedly blunted (g). Hematoxylin and eosin stain (100×).

3.2.2. Liver

Adult worms were found in the portal veins and hepatic sinusoids of 14 birds. In five cases, mild to severe inflammatory reactions were observed around the parasites or eggs in the hepatic parenchyma, with degeneration of the hepatic cells and infiltration of a large number of inflammatory cells in the hepatic sinusoids and the portal triads (Figure 2A,B). Fourteen swans had areas of *bile pigment deposition* (biliverdin) in the liver parenchyma, which stained positively with Hall's stain (Figure 2C). In addition, mild to marked deposition of hemosiderin pigment, positive on Berlin blue staining, was apparent in the liver of 18 swans (Figure 2D).

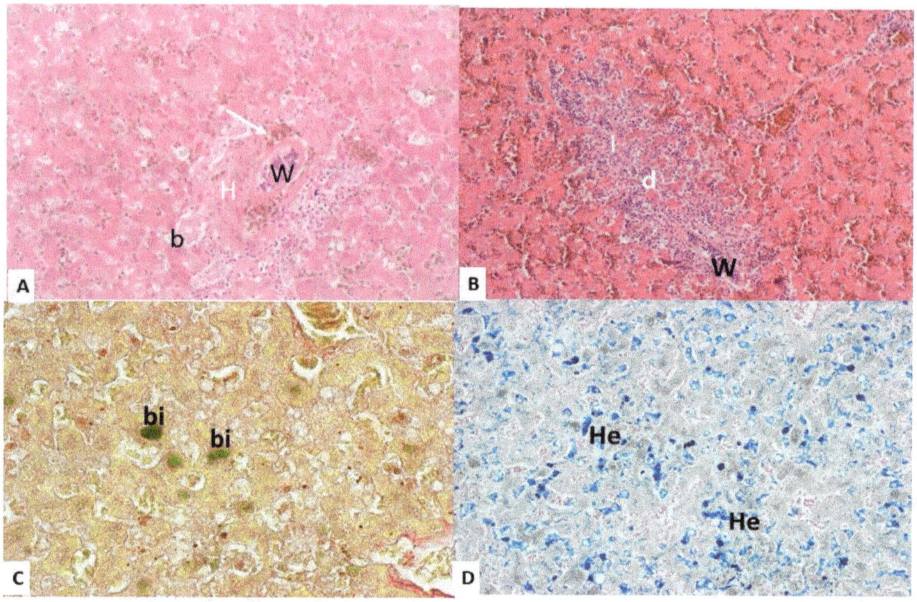

Figure 2. Effect of the parasite in the liver. (**A**) Adult worms (W) present in the thickened walled of the portal vein (H) with hemosiderin pigment deposition (white arrow) and bile duct hyperplasia (b). (**B**) Schistosome parasite (W) found in the hepatic sinusoids surrounded by degenerated hepatocyte (d) and massive inflammatory reaction (I). Hematoxylin and eosin stain (100×). (**C**) Emerald green–colored clumps of bile pigment (bi), Hall stain (400×). (**D**) Macrophages laden with bluish pigment (He), Berlin blue stain (100×).

3.2.3. Adrenal Glands

Numerous sections of adult schistosomes were observed within the adrenal sinusoids of 10 swans, and some sinusoids were completely occluded, resulting in pressure on the surrounding cells (Figure 3A). An inflammatory reaction was seen around the worms in six birds, with infiltration of lymphocytes and plasma cells and degeneration of the adrenal gland cells (Figure 3B).

3.2.4. Spleen

Adult worms were present in the subcapsular sinusoids and splenic veins of 10 swans (Figure 3C). Furthermore, mild to marked deposition of hemosiderin pigment was reported in the spleen of 18 swans (Figure 2D).

3.2.5. Testes

Multiple adult worms were found in the superficial subcapsular veins underneath the tunica albuginea in three swans. In these cases, infiltration of inflammatory cells, predominantly lymphocytes, macrophages, and a few heterophils, was seen in the surrounding parenchyma (Figure 3D).

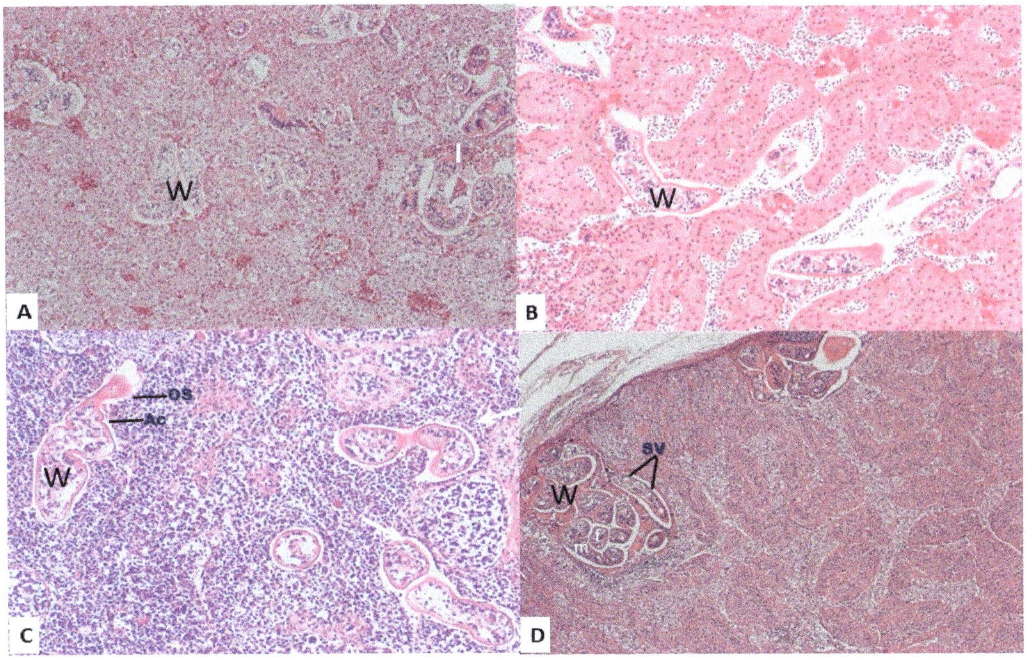

Figure 3. Effect of the parasite in the adrenal gland, spleen, and testis. (**A**, **B**) Multiple cross-sections of adult worms (W) found in the sinusoids of the adrenal gland surrounded by infiltration of mononuclear inflammatory cells (I). (**C**) Adult worms (W) found in the splenic veins. Note the oral sucker (Os) and acetabulum (Ac) of the parasite. (**D**) Multiple cross-sections of adult schistosomes (W) completely occlude the subcapsular veins of the testis and were surrounded by the infiltration of mononuclear inflammatory cells (I). Note the seminal vesicles of the parasite (Sv) and the presence of female (f) in the ventral groove of the male (m) parasite. Hematoxylin and eosin stain (100×).

3.3. Parasitological Findings

Based on the available information, including the species of the affected bird and its location, the morphological characteristics of the schistosome worm and eggs in the intestinal lamina propria, and pathological findings, the schistosomes of the present study were assumed to be *A. visceralis*. The death of the investigated swans was suspected to be due to obstructive phlebitis associated with the suspected parasite. Eggs were found abundantly in the intestinal lamina propria and were mostly ovoid to asymmetrical in shape (Figure 1D); however, confirmation at the species level requires further molecular investigation. Moreover, the schistosome flukes occurred in abundance in the veins of different internal organs with varying morphological characteristics, i.e., oral sucker, posterior sucker, or acetabulum), seminal vesicles, and testis (Figure 3C). Some adult schistosome parasites were found in pairs, with the male carrying the female in its ventral groove or gynecophoric canal (Figure 3D).

4. Discussion

Schistosomes are considered to be highly pathogenic in migratory waterfowl [37]. Because the worm is very small and located in the blood vessels, schistosomes in whooper swans can be overlooked on gross necropsy [9,36]. It should be stressed that Swimmer's itch is considered an emerging disease in various parts of the world, resulting in various nervous or pulmonary symptoms on the basis of the infecting species [38]. Furthermore, avian schistosomes have been considered the most neglected parasitic zoonosis among aquatic birds worldwide [23]. To the best of our knowledge, there are no published studies describing the pathological effects of schistosome infection in whooper swans in Japan. Thus, this study provides a novel contribution to this research topic and adds knowledge on a potentially zoonotic parasite.

We detected adult schistosomes in 43% (23/54) of whooper swans on necropsy; the worms were mostly present in the veins of the large and small intestine, liver, adrenal gland, spleen, and testis.

These findings are consistent with previous studies reporting that vascular lesions caused by avian schistosome infection in birds are comparable with lesions observed in visceral schistosomiasis in mammals [9,13,20]. Given the fact that this study was carried out during the period 2005–2007, we planned to perform molecular characterization of the parasite but there were no available samples to do perform this step. In Japan, Hayashi et al. (2017) [13] detected for the first time *A. visceralis* in the capillaries of several organs of whooper swans using molecular methods, without microscopical or histological evidence of eggs or worm. Meanwhile, studies performed in Iceland [28,29] and North America [30] identified vascular lesions caused by schistosomes in whooper swans and tundra swans, respectively. We believe that emaciation and weakness in all 23 infected swans may have resulted from the severe vascular effects associated with schistosome infection, namely, the obstruction of venous return in the mesenteric, intestinal, splenic, and portal veins as well as enteropathy. Both adult schistosomes and eggs contributed to the enteropathy: the adults caused obliterative vascular lesions, whereas the migration of the eggs led to enteritis with villous atrophy [19]. However, in cases such as these, it is not clear whether the parasites are the cause of emaciation [31,39], as important data, such as bodyweight and parasitic load of healthy birds for comparison, are missing [15]. We did not have data on the body weight and parasitic load of apparently healthy whooper swans from this region for comparison. In the current study, the blood flukes infecting the whooper swan were assumed to likely be *A. visceralis*, on the basis on the species of the affected bird, morphological characteristics of the worm and eggs found in the internal organs, and pathological findings associated with their presence in the blood vessels of different organs in both adult and juvenile birds. This method of identification was previously accepted and is in agreement with the findings of Kolářová et al. (2010) [36]. However, further accurate identification methods (i.e., molecular characterization methods are still needed. We were unable to describe the morphological features of adult worms in this study because of the difficulty in obtaining intact specimens: adult worms are very small and are usually present only in the lumen of affected veins, which is consistent with some previous reports [11,19]. Furthermore, these findings are supported by the results from Hayashi et al. (2017) [13], who did not detect egg-like structures of the schistosome in the swans but there was no any gross abnormality or necrosis in the organs of affected swans and assumed that schistosomes did not cause severe damage to the swans examined. Similarly, a recent study reported unidentified schistosomes and their eggs only by histopathological examination [18]. In this study, flukes were found inside the lumen of blood vessels of the muscular layer and in the mucosa of the esophagus, intestine, and caeca but with a slight inflammatory response in only three cases, represented by hemorrhage and infiltration of some inflammatory cells, such as lymphocytes and heterophiles [18]. In contrast, Brant (2007) [24] detected adult worms and egg-tissue debris in a nodule of the inferior mesenteric vein and suggested that, to identify the species of parasite, it is important to investigate the correlation between the pathological lesions and the general condition of the swans, as well as to determine the presence or absence of eggs. The disease features were similar to those described in several reports of schistosome infection in swans from Europe and Australia, including the black swan (*Cygnus atratus*) and the mute swan (*Cygnus olor*) in Australia [27,40] and the whooper swan in Europe [27]. Our results indicated that the number of young birds affected was higher than the numbers of adults, i.e., 61% (14/23) of affected swans were immature. The higher prevalence of infection in the young birds might be due to lower immunity, as compared with the increased immunity in adults that results from repeated exposure to schistosome parasites [41]. In the present study, most infected swans 78% (18/23) showed endophlebitis of the veins containing adult worms, with infiltration of leukocytes into the surrounding tissues. This may have resulted from the irritation of the vessel walls caused by the worms, which led to myointimal hyperplasia and, in some instances, to occlusion of the affected blood vessels. This concept and previous findings are consistent with the reports of Warren (1977) [42], Bolhuis et al. (2004) [19], and Kolářová et al. (2001) [43], all of whom suggested that viable adult schistosomes cause proliferation of the vascular intima either via mechanical injury to the intima or via the secretion of antigens as an immune (allergic) reaction against the schistosomes. Bolhuis et al. (2004) [19] revealed the occurrence of *Trichobilharzia* sp. in five of eight mute swans, whereas pathological lesions including moderate to severe, diffuse, hyperplastic endophlebitis were reported in the intestinal veins together with splenic and hepatic hemosiderosis [19]. In the current study, we did not find any fibrosis in the portal triad in the birds examined. This is consistent with the findings of Kolářová et al. (2006) [15] but in contrast to those of Bolhuis et al. (2004) [19], who reported mild to extensive fibroplasia of the portal triads in mute swans and attributed this finding to the aberrant localization of female schistosomes in the bile ducts. Similarly, Wojcinski et al. (1987) [44] reported the same lesions in ducks infected with schistosomes but found no evidence of parasites in bile ducts, and Robinson and Maxie (1993) [20] reported that in mammals, severe cases of schistosomiasis might result in occlusion of the lumen of the veins, and lesions may extend to the intrahepatic branches of the portal vein, leading to prominent portal fibrosis. Bolhuis et al. (2004) [19] also reported the development of granulomas due to the severe perivascular inflammatory reaction around the veins harboring the adult parasite in the liver of juvenile and adult birds; in contrast, Brant (2007) [24] did not find any granulomas in the portal triads of infected swans.

In the present work, worm eggs were found multifocally in the lamina propria of the small and/or large intestine, and 35% (8/23) of swans showed mild to severe villous atrophy (villous blunting, fusion, and edema) and superficial enteritis, which might have resulted from the migration of schistosome eggs through the intestinal wall. This explanation is supported by a previous study conducted by Wojcinski et al. (1987) [44]. In addition, in their study, Bolhuis et al. (2004) [19] reported lymphocytic and granulocytic enteritis associated with the presence of eggs of schistosomes in the intestinal mucosa of examined swans. However, Horák et al. (2002) reported that in human schistosomiasis, some eggs fail to reach the intestinal lumen and are instead disseminated through the circulatory system to the liver, lungs, and other organs, where they cause reactions ranging from very mild to marked granulomatous inflammation. Robinson and Maxie (1993) [20] stated that schistosome eggs release antigens that induce a delayed hypersensitivity response and cause the formation of small granulomas, which are characterized by the infiltration of eosinophils, mononuclear leukocytes, and giant cells as well as reactive fibrosis. In the present study, we observed bile pigments and hemosiderin in the liver of 61% (14/23) and 78% (18/23) of whooper swans infected with avian schistosomes, respectively, whereas adult worms and/or eggs were detected in the liver of 61% (14/23) of infected swans. This indicates that cholestatic jaundice may be caused by avian schistosomiasis, as found by Akagami et al. (2010) [16]. Schistosomes were detected in the sinusoids of the adrenal gland in 44% (10/23) of swans in the present study; this finding has not previously been reported, except in one study by Hayashi et al. (2017) [13]. A unique finding of this study is the detection of worms in the sinusoids of the testes in 13% (3/23) of infected swans. We believe that the presence of parasites in the adrenal glands and in the testes was due to the migration of parasites through the vascular system of heavily infected birds.

5. Conclusions

In conclusion, our study provides interesting data that describe the pathological effects of schistosome infection, assumed to be *A. visceralis*, in whooper swans in Japan, which provides a novel contribution to this field of research. It could be suggested that these parasites were the cause of death in the infected swans in this study, because they were found in the blood vessels of all infected swans and caused obstructive phlebitis. Additional molecular studies on schistosome infection in whooper swans and in their snail intermediate hosts are required to better characterize the parasite species.

Author Contributions: M.S.A. and T.Y. involved in the conception of the research idea and methodology design and performed data analysis and interpretation. R.E.K., A.A.-B. and E.K.E. participated of the methodology, sampling, the laboratory work and data analysis and prepared the manuscript for publication. M.S.A., R.E.K., A.A.-B., T.Y. and E.K.E. contributed their scientific advice, prepared the manuscript for publication, and performed the revision. All authors have read and agreed to the published version of the manuscript.

Acknowledgments: The authors sincerely thank the staff members of the rescue/rehabilitation centers for their efforts in the collection of swans. They also thank the members of the Department of Veterinary Pathology, Faculty of Applied Biological Science, Gifu University, and Biomedical Science Examination and Research Center, Okayama University of Science, Japan, for their support. The authors thank Taif University Researchers Supporting Program (Project number: TURSP-2020/151), Taif University, Saudi Arabia for their support.

References

1. Horak, P.; Mikes, L.; Lichtenbergova, L.; Skala, V.; Soldanova, M.; Brant, S.V. Avian schistosomes and outbreaks of cercarial dermatitis. *Clin. Microbiol. Rev.* **2015**, *28*, 165–190. [CrossRef] [PubMed]
2. Turjanicová, L.; Mikeš, L.; Pecková, M.; Horák, P. Antibody response of definitive hosts against antigens of two life stages of the neuropathogenic schistosome Trichobilharzia regenti. *Parasites Vectors* **2015**, *8*, 1–11. [CrossRef] [PubMed]
3. Azimov, D. *Schistosomes of Animals and Man*; Izdatel'stvo 'FAN': Taskhent, Uzbekistan, 1975.
4. Webster, B.L.; Southgate, V.R.; Littlewood, D.T. A revision of the interrelationships of Schistosoma including the recently described Schistosoma guineensis. *Int. J. Parasitol.* **2006**, *36*, 947–955. [CrossRef]
5. Atkinson, C.T.; Thomas, N.J.; Hunter, D.B. *Parasitic Diseases of Wild Birds*; John Wiley & Sons: Hoboken, NJ, USA, 2009.
6. Brant, S.V.; Loker, E.S. Molecular systematics of the avian schistosome genus Trichobilharzia (Trematoda: Schistosomatidae) in North America. *J. Parasitol.* **2009**, *95*, 941–963. [CrossRef] [PubMed]
7. Rudolfová, J. New findings of schistosomes in wildfowl and snails. *Helminthologia* **2001**, *38*, 248–249.
8. Skrjabin, K. Family Schistosomatidae Looss, 1899. *Trematodes Anim. Man* **1951**, *5*, 225–414.
9. Horak, P.; Kolarova, L.; Adema, C.M. Biology of the schistosome genus Trichobilharzia. *Adv. Parasitol.* **2002**, *52*, 155–233.
10. Farley, J. A review of the family Schistosomatidae: Excluding the genus Schistosoma from mammals. *J. Helminthol.* **1971**, *45*, 289–320. [CrossRef]
11. Khalil, L. Family Schistosomatidae Stiles & Hassall, 1898. *Keys Trematoda* **2002**, *1*, 419–432.
12. McLaren, D.J.; Hockley, D.J. Blood flukes have a double outer membrane. *Nature* **1977**, *269*, 147–149. [CrossRef]
13. Hayashi, K.; Ichikawa-Seki, M.; Ohari, Y.; Mohanta, U.K.; Aita, J.; Satoh, H.; Ehara, S.; Tokashiki, M.; Shiroma, T.; Azuta, A.; et al. First detection of Allobilharzia visceralis (Schistosomatidae, Trematoda) from Cygnus cygnus in Japan. *Parasitol. Int.* **2017**, *66*, 925–929. [CrossRef]
14. Randall, C.; Reece, R.L. *Color Atlas of Avian Histopathology*; Mosby-Wolfe: London, UK; Baltimore, MD, USA, 1996.
15. Kolarova, L.; Rudolfova, J.; Hampl, V.; Skirnisson, K. Allobilharzia visceralis gen. nov., sp. nov. (Schistosomatidae-Trematoda) from Cygnus cygnus (L.) (Anatidae). *Parasitol. Int.* **2006**, *55*, 179–186. [PubMed]
16. Akagami, M.; Nakamura, K.; Nishino, H.; Seki, S.; Shimizu, H.; Yamamoto, Y. Pathogenesis of venous hypertrophy associated with schistosomiasis in whooper swans (Cygnus cygnus) in Japan. *Avian Dis.* **2010**, *54*, 146–150. [CrossRef] [PubMed]
17. Paré, J.A.; Black, S.R. Schistosomiasis in a collection of captive Chilean flamingos (Phoenicopterus chilensis). *J. Avian Med. Surg.* **1999**, 187–191.
18. Oyarzún-Ruiz, P.; Muñoz, P.; Paredes, E.; Valenzuela, G.; Ruiz, J. Gastrointestinal helminths and related histopathological lesions in black-necked swans Cygnus melancoryphus from the Carlos Anwandter Nature Sanctuary, Southern Chile. *Rev. Bras. De Parasitol. Vet.* **2019**, *28*, 613–624. [CrossRef] [PubMed]
19. van Bolhuis, G.H.; Rijks, J.M.; Dorrestein, G.M.; Rudolfova, J.; van Dijk, M.; Kuiken, T. Obliterative endophlebitis in mute swans (Cygnus olor) caused by Trichobilharzia sp. (Digenea: Schistosomatidae) infection. *Vet. Pathol.* **2004**, *41*, 658–665. [PubMed]
20. Robinson, W.F.; Maxie, M.G. The cardiovascular system. In *Pathology of Domestic Animals*, 4th ed.; Jubb, K.V.F., Kennedy, P.C., Palmer, N., Eds.; Academic Press: San Diego, CA, USA, 1993; Volume 3, pp. 1–100.
21. Pence, D.B.; RHODES, M.J. Trichobilharzia physellae (Digenea: Schistosomatidae) from endemic waterfowl on the high plains of Texas. *J. Wildl. Dis.* **1982**, *18*, 69–74. [CrossRef]
22. Leedom, W.S.; Short, R.B. Cercaria pomaceae sp. n., a dermatitis-producing schistosome cercaria from Pomacea paludosa, the Florida apple snail. *J. Parasitol.* **1981**, 257–261. [CrossRef]

23. Lashaki, E.K.; Teshnizi, S.H.; Gholami, S.; Fakhar, M.; Brant, S.V.; Dodangeh, S. Global prevalence status of avian schistosomes: A systematic review with meta-analysis. *Parasite Epidemiol. Control* **2020**, *9*, e00142. [CrossRef]
24. Brant, S.V. The occurrence of the avian schistosome Allobilharzia visceralis Kolakrova, Rudolfova, Hampl et Skirnisson, 2006 (Schistosomatidae) in the tundra swan, Cygnus columbianus (Anatidae), from North America. *Folia Parasitol (Praha)* **2007**, *54*, 99–104. [CrossRef]
25. Jouet, D.; Ferte, H.; Hologne, C.; Kaltenbach, M.L.; Depaquit, J. Avian schistosomes in French aquatic birds: A molecular approach. *J. Helminthol.* **2009**, *83*, 181–189. [CrossRef] [PubMed]
26. Chamot, E.; Toscani, L.; Rougemont, A. Public health importance and risk factors for cercarial dermatitis associated with swimming in Lake Leman at Geneva, Switzerland. *Epidemiol. Infect.* **1998**, *120*, 305–314. [CrossRef] [PubMed]
27. Kolárová, L. Avian schistosomes of the genus Trichobilharzia in final hosts in Europe. *Bull. Scand. Soc. Parasitol.* **2005**, *14*, 85–86.
28. Kolarova, L.; Skirnisson, K.; Horak, P. Schistosome cercariae as the causative agent of swimmer's itch in Iceland. *J. Helminthol.* **1999**, *73*, 215–220. [CrossRef] [PubMed]
29. Huelsenbeck, J.P.; Ronquist, F. MRBAYES: Bayesian inference of phylogenetic trees. *Bioinformatics* **2001**, *17*, 754–755. [CrossRef]
30. Petersen, A. *Íslenskir Fuglar (Icelandic Birds.)*; Vaka-Helgafell: Reykjavík, Iceland, 1998.
31. Wobeser, G.A. *Diseases of Wild Waterfowl*; Springer Science & Business Media: New York, NY, USA, 2012.
32. Blankespoor, H.; Reimink, R. The Control of Swimmer's Itch in Michigan: Past, Present, and Future. *Mich. Acad.* **1991**, *24*, 7–23.
33. Cramp, S.; Perrins, C. *The Birds of the Western Palearctic*; Oxford University Press: Oxford, UK, 1977; Volumes 1–9.
34. Bancroft, J.D.; Gamble, M. *Theory and Practice of Histological Techniques*; Elsevier Health Sciences: Amsterdam, The Netherlands, 2008.
35. Watanaba, Y.; Sakaguchi, H.; Hosoda, Y. *The Methods of Preparing Histologic Sections*, 6th ed.; Igaku Shoin Company Ltd.: Tokyo, Japan, 1992; pp. 81–140.
36. Kolarova, L.; Horak, P.; Skirnisson, K. Methodical approaches in the identification of areas with a potential risk of infection by bird schistosomes causing cercarial dermatitis. *J. Helminthol.* **2010**, *84*, 327–335. [CrossRef]
37. Soulsby, E. *Helminths Arthropods and Protozoa of Domesticated Animals*; Baillière Tindall: London, UK, 1982.
38. Picot, H.; Bourdeau, P.; Bardet, R.; Kerjan, A.; Piriou, M.; Le, A.G.; Bayssade-Dufour, C.; Chabasse, D.; Mott, K. Cercarial dermatitis in Europe: A new public health problem? *Bull. World Health Organ.* **1996**, *74*, 159–163.
39. Pennycott, T.W. Lead poisoning and parasitism in a flock of mute swans (Cygnus olor) in Scotland. *Vet. Rec.* **1998**, *142*, 13–17. [CrossRef] [PubMed]
40. Palmer, D.; Ossent, P. Nasal schistosomiasis in mute swans in Switzerland. *Rev. Suisse De Zool.* **1984**, *91*, 709–715. [CrossRef]
41. Guth, B.; Blankespoor, H.; Reimink, R.; Johnson, W. Prevalence of dermatitis-producing schistosomes in natural bird populations of lower Michigan. *Proc. Helminthol. Soc. Wash.* **1979**, *46*, 58–63.
42. Warren, K.S. Modulation of immunopathology and disease in schistosomiasis. *Am. J. Trop. Med. Hyg.* **1977**, *26*, 113 119. [CrossRef] [PubMed]
43. Kolarova, L.; Horak, P.; Cada, F. Histopathology of CNS and nasal infections caused by Trichobilharzia regenti in vertebrates. *Parasitol. Res.* **2001**, *87*, 644–650. [PubMed]
44. Wojcinski, Z.W.; Barker, I.K.; Hunter, D.B.; Lumsden, H. An outbreak of schistosomiasis in Atlantic brant geese, Branta bernicla hrota. *J. Wildl. Dis.* **1987**, *23*, 248–255. [CrossRef]

8

Comparison of Two DNA Extraction Methods and Two PCRs for Detection of *Echinococcus multilocularis* in the Stool Samples of Naturally Infected Red Foxes

Katarzyna Skrzypek, Jacek Karamon *, Małgorzata Samorek-Pieróg, Joanna Dąbrowska, Maciej Kochanowski, Jacek Sroka, Ewa Bilska-Zając and Tomasz Cencek

Department of Parasitology and Invasive Diseases, National Veterinary Research Institute, Partyzantów Avenue 57, 24-100 Puławy, Poland; katarzyna.skrzypek@piwet.pulawy.pl (K.S.); malgorzata.samorek-pierog@piwet.pulawy.pl (M.S.-P.); Joanna.dabrowska@piwet.pulawy.pl (J.D.); maciej.kochanowski@piwet.pulawy.pl (M.K.); jacek.sroka@piwet.pulawy.pl (J.S.); ewa.bilska@piwet.pulawy.pl (E.B.-Z.); tcencek@piwet.pulawy.pl (T.C.)

* Correspondence: j.karamon@piwet.pulawy.pl.

Simple Summary: The goal of the study was to compare the efficiency of two commercial DNA extraction kits together with two different Polymerase Chain Reaction (PCR) protocols in the detection of *Echinococcus multilocularis* in the feces of naturally infected foxes. Stool samples from red foxes were collected in a highly endemic area in Poland. Sedimentation and counting technique (SCT) was used as a reference method. From 48 samples, 35 were positive in SCT. Further investigations showed that 40.0% of samples (from those with SCT positive result) after Z—DNA extraction and 45.7% after Q—DNA extraction gave positive results in nested PCR. In multiplex PCR, positive results were obtained in 54.3% of samples after Z isolation and 48.6% of samples after Q. Additionally, one sample negative in SCT gave a positive result in PCR. The number of worms detected in the intestines had no influence on the PCR results. Both of the extraction methods showed similar efficiency in DNA isolation and dealing with inhibitors; however, they showed relatively low sensitivity.

Abstract: (1) Background: Due to the increasing distribution of *Echinococcus multilocularis* infections in final hosts, epidemiological investigations are important for recognizing the spreading pattern of this parasite and also to estimate risk infection for humans. (2) Methods: Investigations were conducted with two commercial kits dedicated for DNA extraction from feces: ZR Fecal DNA Mini Prep (Zymo Research, Freiburg, Germany) and QIAamp FAST DNA Stool Mini Kit (Qiagen, Hilden, Germany) (marked as Z and Q), together with two common PCR protocols (nested PCR and multiplex PCR). The goal was to compare their efficiency in detecting the genetic material of *E. multilocularis* in the samples of feces. Stool samples from red foxes were collected in a highly endemic area in Poland. Sedimentation and counting technique (SCT) was used as a reference method. (3) Results: From 48 samples, 35 were positive in SCT. Further investigations showed that 40.0% of samples (from those with SCT positive result) after Z-DNA extraction and 45.7% after Q-DNA extraction gave positive results in nested PCR. In multiplex PCR, positive results were obtained in 54.3% of samples after Z isolation and 48.6% of samples after Q. Additionally, one sample that resulted in being negative in SCT gave a positive result in PCR. The number of worms detected in the intestines had no influence on PCR results. (4) Conclusions: Both of the extraction methods showed similar efficiency in DNA isolation and dealing with inhibitors; however, they showed relatively low sensitivity. This was probably caused by degradation of genetic material in the field-collected samples.

Keywords: *Echinococcus multilocularis*; PCR; DNA extraction; feces

1. Introduction

Echinococcus multilocularis is a zoonotic cestode belonging to the Taenidae family. Circulation of this parasite occurs mostly in the sylvatic cycle, based on predator–prey relationship. Typical definitive hosts for this tapeworm are canids—in Europe, mainly red foxes (*Vulpes vulpes*) but also raccoons, dogs, arctic foxes and wolves. Its intermediate hosts are small rodents, mainly from the Cricetidae family [1,2]. Humans can become an incidental intermediate host; as a consequence, this infection leads to the development of alveolar echinococcosis disease caused by larval stage of *E. multilocularis*, which is one of the most dangerous parasitic zoonosis in Europe [2]. This happens through accidental ingestion of the tapeworm's eggs shed into the environment with feces of infected final hosts. It has been shown that domestic animals, i.e., dogs and cats, can be infected with this parasite and can become a potential source of human infections. Nevertheless, the red fox is still the crucial species responsible for contamination of the environment [2–5]. In light of the recent studies, the distribution pattern of *E. multilocularis* and prevalence in previously known areas have increased. Thus, it is important to conduct monitoring among populations of final hosts. The "gold standard" in detection of adult worms in definitive host is sedimentation and counting technique (SCT). However, since the SCT technique is applied postmortem, it is impractical for use in domestic animals. There are many alternative methods developed for recognizing *E. multilocularis* infection in definitive hosts, i.e., coproantigen detection by ELISA [6] or different PCR techniques designed for detection of the parasite's DNA (from eggs or copro-DNA) in animal feces [7–12]. One of the advantages of the abovementioned molecular methods is their sensitivity; however, it is possible that inhibitors present in the feces may prevent the successful PCR reaction. Consequently, reported results can be false negative. In order to avoid the negative influence of inhibitors on the amplification process, there are several methods of removing them from the samples, e.g., using the inhibitor-binding substances included in commercial kits dedicated for DNA extraction from stool or using the magnetic capture (MC) technique that binds the target DNA on the magnetic beads in a very specific way [9,10].

The aim of this study was to compare two commercial DNA extraction kits combined with two PCR techniques commonly used for detection of *E. multilocularis* DNA. We evaluate their effectiveness and ability of dealing with inhibitors present in feces.

2. Materials and Methods

The material for this study (48 stool samples) was collected from the large intestine of red foxes shot by hunters in the area of Podkarpackie province in Southeastern Poland. Intestines were kept in −80 °C for 7 days, for safety reasons, before examination. In a further stage, they were taken out to thaw overnight, and the next day, sedimentation and counting technique (SCT) was performed [13,14]. SCT results were treated as reference data for analyzing PCR results. During SCT protocol, stool samples were collected from posterior part of the rectum and then frozen at −20 °C, for further molecular analysis.

2.1. DNA Extraction

DNA extraction was carried out for all stool samples with two extraction kits:

Z—ZR Fecal DNA Mini Prep (Zymo Research, Freiburg, Germany): An isolation was conducted in accordance with the standard manufacturer's protocol.

Q—QIAamp FAST DNA Stool Mini Kit (Qiagen, Hilden, Germany): The isolation was performed in accordance with the special manufacturer's protocol for DNA isolation from large volume of stool with few modifications. In the first step, 1 g of stool sample diluted in 10 mL of InhibitEX Buffer was vortexed vigorously in 50 mL centrifuge tube containing glass beads. In the first incubation, the suspension was heated at 95 °C (5 min), according to manufacturer's recommendation for samples difficult to lyse. Second incubation was carried out at 70 °C for 20 min. In the last step, after adding ATE buffer, samples were left at room temperature for 5 min. Then, the isolates were kept in −20 °C, until further analysis.

2.2. Polymerase Chain Reactions (PCRs)

PCR was performed simultaneously with two different PCR methods for all DNA samples. Multiplex PCR [8] was accomplished for amplification of NADH dehydrogenase subunit 1 (nad1) of *E. multilocularis*, small subunit of ribosomal RNA (rrnS) of *Taenia* spp. and rrnS of *E. granulosus*. Nested PCR [7], with some modifications [15], was conducted for amplification of mitochondrial 12S ribosomal RNA (12S rRNA) of *E. multilocularis*. Each DNA sample was tested in undiluted (1/1) and tenfold diluted (1/10) variant. Moreover, each variant of DNA sample was tested in repetition. Internal control (DNA extracted from *E. multilocularis* adult worms) was added to one of two repeated samples, to make sure that no inhibition occurred. There was no inhibition if the specific band was present on the gel after electrophoresis.

2.3. Statistical Analysis

Differences in numbers of positive PCR results among two isolation methods (Z and Q) in each PCR variant were estimated by a chi-square test (or chi-square with Yates correction). The distribution of quantitative variables was tested by the Shapiro–Wilk test, and the normality hypothesis of the data was rejected. The relationship between the intensity of infection (number of *E. multilocularis* worms in the intestine assessed with SCT) and PCR results was calculated with Spearman's rank-order correlation. The differences were considered statistically significant when $p < 0.05$. The statistical analysis was performed by using Statistica 9.1 (StatSoft Inc., Tulsa, OK, USA).

3. Results

SCT examination showed the presence of *E. multilocularis* tapeworms in 35 of the 48 tested samples. The intensity of infection ranged from 1 to 75,000 tapeworms per intestine.

The PCR results (for *E. multilocularis*) were compared to the results of SCT. Out of 35 samples positive for *E. multilocularis* in SCT, 23 gave a positive result, simultaneously in nested and multiplex PCR. Nested PCR showed the presence of *E. multilocularis* genetic material in 14 (after Z isolation) and 16 (after Q isolation) stool samples in total, 40.0% and 45.7%, respectively (Table 1). In multiplex PCR, 19 samples (Z) and 17 (Q) gave positive results, 54.3% and 48.6%, respectively (Table 1). There were no significant differences between Z and Q extraction methods in any variant of PCR and dilution. Twelve SCT positive samples did not give a band specific for *E. multilocularis* DNA in any of the PCRs applied, regardless of the intensity of the infection. Additionally, one negative sample in SCT, gave a positive result in multiplex PCR (only in undiluted DNA) (Q).

Table 1. Percentages of PCR *Echinococcus multilocularis* positive results among fecal samples obtaining from *Echinococcus multilocularis* sedimentation and counting technique (SCT) positive intestines.

Method of Isolation	Percentage of Positive Results in *Echinococcus multilocularis*									
	Nested PCR					Multiplex PCR				
	Total	1/1	1/10	Only 1/1	Only 1/10	Total	1/1	1/10	Only 1/1	Only 1/10
Z	40.0	40.0	34.3	5.7	-	54.3	51.4	42.9	11.4	2.9
Q	45.7	45.7	25.7	20.0	-	48.6	45.7	28.6	22.9	2.9

1/1—results obtained in undiluted DNA variant; 1/10—results obtained in tenfold diluted DNA variant; only 1/1—positive results obtained only in undiluted variants (while diluted variants were negative); only 1/10—positive results obtained only in diluted variants (while undiluted variants were negative); Z—ZR Fecal DNA Mini Prep (Zymo Research, Freiburg, Germany); Q—QIAamp FAST DNA Stool Mini Kit (Qiagen, Hilden, Germany).

The analysis of relationship between number of *E. multilocularis* worms in the intestine and PCR results showed modern positive correlation for Z extraction ($r_s = 0.5429$ for nested PCR; $r_s = 0.4629$ for multiplex PCR) and low positive correlation for Q extraction ($r_s = 0.3436$ for nested PCR; $r_s = 0.3680$ for multiplex PCR).

Figure 1 presents percentages of positive PCR results grouped in three levels of intensity estimated with SCT: low (1–10 worms) ($n = 6$), medium (11–1000) ($n = 17$) and high (>1000) ($n = 12$) intensity. We observed that only the Q extraction allowed for positive PCR results in low number of worms in the intestine. Moderate- and high-intensity infection percentages of positive PCR results were similar in both extraction methods. The highest number of PCR positive results in each variant was detected in feces coming from intestines infected with a high number of worms (>1000).

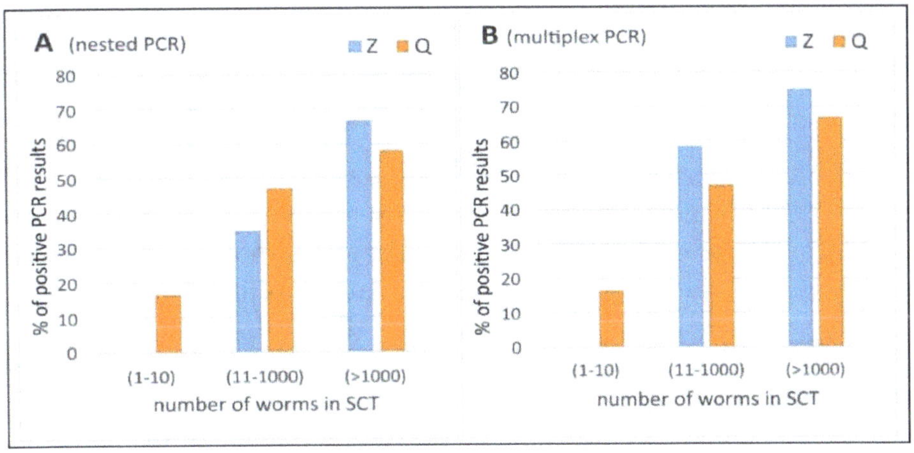

Figure 1. Percentages of *Echinococcus multilocularis* positive PCR results in samples of feces coming from intestines with different number of worms estimated with sedimentation and counting technique (SCT)—grouped in three levels of intensity: low (1–10 worms), medium (11–1000) and high (>1000) intensity. Z—ZR Fecal DNA Mini Prep (Zymo Research, Freiburg, Germany); Q—QIAamp FAST DNA Stool Mini Kit (Qiagen, Hilden, Germany); (**A**) nested PCR and (**B**) multiplex PCR.

Internal control gave negative results (both in diluted and undiluted DNA) only in one sample after Q isolation tested with nested PCR (in multiplex PCR it was positive). This sample after DNA extraction with the Z method gave positive results in both PCRs. Additionally, in nested PCR, undiluted samples with added internal control gave significantly more positive results after Z isolation (97.9%) than Q (83.3%) (Table 2)

Table 2. Results in *Echinococcus multilocularis* internal controls obtained in nested PCR and multiplex PCR.

Method of Isolation	Percentage of Positive Results in *Echinococcus multilocularis* Internal Controls									
	Nested PCR					Multiplex PCR				
	Total	1/1	1/10	Only 1/1	Only 1/10	Total	1/1	1/10	Only 1/1	Only 1/10
Z	100.0	97.9 [a]	100.0	0.0	2.1	100.0	100.0	100.0	0.0	2.1
Q	97.9	83.3 [b]	97.9	0.0	14.6	100.0	100.0	97.9	0.0	0.0

[a,b] Different letters in superscript indicate statistically significant differences among methods of isolation in individual variants ($p < 0.05$). 1/1—results obtained in undiluted DNA variant; 1/10—results obtained in tenfold diluted DNA variant; only 1/1—positive results obtained only in undiluted variants (while diluted variants were negative); only 1/10—positive results obtained only in diluted variants (while undiluted variants were negative); Z—ZR Fecal DNA Mini Prep (Zymo Research, Freiburg, Germany); Q—QIAamp FAST DNA Stool Mini Kit (Qiagen, Hilden, Germany).

Taenia spp. band in multiplex PCR gave a total of 42 out of 48 isolates (87.5%) after Z isolation and 91.7% after Q isolation (Table 3). There were no significant differences between method of DNA extraction in detection of *Taenia* spp. in any variant.

Table 3. Percentages of PCR *Taenia* spp. positive results (multiplex PCR).

Method of Isolation	Percentage of Positive Results for *Taenia* spp.				
	Multiplex PCR				
	Total	1/1	1/10	only 1/1	only 1/10
Z	87.5	87.5	77.1	10.4	-
Q	91.7	89.6	64.6	27.1	2.1

1/1—results obtained in undiluted DNA variant; 1/10—results obtained in tenfold diluted DNA variant; only 1/1—positive results obtained only in undiluted variants (while diluted variants were negative); only 1/10—positive results obtained only in diluted variants (while undiluted variants were negative); Z—ZR Fecal DNA Mini Prep (Zymo Research, Freiburg, Germany); Q—QIAamp FAST DNA Stool Mini Kit (Qiagen, Hilden, Germany).

Product specific for *E. granulosus* was not obtained in any of tested samples by multiplex PCR.

4. Discussion

The present study was undertaken to compare two widely used commercial DNA extraction kits, together with two PCR protocols, i.e., multiplex PCR [8] and nested PCR [7]. We determined the efficiency of detecting *E. multilocularis* infection in final hosts by molecular detection of copro-DNA.

Some authors reported higher sensitivity of molecular methods over widely used reference standards such as SCT or intestinal scraping technique (IST) [10,16]. Isaksson et al. [9] estimated sensitivity of magnetic capture (MC)-PCR to be 88.2%, and Dinkel et al. [7] estimated sensitivity of 89% for nested PCR. In our study, from all of the samples confirmed as positive by SCT, only 40.0–54.3% of them gave positive results in molecular tests (maximum with combination of Z extraction and multiplex PCR). A similar percentage of positive results (52%) was obtained by Maksimov et al. [17] in the stool samples from *E. multilocularis* naturally infected foxes. In Dinkel et al.'s [7] study, they showed correlation of *E. multilocularis* gravid worm number in IST and PCR sensitivity. It was on a level of 100% for samples containing 1000 and more adult tapeworms and 70% for 10 or less of immature ones. Similar dependency was observed by Maksimov et al. [17]. In their studies, PCR sensitivity was 90% for the samples taken from foxes with intense infection and only 30% for those with low infection level. In our study, we observed moderate or low positive correlation between number of worms detected in SCT and PCR results. However, it must be stressed that some of the SCT positive samples did not show positive PCR results, even though they were extracted from the stool taken from intestines of foxes with very differential number of tapeworms (from 1 to more than 1000 per sample). We obtained negative results in molecular tests both for samples with less than 10, as well as a few thousands of adult worms. Among all of the SCT negative samples, only one sample was PCR positive. In contrast, Dinkel et al. [7] used IST as a reference method. IST has been proven to be less sensitive than SCT [18,19]. Therefore, this could be a reason for the higher PCR sensitivity (compared to IST) in Dinkel's study than in presented investigation, where SCT was used as a standard. The other factor that might have affected the detection of *E. multilocularis* DNA with PCR is that all intestine samples in this study were collected by hunters in the field. Thus, the storage and transport conditions could not be controlled in detail. With conventional PCR, Maksimov et al. [17] obtained much better sensitivity results for samples experimentally spiked with tapeworm eggs in the laboratory conditions than from naturally infected foxes. Natural conditions and DNase enzymes in the feces may influence or even damage DNA [20], resulting in a negative PCR outcome even in samples positive in SCT.

PCR amplification of genetic material extracted from stool samples can be disrupted by inhibitors present in the feces, giving false negative results. There are two most common approaches for sample treatment that can be applied in order to limit inhibitors presence and lower the risk of amplification disturbance. One of these approaches is to perform extraction not directly from stool but from tapeworm eggs separated from the sample prior to extraction [21,22]. This method is useful especially for experiments with small amounts of stool samples [22]. However, it is time-consuming, laborious and carries the risk of losing the positive material. Additionally, flotation is not so highly efficient in detecting tapeworm eggs; thus, this method may eliminate some of the potentially positive samples [23]. It is also limited because there are no eggs in the stool in early stage infections with immature worms [7]. The second approach is conducting DNA extraction from the stool and then diluting the isolate [23]. Extracting genetic material directly from feces lowers the risk of losing positive material. Diluting the DNA helps to lower the concentration of inhibitors in the final sample volume, decreasing the possibility of their influence on the amplification process. It leads not only to lower the concentration of inhibitors but also a specific DNA, so it is important to use sensitive and specific PCR protocol in order to obtain satisfactory results. Additionally, the use of an extraction method suitable for feces is a key factor. In Al-Sabi et al.'s [21] study, they obtained results with sensitivity on a very low level, by using a commercial kit dedicated for tissues. However, they isolated the genetic material from stool samples with no inhibitors eliminating step. In Karamon's [23] study, two stool dedicated extraction kits gave significantly more positive results in comparison to the method dedicated for tissues. In order to determine if any DNA inhibition occurred, each sample was tested in repetition with internal control. In one variant (extraction kit Q combined with nested PCR), there were eight negative results of internal controls in undiluted DNA samples, while there was only one in diluted DNA. This confirms the need to examine additional diluted variants of samples, to avoid false negative results.

The impact of freezing-and-thawing process on the quality of DNA occurring in feces should also be presented. In this study, all of the intestines were frozen at −80 °C, for one week, due to safety reasons. Then, stool samples taken from the intestines during SCT preparation were frozen at −20 °C and kept for further analysis. Klein et al.'s [16] study shows that freeze–thawing cycles significantly increase PCR sensitivity, possibly by mechanical disruption of egg shells, which helps release DNA. In this method, the number of eggs prevalent in the feces influenced the result. On the other hand, repeated freezing and thawing degrades "free" DNA (DNA from tissue fragments or the whole worms shed with feces), which negatively affects the sensitivity of further molecular analysis when there are no or few parasite eggs in the sample [7,23]. False negative results may be also due the fact that, even if the eggs are present in stool, they may contain too little DNA for efficient amplification [24].

5. Conclusions

Our investigation showed similar effectiveness of two DNA extraction kits dedicated for stool samples in *E. multilocularis* detection. Moreover, the presented methods were found to be good at eliminating of copro-inhibitors. The study indicated the problem with relatively low sensitivity of PCRs in the examination of field samples from naturally infected animals (in comparison to microscopic examination of intestine), what was probably connected with degradation of genetic material in feces.

Author Contributions: Conceptualization, K.S., J.K. and T.C.; methodology, J.K., M.S.-P. and J.S.; software, J.K.; investigation, J.K., J.D. and M.K.; data curation, J.S. and E.B.-Z.; writing—original draft preparation, K.S., J.K. and M.S.-P.; writing—review and editing, J.K. and T.C.; visualization, M.K.; supervision, T.C. All authors have read and agreed to the published version of the manuscript.

References

1. Nakao, M.; Xiao, N.; Okamoto, M.; Yanagida, T.; Sako, Y.; Ito, A. Geographic pattern of genetic variation in the fox tapeworm *Echinococcus multilocularis*. *Parasitol. Int.* **2009**, *58*, 384–389. [CrossRef] [PubMed]
2. Oksanen, A.; Siles-Lucas, M.; Karamon, J.; Possenti, A.; Conraths, F.J.; Romig, T.; Wysocki, P.; Mannocci, A.; Mipatrini, D.; La Torre, G.; et al. The geographical distribution and prevalence of *Echinococcus multilocularis*

in animals in the European Union and adjacent countries: A systematic review and meta-analysis. *Parasites Vectors* **2016**, *9*, 1–23. [CrossRef] [PubMed]

3. Kapel, C.M.O.; Torgerson, P.R.; Thompson, R.C.A.; Deplazes, P. Reproductive potential of *Echinococcus multilocularis* in experimentally infected foxes, dogs, raccoon dogs and cats. *Int. J. Parasitol.* **2006**, *36*, 79–86. [CrossRef] [PubMed]
4. Romig, T. *Echinococcus multilocularis* in Europe—state of the art. *Vet. Res. Commun.* **2009**, *33*, S31–S34. [CrossRef] [PubMed]
5. Hegglin, D.; Deplazes, P. Control of *Echinococcus multilocularis*: Strategies, feasibility and cost-benefit analyses. *Int. J. Parasitol.* **2013**, *43*, 327–337. [CrossRef]
6. Deplazes, P.; Alther, P.; Tanner, I.; Thompson, R.C.A.; Eckert, J. *Echinococcus multilocularis* coproantigen detection by enzyme-linked immunosorbent assay in fox, dog, and cat populations. *J. Parasitol.* **1999**, *85*, 115–121. [CrossRef]
7. Dinkel, A.; Von Nickisch-Rosenegk, M.; Bilger, B.; Merli, M.; Lucius, R.; Romig, T. Detection of *Echinococcus multilocularis* in the definitive host: Coprodiagnosis by PCR as an alternative to necropsy. *J. Clin. Microbiol.* **1998**, *36*, 1871–1876. [CrossRef]
8. Trachsel, D.; Deplazes, P.; Mathis, A. Identification of taeniid eggs in the faeces from carnivores based on multiplex PCR using targets in mitochondrial DNA. *Parasitology* **2007**, *134*, 911–920. [CrossRef]
9. Isaksson, M.; Hagstrom, A.; Armua-Fernandez, M.T.; Wahlstrom, H.; Agren, E.O.; Miller, A.; Holmberg, A.; Lukacs, M.; Casulli, A.; Deplazes, P.; et al. A semi-automated magnetic capture probe based DNA extraction and real-time PCR method applied in the Swedish surveillance of *Echinococcus multilocularis* in red fox (*Vulpes vulpes*) faecal samples. *Parasites Vectors* **2014**, *7*, 583. [CrossRef]
10. Maas, M.; Van Roon, A.; Dam-Deisz, C.; Opsteegh, M.; Massolo, A.; Deksne, G.; Teunis, P.; Van der Giessen, J. Evaluation by latent class analysis of a magnetic capture based DNA extraction followed by real-time qPCR as a new diagnostic method for detection of *Echinococcus multilocularis* in definitive hosts. *Vet. Parasitol.* **2016**, *230*, 20–24. [CrossRef]
11. Dinkel, A.; Kern, S.; Brinker, A.; Oehme, R.; Vaniscotte, A.; Giraudoux, P.; Mackenstedt, U.; Romig, T. A real-time multiplex-nested PCR system for coprological diagnosis of *Echinococcus multilocularis* and host species. *Parasitol. Res.* **2011**, *109*, 493–498. [CrossRef] [PubMed]
12. Knapp, J.; Umhang, G.; Poulle, M.-L.; Millon, L. Development of a Real-Time PCR for a Sensitive One-Step Coprodiagnosis Allowing both the Identification of Carnivore Feces and the Detection of *Toxocara* spp. and *Echinococcus multilocularis*. *Appl. Environ. Microbiol.* **2016**, *82*, 2950–2958. [CrossRef] [PubMed]
13. Hofer, S.; Gloor, S.; Muller, U.; Mathis, A.; Hegglin, D.; Deplazes, P. High prevalence of *Echinococcus multilocularis* in urban red foxes (*Vulpes vulpes*) and voles (*Arvicola terrestris*) in the city of Zurich, Switzerland. *Parasitology* **2000**, *120*, 135–142. [CrossRef] [PubMed]
14. OIE. Echinococcosis/hydatidosis (infection with *Echinococcus granulosus* and *E. multilocularis*). In *Manual of Diagnostic Tests and Vaccines for Terrestrial Animals*, 6th ed.; Office International des Epizooties: Paris, France, 2008; Volume 1, pp. 1–15.
15. Karamon, J.; Sroka, J.; Cencek, T. The first detection of *Echinococcus multilocularis* in slaughtered pigs in Poland. *Vet. Parasitol.* **2012**, *185*, 327–329. [CrossRef] [PubMed]
16. Klein, C.; Liccioli, S.; Massolo, A. Egg intensity and freeze-thawing of fecal samples affect sensitivity of *Echinococcus multilocularis* detection by PCR. *Parasitol Res* **2014**, *113*, 3867–3873. [CrossRef] [PubMed]
17. Maksimov, P.; Schares, G.; Press, S.; Frohlich, A.; Basso, W.; Herzig, M.; Conraths, F.J. Comparison of different commercial DNA extraction kits and PCR protocols for the detection of *Echinococcus multilocularis* eggs in faecal samples from foxes. *Vet. Parasitol.* **2017**, *237*, 83–93. [CrossRef]
18. Karamon, J.; Sroka, J.; Cencek, T.; Kochanowski, M.; Dąbrowska, J. Efficacy of intestinal scraping technique in the detection of *Echinococcus multilocularis*—Estimation of the limit of the detection and comparison with sedimentation and counting technique. *Bull. Vet. Inst. Pulawy* **2012**, *56*, 535–538. [CrossRef]
19. EFSA. The EU summary Report on Trends and Sources of Zoonoses, Zoonotic Agents and Food-borne Ourbreaks in 2013. *EFSA J.* **2015**, *13*, 3991.
20. Irie, T.; Ito, T.; Kouguchi, H.; Yamano, K.; Uraguchi, K.; Yagi, K.; Nonaka, N. Diagnosis of canine *Echinococcus multilocularis* infections by copro-DNA tests: Comparison of DNA extraction techniques and evaluation of diagnostic deworming. *Parasitol. Res.* **2017**, *116*, 2139–2144. [CrossRef]

21. Al-Sabi, M.N.S.; Kapel, C.M.O.; Deplazes, P.; Mathis, A. Comparative copro-diagnosis of *Echinococcus multilocularis* in experimentally infected foxes. *Parasitol. Res.* **2007**, *101*, 731–736. [CrossRef]
22. Mathis, A.; Deplazes, P.; Eckert, J. An improved test system for PCR-based specific detection of *Echinococcus multilocularis* eggs. *J. Helminthol.* **1996**, *70*, 219–222. [CrossRef] [PubMed]
23. Karamon, J. Detection of *Echinococcus multilocularis* in faeces by nested PCR with the use of diluted DNA samples. *Pol. J. Vet. Sci.* **2014**, *17*, 79–83. [CrossRef] [PubMed]
24. Oines, O.; Isaksson, M.; Hagstrom, A.; Tavornpanich, S.; Davidson, R.K. Laboratory assessment of sensitive molecular tools for detection of low levels of *Echinococcus multilocularis*-eggs in fox (*Vulpes vulpes*) faeces. *Parasites Vectors* **2014**, *7*, 246. [CrossRef] [PubMed]

9

Seasonal Pattern of Prevalence and Excretion of Eggs of *Baylisascaris transfuga* in the Brown Bear (*Ursus arctos*)

Ladislav Molnár [1], Alžbeta Königová [2,*], Peter Major [1], Zuzana Vasilková [2], Martina Tomková [3] and Marián Várady [2]

1 Clinic for Birds and Exotic Animals, University of Veterinary Medicine and Pharmacy, 040 01 Košice, Slovakia; ladislav.molnar@uvlf.sk (L.M.); major.dr@gmail.com (P.M.)
2 Institute of Parasitology of the Slovak Academy of Sciences, 040 01 Košice, Slovakia; vasilko@saske.sk (Z.V.); varady@saske.sk (M.V.)
3 Slovak Hydrometeorological Institute, Ďumbierska 26, 041 17 Košice, Slovakia; martina.tomkova@shmu.sk
* Correspondence: konig@saske.sk.

Simple Summary: The main goal of this study was to monitor the seasonal dynamics of faecal egg counts (FEC) expressed as eggs per gram (EPG) and intensity of excretion of the egg nematode *Baylisascaris transfuga* in the European brown bear over three years. The number of nematode eggs in the faecal samples began to rise in the spring and peaked in the autumn throughout the study period. Presence of nematode eggs in the samples was also observed in the winter season. Of the environmental factors, the seasonal dynamics and intensity of the infection were most influenced by temperature, while humidity and mean precipitation did not affect it. Increasing mean temperatures during the winter and short or no hibernation together with the presence of *B. transfuga* infection may negatively affect the health of infected bears. Due to the zoonotic potential of the parasite and the increased occurrence of bears in the vicinity of human dwellings, the dissemination of propagative stages may also pose a threat to human health.

Abstract: The seasonal dynamics of the prevalence, abundance, and mean intensity of egg excretion by the nematode parasite *Baylisascaris transfuga* in the European brown bear (*Ursus arctos*) were monitored relative to environmental factors (mean temperature, humidity, and temperature) over three years. The prevalence, abundance, and mean intensity of egg excretion tended to increase from spring to autumn throughout the monitoring period. The seasonal prevalence (84.2–90.6%), abundance (470.2–545.3 eggs per gramme (EPG) of faeces), mean intensity of excretion (558.3–602.1 EPG), and number of eggs (1150 EPG) were highest in autumn. The prevalence of eggs (up to 48.5%), abundance (37.8–60.6 EPG), and mean intensity of excretion (94.4–125.0 EPG) were high in winter, despite the period of hibernation. The seasonal dynamics of *B. transfuga* abundance in bears, the mean temperature between spring and autumn, and the seasonal trend of increase in intensity of egg excretion with temperature from winter to summer were interrelated. Abundance differed significantly between winter and autumn, spring and autumn, and summer and autumn ($p < 0.0001$) in all years and between spring and summer in 2016 ($p < 0.005$), 2017 ($p < 0.05$). *B. transfuga* abundance differed significantly between the seasons over the three years only in spring ($p \leq 0.0001$).

Keywords: European brown bear; *Baylisascaris transfuga*; prevalence; seasonal dynamics

1. Introduction

The European brown bear (*Ursus arctos*) is present in 22 European countries, with an estimated total number of approximately 17,000 individuals [1]. Most of these populations are strictly protected and are currently increasing [2]. The Carpathian population includes brown bears in Slovakia, Poland, the Ukraine, and Romania. The population in the Carpathian Mountains is estimated at about 8100 bears, and is the second largest in Europe. More than 90% of bears in Slovakia belong to the West Carpathian subpopulation, which is no longer isolated, but is again contiguous with that in the East Carpathian subpopulation in north-eastern Slovakia, south-eastern Poland, and the Ukrainian Carpathians. Some of these bears also likely have transborder home ranges [3]. Data from the State Nature Conservancy indicate that brown bears in Slovakia inhabit about 33% of the area, covering 16,000 km^2 [4,5]. Štofik et al. [5] documented significant growth of the bear population over the last decades. Estimated population density was one bear per < 850 ha in 2001 and one bear per < 380 ha in 2014, i.e., a 2.2-fold increase in density. The estimated density in 2019 was one bear per < 310 ha [4]. The estimated population in 2014 based on faecal genetic analyses was 1256 individuals, and the current number of brown bears in Slovakia is about 1500–1600 individuals [6,7]. This bear population growth can be explained by the reduction of human settlements and increasing forestation and food sours [8], and by the protection of the brown bear. According to the Habitats Directive (Annex IV of 92/43/EEC Directive), the Slovak Act on Nature and Landscape Protection (No. 543/2002) and the Decree of the Ministry of Environment (No. 24/2003), the brown bear is a species of European importance with a high protection priority. Conservation and management are guided by the accepted management plan for large carnivores in Slovakia. The bear population has been increasing from the long-term perspective [5]. Since bears utilize food sources provided by a man for wild boar, we presume that the population growth of brown bears in region [5] can also be stimulated by supplementary feeding by hunters. This leads to sufficient food source for non-denning bears and subsequently decreased winter home range.

The changing living conditions of wild bears, their shrinking home ranges, the impact of urbanization (human density, or human agricultural land use, developed and forested) are factors supporting the transmission of infective stages of nematodes, which have the potential to cause parasitic zoonoses in humans [9]. All species of *Baylisascaris* nematodes in wild carnivores can be regarded as potentially zoonotic [10]. Kazacos [11] stated that all *Baylisascaris* species could be considered potential etiological agents of larva migrans depending on the dose of infective eggs, although *B. procyonis* and *B. columnaris* in common raccoons are the primary causative agents of zoonoses associated with wild carnivores. *B. transfuga* is a widespread pathogen in populations of free-ranging bears in many areas of the world [12,13]. Adult *B. transfuga* are first detected in bear cubs from five months of age [14], and infection decreases with age. Partridge [15] and Moran et al. [16] reported that young and immature bears were more susceptible. The pathogenicity of intestinal infection with *B. transfuga* is low in bears; one case of granulomatous peritonitis caused by nematodes was described in a cub [17]. Little information is available about the life cycle of *B. transfuga* in wild bears. The complete life cycles of most species of *Baylisascaris* are unknown [18]. Moran et al. [16] stated that infection with *B. transfuga* could be direct or via a paratenic host, such as wild rodents. Encapsulated larvae of *B. transfuga* have been detected in the mesentery and the wall of the large intestine of the grey-sided vole (*Myodes rufocanus*) and the tundra vole (*M. oeconomus*) [19]. Abdelrasoul and Fowler [20] found that the life cycle was direct, but could also be indirect via encysted larvae using various rodents, birds, or insects as intermediate hosts. Transmammary and transplacental transmission are apparently unlikely [11]. In contrast, larvae migrate through various tissues in rodents, e.g., white mice and Mongolian gerbils, which are susceptible to experimental infection with *B. transfuga*, growing and developing to the third stage and causing various degrees of visceral, neural, or ocular larva migrans [21]. Larva migrans are the most serious complication associated with *Baylisascaris*, mainly caused by larvae of the common raccoon parasite *B. procyonis* in intermediate and occasional hosts. *Baylisascaris procyonis* is the most common clinical larva migrans in animals, in which it is usually associated with fatal or severe neurological disease. It is known for aggressive somatic migration, larval invasion of the central nervous system, and the capability for continued larval growth within intermediate hosts [22]. A single larva in the brain of a rodent is enough to cause clinical signs, even death [11,23]. In infants and young children, in its most severe form, *B. procyonis* is a rare cause of fatal or neurologically devastating neural larva migrans [22].

Definitive hosts of *B. transfuga* rarely show clinical signs unless heavy infections of adult worms block the digestive tract. Wallach and Boever [24] reported symptoms of diarrhoea, anorexia, and dry and severe cough, with the occasional presence of parasites in the faeces. Heavy infestation can lead to intestinal obstruction and subsequently to death [24,25]. Foster et al. [14] reported that black bear cubs harboured 1–39 nematodes in their intestines. Infected captive bears may shed as many as 10,000–20,000 eggs per gramme (EPG) of faeces [26] and thereby heavily contaminate their domestic areas.

Most information about the prevalence of *B. transfuga* in populations of wild bears has been from the American, Canadian, and Russian populations of black, brown, grizzly, and polar bears, respectively [14,27–33]. Information about the prevalence of *B. transfuga* in populations of wild brown bears in Europe is limited [1,34–39], and little is known about the seasonal dynamics of *B. transfuga* in these populations [36–38,40]. The seasonal dynamics of *B. transfuga* in wild carnivores can also be influenced by external factors such as temperature, humidity, and rainfall. Sufficient humidity and optimal temperature support the growth and survival of infective stages of nematodes, leading to higher contamination of carnivore environments. Climatic factors can impact the growth and survival of infective stages of *Baylisascaris* nematode. Temperature, humidity, and rainfall can affect environmental moisture retention of soils that were associated with transmission to paratenic hosts by improving viability at or near the surface [9]. Moisture and particle size also can affect egg viability, keeping viable eggs and can increase the potential risk of infection [41].

The present study determined the seasonal changes during a three-year period in the prevalence of *B. transfuga* eggs in faecal samples of the brown bear in Poloniny National Park, Eastern Carpathians, in Slovakia.

2. Materials and Methods

Permission for conducting a study was granted by the Administration of the Poloniny National Park. According to national law, formal ethical approval is not required for studies based on the monitoring of indirect signs of animals, such as collection of faecal samples.

2.1. Study Area

The study was conducted at the East Carpathians Biosphere Reserve (ECBR, UNESCO Man and Biosphere), the first European trilateral Man and Biosphere reserve (Slovakia/Poland/Ukraine) and the second largest biosphere reserve in Europe. The reserve covers an area of 208,089 ha (the Polish, Slovak, and Ukrainian parts occupy 52.2%, 19.59%, and 28.16%, respectively) includes six large protected areas, and contains the largest European complexes of original beech forests, and East Carpathian montane meadows. Poloniny National Park, part of ECBR, is the largest forest complex in Slovakia, with an area of 29,805 ha (a buffer zone of 10,973 ha). Endemic communities are predominant, with a large local population of European brown bears. The estimated density varies between 5 and 11 bears per 100 km^2.

2.2. Parasitological Examinations

A total of 524 faecal samples from brown bears were collected at the Poloniny National Park in north-eastern Slovakia from January 2016 to December 2018. The samples were collected with the assistance of the staff of the national park from several bear territories with presumed or reported occurrences of the animals (Figure 1). The national management plan for large carnivores estimates that the population size consists of around 35 bear individuals in the present time (2016–2018). Collection of bear faeces was roughly in the same point of an area usually correlated with hunters' feeding places, salt lick sites, or snow tracking in the winter period. During the snow season, bear tracks were followed in opposite direction of the bear movement to avoid disturbing the animal. Length and width of the footprint was recorded, if possible, on the snow or mud to identify individual bears. In the periods without snow cover, the faeces were collected systematically during the whole period following the method of Persson [42] et al. (2001) from the areas with reported and suspected occurrence of bears (orchards, roads, feeding racks). A GPS device (Garmin eTrex Vista H) was used to store the position and altitude of exact localities to avoid multiple sampling from the same scats. The numbers of faecal sampled was determined monthly.

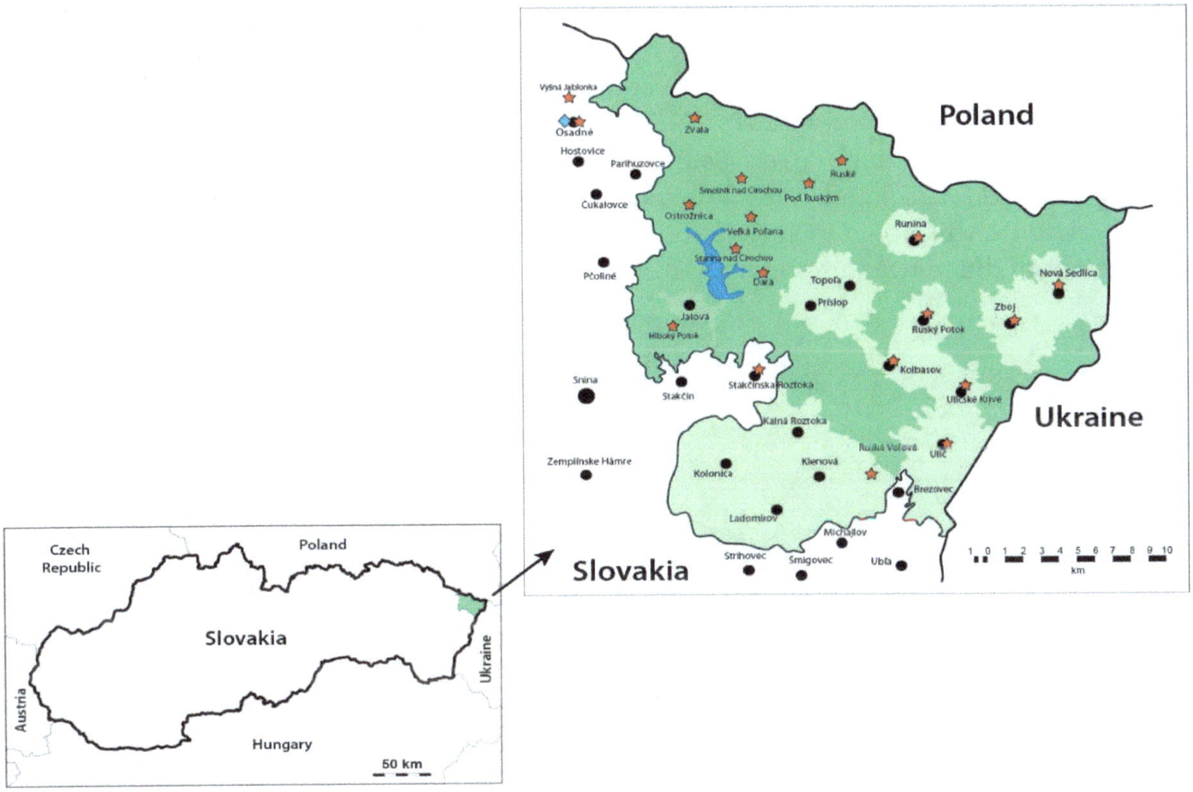

Figure 1. Distribution of the brown bear faecal samples in the study area in Poloniny National Park, Slovakia (★—sampling sites; ◇—Hydrometeorological station, National Park Poloniny in Osadné).

Each faecal sample was stored in a plastic container at 4 °C and subsequently frozen until further processing. Frozen samples were thawed 24 h prior to coprological examination. All samples were analysed no later than two weeks after collection. The faecal egg count (FEC) was used to monitor the prevalence of the nematode *B. transfuga* in brown bears. Baylisascaris FEC were performed using the coprological McMaster technique according Coles et al. [43] with Sheather's sugar flotation solution (1.25 specific gravity) and expressed as EPG (eggs per gram). Identification of *Baylisascaris transfuga* eggs was performed based on the morphology of the eggs by Sprent [44], and Kazacos and Turek [45]. The data on *B. transfuga* eggs were used to estimate prevalence, based the recommendations of Margolis et al. [46]: Prevalence (%), number of bears infected with *B. transfuga* eggs excreted in faecal samples divided by total number of bears examined. Mean excretion of eggs (EPG), total number of excreting of *B. transfuga* eggs in a bear faecal sample divided by number of infected bears; and abundance (EPG), total number of excreting of *B. transfuga* eggs in a bear faecal sample divided by total number of bears examined.

Basic climatological data, mean air temperature, minimum and maximum air temperatures, mean rainfall, and mean relative air humidity for 2016–2018 were obtained from the Slovak Hydrometeorological Institute (SHI), from the particular Hydrometeorological station, National Park

Poloniny in Osadné (Figure 1). The data were analysed for the four seasons to assess the influence of meteorological factors: Spring (March–May), summer (June–August), autumn (September–November), and winter (December–February). The Kruskal–Wallis test (nonparametric ANOVA) was used to identify significant differences between seasonal prevalences (spring, summer, autumn, and winter) at $p < 0.05$ (GraphPad Software, San Diego, CA, USA).

3. Results

3.1. Seasonal Prevalence of *B. transfuga* in the European Brown Bear

The seasonal dynamics of the prevalence of *B. transfuga* eggs in brown bears (a total of 524 faecal samples) in connection to temperature for three years is shown in Figure 2. The prevalence of baylisascariasis steadily increased over the years from spring to autumn. The difference of prevalence in spring is not statistically significant between 2016 (10.3%) and 2017 (19.1%), but significantly higher prevalence was observed in 2018 (59.5%). Prevalence in summer was similar (59.6–63.6%). Prevalence was highest in autumn (from 84.2 to 90.6%). Prevalence in winter was high (38.1–48.5%) in non-denning bears. Similar patterns of variation were observed between the dynamics and variations in mean temperature was noted in spring and autumn (temperature was recorded in the same range and no interannual differences among temperature a same season were determined) (Figure 2).

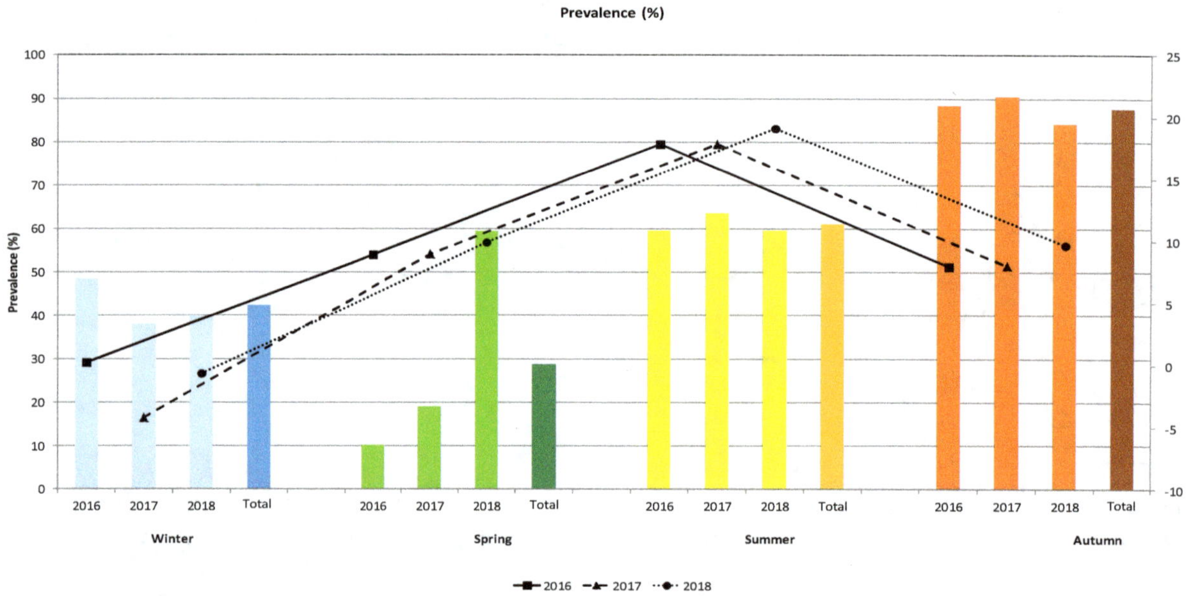

Figure 2. Prevalence of eggs of the nematode *B. transfuga* in the faecal samples of the brown bear (*Ursus arctos*) and mean temperature (°C) during different seasons of the three-year survey.

3.2. Seasonal Abundance of *B. transfuga* in the European Brown Bear

Figure 3 shows the seasonal dynamics of the abundance of baylisascariasis in bear faecal samples and the variations in mean temperature during the three-year period, with an increasing trend from spring to autumn. Abundance was lowest in spring (11.5 ± 43.6 EPG ± SD), with a maximum EPG of 250 (Table 1). Abundance in summer varied from 110.0 ± 135.9 to 149.0 ± 178.6 EPG during the study period. Although abundance was higher in winter (37.8 ± 70.0 to 60.6 ± 93.3 EPG) than in spring, abundance was not so high in the other season. The similar patterns of variation between the abundance of *B. transfuga* and variations in mean temperature were recorded from winter to summer. The abundance of baylisascariasis increased with temperature from winter to summer for the three years, except in spring 2016 and 2017, when EPGs were lower (11.5 ± 43.6 and 22.6 ± 57.6). Abundance increased rapidly in autumn (470.2 ± 268.9 to 545.3 ± 304.2 EPG) (Figure 3), similar to the autumn prevalence rates (84.2–90.6%) (Figure 2).

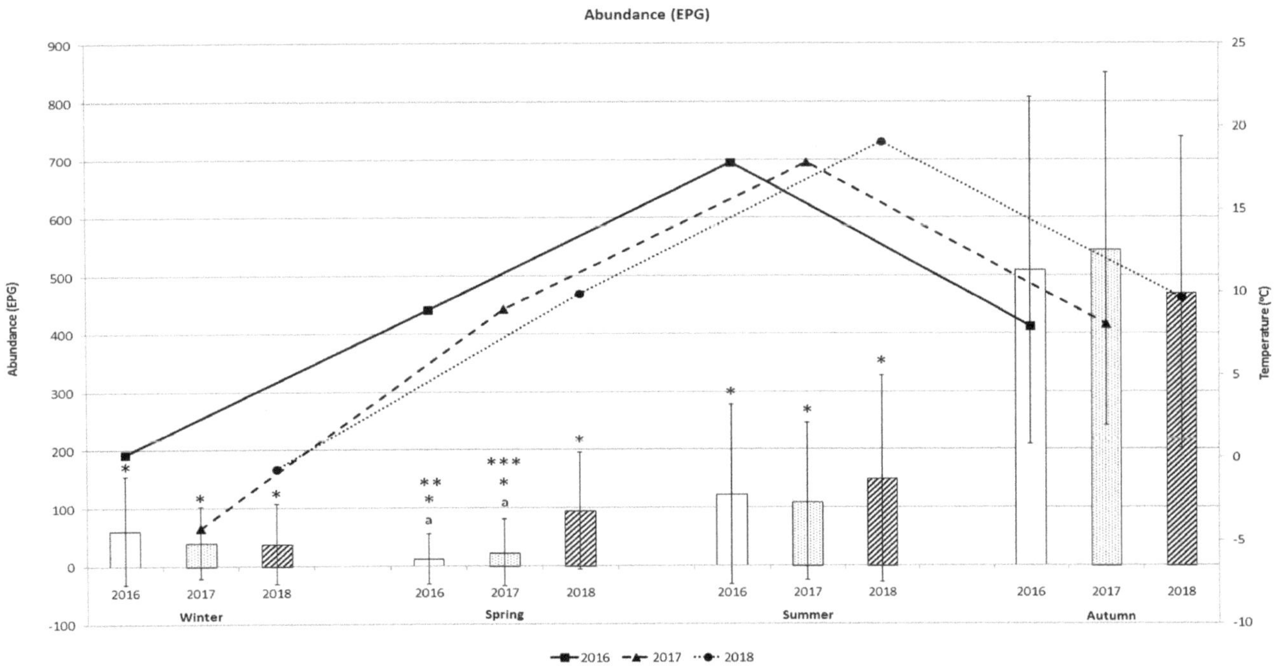

Figure 3. Abundance (mean EPG) of *B. transfuga* eggs in the faecal samples of the brown bear (*Ursus arctos*) and mean temperature (°C) during different seasons of the three-year survey; a significant difference between spring 2016 and 2017, and spring 2018, $p < 0.0001$; *, significant differences between autumn and winter, spring, and summer 2016, 2017, and 2018; $p < 0.0001$; **, significant difference between spring and summer 2016, $p < 0.005$; ***, significant difference between spring and summer 2017, $p < 0.05$.

Seasonal *B. transfuga* eggs' abundance in brown bears differed significantly only between spring 2016 and 2018 ($p < 0.0001$), and spring 2017 and 2018 ($p = 0.0001$). *B. transfuga* eggs' abundance in brown bears differed significantly between winter and autumn ($p < 0.0001$), spring and autumn ($p < 0.0001$), summer and autumn ($p < 0.0001$), and spring and summer 2016–2017 ($p < 0.005$; $p < 0.05$) (Figure 3).

3.3. Seasonal Mean Excretion of B. transfuga Eggs in the European Brown Bear

The seasonal dynamics of mean excretion of *B. transfuga* eggs in the faecal samples from brown bears and the variations in mean temperature during the three years are shown in Figure 4. Mean excretion of *B. transfuga* eggs in bears seasonally increased from winter to autumn in all three years. The excretion of eggs in 2016 differed significantly between winter and autumn ($p < 0.0001$), spring and autumn ($p < 0.005$), and summer and autumn ($p < 0.0001$). The excretion of eggs in 2017 differed significantly between winter and autumn, spring and autumn, and summer and autumn ($p < 0.0001$ in all cases). Mean excretion did not differ significantly between the seasons over the three years. The intensity of excretion in 2018 differed significantly between winter and summer and winter and autumn ($p < 0.005$ in both cases). Mean excretion was lowest in winter (94.4 ± 83.8 to 125.0 ± 100.0 EPG ± SD), with a maximum of 400 EPG (winter 2018). Mean excretion was low in spring 2016 (112.5 ± 94.7 EPG), with a maximum of 250 EPG. Mean excretion increased in summer, with EPGs varying between 172.9 ± 134.7 and 205.4 ± 152.4 EPG, with a maximum of 550 EPG. Mean excretion was highest in autumn (from 558.3 ± 189.4 to 602.1 ± 259.7 EPG), with a maximum of 1550 EPG (2017).

Table 1. Number of examined and infected faecal samples, minimum and maximum eggs per gram (EPG) of faeces, abundance, mean intensity of excretion, and prevalence of *B. transfuga* eggs in the brown bear (*Ursus arctos*) during different seasons of the three-year survey.

Season	Year	Number of Examined	Number of Infected	Minimum EPG	Maximum EPG	Abundance (EPG ± SD)	Mean Intensity of Excretion (EPG ± SD)	Prevalence (%) 95% CI
Winter	2016	33	16	0	350	60.6 ± 93.3	125.0 ± 100.0	48.5 (0.308–0.664)
	2017	21	8	0	200	40.5 ± 62.5	106.3 ± 56.3	38.1 (0.181–0.616)
	2018	45	18	0	400	37.8 ± 70.0	94.4 ± 83.8	40.0 (0.257–0.557)
Spring	2016	39	4	0	250	11.5 ± 43.6	112.5 ± 94.7	10.3 (0.029–0.242)
	2017	42	8	0	250	22.6 ± 57.6	118.8 ± 79.9	19.0 (0.086–0.341)
	2018	37	22	0	350	94.6 ± 101.2	159.1 ± 82.6	59.5 (0.421–0.753)
Summer	2016	47	28	0	500	122.3 ± 154.9	205.4 ± 152.4	59.6 (0.443–0.736)
	2017	55	35	0	500	110.0 ± 135.9	172.9 ± 134.7	63.6 (0.496–0.762)
	2018	52	31	0	550	149.0 ± 178.6	250 ± 167.8	59.6 (0.451–0.73)
Autumn	2016	43	38	0	1300	508.1 ± 299	575.0 ± 249.0	88.4 (0.749–0.961)
	2017	53	48	0	1550	545.3 ± 304.2	602.1 ± 259.7	90.6 (0.793–0.968)
	2018	57	48	0	950	470.2 ± 268.9	558.3 ± 189.4	84.2 (0.721–0.925)

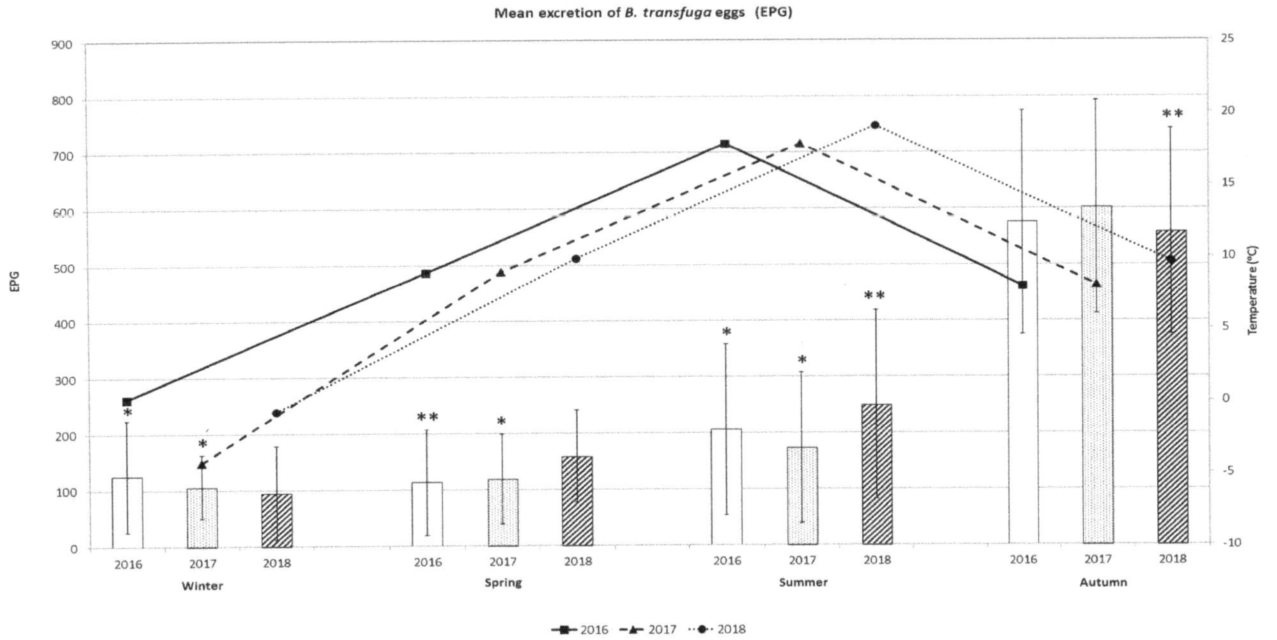

Figure 4. Mean excretion of *B. transfuga* eggs (EPG) in the brown bear (*Ursus arctos*) and mean temperature (°C) during different seasons of the three-year survey; *, significant differences between autumn, winter, and summer 2016 and between winter, spring, and summer 2017; $p < 0.0001$; **, significant differences between spring and autumn 2016 and between winter, summer, and autumn 2018, $p < 0.00$.

The excretion of parasitic eggs was highest in autumn, with the maximum EPG over the three years. Mean excretion tended to increase with temperature from winter to summer.

Any relationship was not observed between data on precipitation and humidity and seasonal results of FEC. In our study, we also investigated the relationship between the occurrence of *B. transfuga* and mean precipitation and humidity (Table 2). We did not observe any relationship between our findings and any of the mentioned climatic parameters.

Table 2. Basic climatological parameters, mean temperature, minimum and maximum temperatures, mean rainfall, and mean humidity, during the three-year survey (2016–2018).

Season	Temperature (°C)									Mean Rainfall (mm)			Mean Humidity (%)		
	2016			2017			2018			2016	2017	2018	2016	2017	2018
	Mean	Min	Max	Mean	Min	Max	Mean	Min	Max						
Winter	0.2	−16.6	14.5	−4.2	−20.5	12.5	−0.7	−14.2	10.5	90.8	56.3	66.8	83.1	85.5	83.2
Spring	8.9	−6.2	26.9	9.0	−3.4	26.3	9.9	−18.0	27.6	53.9	62.1	70.9	76.9	74.2	73.7
Summer	17.8	3.1	32.2	17.8	4.2	32.0	19.1	4.7	30.7	118.4	88.1	105.6	72.9	75.6	77.8
Autumn	7.9	−8.9	28.0	8.0	−7.2	28.5	9.7	−13.0	28.6	87.7	99.8	40.3	82.8	85.5	79.7

Source: SHI, Bratislava, Hydrometeorological station Osadné, SR.

4. Discussion

Our study describes seasonal patterns of mean excretion, abundance, and prevalence of *B. transfuga* eggs by brown bears in a Central Europe area. The prevalence, intensity, and geographic distribution of *B. transfuga* infections have been confirmed worldwide in free-ranging bears such as the American black bear and grizzly bear, the European brown bear, and the polar bear. The seasonal dynamics of *B. transfuga* infections in populations of wild bears could also be influenced by the large differences between bear species and the genetic variability and adaptability of nematodes to a wide range of external temperature differences. Further studies would be useful to clarify the intra- and interspecific relationships amongst *B. transfuga* from different geographic areas and bear species and to address epidemiological and zoonotic patterns of this bear nematode.

Only limited data has been reported for the seasonal dynamics of *B. transfuga* prevalence in populations of free-ranging bears, with some conflicting results. The prevalence of *B. transfuga* in American and Canadian populations of wild bears has been reported in several studies [14,25,28–30,32,47–50], but only a few studies have attempted to investigate seasonal trends in prevalence. One of the studies comparing the incidence of eggs confirmed a higher prevalence in spring (42%) compared to autumn prior to denning (13%) in black bears in Canada [29]. Such an opposite trend to our findings may have been due to the development of larvae surviving hibernation [29]. Several studies have provided evidence that intestinal parasites that feed directly on the host organism pass from the gastrointestinal tract before the onset of hibernation [28,49]. Choquette et al. [49] and Rausch [47] also hypothesised that nematodes were eliminated prior to hibernation in bears. Rogers [28] found that bears excreted *B. transfuga* eggs in the spring soon after hibernation and found evidence of egg excretion immediately prior to denning, so whether or not parasitic infections are cleared during winter hibernation remains unclear, and the apparent elimination of *B. transfuga* during hibernation is poorly understood. Rogers [28], however, confirmed that baylisascariasis in a population of wild bears occurred mainly in summer (75%). Similarly, Manville [50] reported the highest prevalence of *B. transfuga* eggs (64%) and adult parasites (89%) of American black bears (*Ursus americanus*) in summer based on faecal floatation and necropsy. Additionally, Clark et al. [48] found that the incidence of *B. transfuga* infection peaked from June to August and was lower during autumn and winter. Gau et al. [30] and Catalano et al. [32], however, observed the opposite seasonal trend, with peaks in autumn in black bears and grizzly bears in Canada, consistent with our results. Gau et al. [30] reported that the prevalence of gastrointestinal parasites, including *Baylisascaris*, in grizzly bear faeces was low in spring (31%) and high in autumn (58%) based on faecal floatation. Such dynamics may have been due to the expulsion of adult nematodes before hibernation and subsequent reinfection in spring, because bears restrict their food intake and evacuate their bowels shortly before hibernation. Catalano et al. [32] observed the seasonal trend in prevalence based on the collection of nematodes at necropsy, with peaks in autumn (87.5%) in grizzly and black bears.

Little information is available on the prevalence of *B. transfuga* in populations of wild brown bears in Europe [1,35–40]. Only a few of these studies have attempted to evaluate the seasonal dynamics of this nematode. De Ambrogi et al. [39] described *B. transfuga* prevalence (13.5%) in free-ranging European brown bears in Croatia based on a coprological study. Goldova et al. [36] identified gastrointestinal parasites in faecal samples in Slovakia, with a predominant prevalence of *B. transfuga* (72.34%). The prevalence of baylisascariasis defined by FEC coprological method in brown bears during the three years of our study was highest in autumn. The FEC coprological non-invasive method is routinely used for detecting *Baylisascaris* in raccoon faeces and in the environment [51,52]. Limitation of this coprological non-invasive method could be false-negative stool examination results [51,52]. Despite the large number of eggs that are eliminated, it is recommended that three daily faecal samples be examined for *Baylisascaris* in raccoons [51], but it was not possible in wild bears. The highest prevalence in autumn in our study may be highly influenced by interactions such as age and sex of the examined bears. The intensity of egg excretion at one sampling site may be influenced by the fact that the source of the samples may be individuals of different ages. Among other factors, the age composition of the studied bears may have had a significant effect on the high prevalence of *B. transfuga* in our results. As is well known, juvenile raccoons are susceptible to infection through ingestion of eggs, while the older bears become infected through paratenic hosts [11], and immunity to larvae is developed following primary exposure in young animals, which decreases the burdens of parasites in future infections [51]. Young racoons can produce an egg output of 115,000–179,000 eggs per day [53]. Differences in prevalence between the sexes were also confirmed in raccoons, where higher prevalence was recorded in males than in females. Transplacental and transmammary transmission has been described in raccoon females [11,54]. Previous ingestion of larvated eggs is probably cumulative and may be affected by factors such as prepatent period (a prepatent period of 7–10 weeks), and also bear physiology changes as hyperphagia before hibernation.

The seasonal dynamics of *B. transfuga* prevalence in bears could be more influenced by internal factors such as hormonal and metabolic changes occurring before, during, and after bear hibernation. The occurrence of roundworms in hibernating bears in spring could be related to brown fat and the hypothalamic hormone, which affect the bear's carbohydrate metabolism by up to 75%. Bear hibernation could affect the metabolism of intestinal nematodes. Glycogen is apparently synthesized from hexoses and plays an important role in supplying energy to nematodes [37]. Hibernation in relation to parasite metabolism has been described by several authors [28,49]. Finnegan [37] hypothesised that adult parasites usually died during hibernation in winter due to carbohydrate deficiency and subsequently disintegrated. Bears accumulate large stores of body fat during late summer and autumn necessary for winter hibernation. They have a hyperphagic phase in which food intake increases 2–3-fold, and their body weight can increase by 30–35% [55]. Hyperphagia provides a sufficient source of carbohydrates for the survival and reproduction of nematodes [37]. Adult nematodes accumulate in the intestinal tracts of bears beginning in spring, which could be correlated with the highest seasonal peak in the prevalence of *B. transfuga* in bears in autumn. However, the mechanism of hibernation in bears is not well known, but is likely to be influenced by the interaction of several stimuli, including reduced food availability, low temperature, snowfall, daylight, physical conditions, sex, age, and reproductive status, and may also be influenced by bear species [56].

The high seasonal prevalence of *B. transfuga* in non-denning bears in winter is a concern and may be a consequence of the increase in mean temperatures due to global warming or to supplemental food sources provided by hunters in winter. Insufficient hibernation time due to warm winters and the consequent high prevalence of *Baylisascaris* infection can negatively affect the health of infected bears. The bear's carbohydrate metabolism in non-denning bears in winter is still built up. Is it assumed that bear hibernation could be negatively affected by the metabolism of intestinal nematodes and lead to "clearing up". This hypothesis can mainly affect juvenile subadults in bears which did not build up sufficient fat deposits and contribute to worsening body condition in spring time. Hibernation in relation to parasite metabolism has been described by several authors [28,49]. Bears, however, may not hibernate in mild winters [57]. The immobilisation of bears could be associated with mild winter temperatures due to global warming. The availability of sufficient food sources until late autumn and winter is another important factor associated with the delay or elimination of bear hibernation. Additionally, intensive feeding of wild bears with maize, as a source of carbohydrates, led to the activity of bears during winter [58,59].

The prevalence of baylisascariasis in brown bears during the three years of our study was highest in autumn. Our findings are consistent with most studies that have investigated the seasonal dynamics of *B. transfuga* in bears [38,40]. These studies found that the prevalence was highest in autumn or winter and lowest in spring. Orosová et al. [40], however, found that the prevalence of *Baylisascaris* was highest in autumn (85.71%) and early winter (100%). Similar results were reported by Major et al. [38] in their coprological study, who also observed that the prevalence of *B. transfuga* was highest in autumn and winter and lowest in spring, which corresponds to the results of our study. Several studies have confirmed the occurrence of parasites in bears during the winter, when bears should hibernate [36,38,40].

We also observed a seasonal occurrence of nematode eggs in bear faeces during the winter. Our study recorded the prevalence of *B. transfuga* excreted eggs in faecal samples in the bears up to 48.5%. Štrkolcová et al. [34] suggested that the high prevalence of endoparasites in winter was associated with relatively warm winters, which shortened or eliminated hibernation. However, it has been reported that seasonal pattern of *B. procyonis* in racoons may be disturbed in warmer southern regions of the United States [60,61]. So, the goal of our study was to confirm or refute this temporal seasonal pattern in the conditions of mild climate in Central Europe. The increase in temperatures during the winter has been observed in the mild climatic conditions of Central Europe in recent years.

For this reason, we decided to monitor the prevalence of *B. transfuga* and the nematode egg excretion in brown bears' faecal samples during all seasons at monthly intervals over 3 years. To a lesser extent, soil type, habitat fragmentation, and other environmental components, such as road density, have been assessed as risk factors for parasitic infection [9]. Increased risk of transmitting *Baylisascaris* infection to paratenic hosts may affect the factors such as moisture retention and size of particles of the soil. Moisture and particle size also can affect egg viability [41]. For this reason, we decided to compare climatic parameters (temperature, humidity, rainfall) with the nematode egg excretion in brown bears in the same period. Environmental factors are related to the secretion of eggs in the same period of time, but mainly affect the accumulation of infectious stages in previous periods. Additionally, since eggs can remain present and viable for many years following deposition [62], seasonal or annual trends may be masked. However, our results confirmed the temporal pattern with a peak FEC in the autumn and a subsequent winter decline without proving the influence of climatic factors.

Our results did not confirm the effect of temperature, precipitation, and humidity on excretion of *Baylisascaris transfuga* eggs in brown bears in the mild climate of Central Europe. Prevalence, abundance, and mean egg excretion may be highly influenced by interactions such as age, sex, hyperphagia before hibernation, and previous larvated eggs ingestion, which are most probably cumulative during the prepatent period.

B. transfuga was not studied in wild brown bears in Europe as *B. procyoonis* in racoons in America. In general, information about the prevalence of *B. transfuga* in wild European bears is limited, and there is no data on environmental effects on the seasonal dynamics of *B. transfuga* in wild bears in Europe.

A national brown bear management plan has yet to be established, despite repeated calls by the Standing Committee of the Bern Convention and the Council of Europe. There has been little meaningful cooperation with neighbouring states sharing the same bear population (Czech Republic, Poland, Ukraine) and so consideration of management at population level, also emphasised by international experts, has been inadequate. Loss, fragmentation, and disturbance of habitat are potentially major threats to wildlife in the Carpathian Mountains. Adequate steps need to be taken to prevent permanent isolation of habitat and wildlife, including bears [63]. Research on ecology is very important to allow better understanding of the needs of bears as well as the causes of bear–human conflicts. Habitat use, social organisation, and dispersal are especially pertinent. Studies focused on the ecology and management of the brown bear in Central/Eastern Europe are needed in the future.

5. Conclusions

The prevalence, abundance, and mean excretion of *B. transfuga* eggs in bears were highest in autumn in all three years. We observed a relationship between the dynamics of *B. transfuga* prevalence in bears and changes in mean temperature in spring and autumn, and a seasonal trend of increasing intensity of parasitic infection from spring to autumn. The increase in the bear population, shrinking territories, and the increase in occurrence in urban areas, however, are also alarming. The dissemination of the propagative stages of bear nematodes in both urban and rural ecosystems near human dwellings could pose a risk to human health.

Author Contributions: Conceptualization, L.M. and A.K.; data curation, P.M.; formal analysis, Z.V. and M.T.; investigation, L.M., A.K., Z.V. and M.V.; methodology, L.M. and P.M.; visualization, Z.V.; writing—original draft, A.K.; writing—review & editing, L.M., A.K. and M.V. All authors have read and agreed to the published version of the manuscript.

Acknowledgments: We thank Jozef Štofík and Jozef Blaško for their professional assistance.

References

1. Aghazadeh, M.; Alson-Riggins, J.; Reljić, S.; de Ambrogi, M.; Huber, D.; Majnarić, C.; Hermosilla, C. Gastrointestinal parasites and the first report of *Giardia* spp. in a wild population of European brown bears (*Ursus arctos*) in Croatia. *Vet. Arhiv.* **2015**, *85*, 201–210.
2. Kaczensky, P.; Chapron, G.; Von Arx, M.; Huber, D.; Andrén, H.; Linnell, J.D. Status, management and distribution of large carnivores—Bear, lynx, wolf and wolverine—In Europe. Part 1. In *IUCN/SSC Large Carnivore Initiative for Europe and Istituto di Ecologia Applicata*; European Commission: Rome, Italy, 2013; p. 72.
3. Rigg, R. Status of brown bears in the Ukraine. *Int. Bear News* **2005**, *14*, 20.
4. Pravda o Medveďoch: Stavy medveďov v Chránenej Poľovnej Oblasti Poľana a Priľahlých Poľovných Revíroch [The Truth about Bears: The Number of Bears in Protected Hunting Area Poľana and Adjacent Hunting Areas]. Available online: https://www.pravdaomedvedoch.sk/stavy-medvedov-v-chpo-polana-a-prilahlych-polovnych-reviroch/ (accessed on 9 September 2019).
5. Štofík, J.; Buraľ, M.; Paule, L.; Straka, M. Zhodnotenie historického rozšírenia medveďa hnedého (*Ursus arctos*) v Bukovských vrchoch a na priľahlých územiach [Evaluation of the historical distribution of the brown bear in the Bukovské vrchy and in the adjacent areas]. *Natura Carpatica* **2010**, *51*, 65–74. (In Slovak)
6. Paule, L. Rozšírenie a početnosť veľkých šeliem na Slovensku [Distribution and population size of large carnivores in Slovakia]. In *Ochrana a Manažment Veľkých šeliem na Slovensku [Conservation and Management of Large Carnvivores in Slovakia]*; Lešová, A., Antal, V., Eds.; Štátna Ochrana Prírody SR: Banská Bystrica, Slovakia, 2016; pp. 73–85. (In Slovak)
7. Králik, T. Medvede a ľudia. Ako ďalej [Bears and people. How to continue]. *Chránené Územia Slovenska* **2019**, *93*, 44–60. (In Slovak)
8. Olah, B.; Boltižiar, M.; Petrovič, F. Land use changes' relation to georelief and distance in the East Carpathians biosphere reserve. *Ekológia* **2006**, *25*, 68–81.
9. French, S.K.; Pearl, D.L.; Peregrine, A.S.; Jardine, C.M. *Baylisascaris procyonis* infection in raccoons: A review of demographic and environmental factors influencing parasite carriage. *Vet. Parasitolol. Reg. Stud. Rep.* **2019**, *16*, 100275. [CrossRef]
10. Samuel, W.M.; Pybus, M.J.; Kocan, A.A. *Parasitic Diseases of Wild Mammals*, 2nd ed.; Iowa State University Press: Iowa City, IA, USA, 2001; p. 559.
11. Kazacos, K.R. *Baylisascaris procyonis* and related species. In *Parasitic Diseases of Wild Mammals*; Samuel, W.M., Pybus, M.J., Kocan, A.A., Eds.; Iowa State University Press: Iowa City, IA, USA, 2001; pp. 301–341.
12. Bauer, C. Baylisascariosis—Infections of animals and humans with 'unusual'roundworms. *Vet. Parasitol.* **2013**, *193*, 40–412. [CrossRef]
13. Sapp, S.G.H.; Gupta, P.; Martin, M.K.; Murra, M.H.; Niedringhaus, K.D.; Pfaff, M.A.; Yabsley, M.J. Beyond the raccoon roundworm: The natural history of non-raccoon *Baylisascaris* species in the New World. *IGP Parasites Wildl.* **2017**, *6*, 85–99. [CrossRef]
14. Foster, G.W.; Cunningham, M.W.; Kinsella, J.M.; Forrester, D.J. Parasitic helminths of black bear cubs (*Ursus americanus*) from Florida. *J. Parasitol.* **2004**, *90*, 173–175. [CrossRef]
15. Partridge, J. *Management Guidelines for Bears and Raccoons*; The Association of British Wild Animal Keepers: Bristol, UK, 1992.
16. Moran, J.F.; Feliu, C.; Gomez, M.S. *Baylisascaris transfuga* (Rudolphy 1819), (Nematoda, Ascarididae); a common parasite of bears. Ecological aspects and treatment. In Proceedings of the International Conference of Aspects of Bear Conservation, Bursa, Turkey, 31 May–5 June 1994; pp. 121–124.
17. Szczepaniak, K.; Listos, P.; Lopuszynski, W.; Skrzypek, T.; Kazimierczak, W. Granulomatous peritonitis in a European brown bear caused by *Baylisascaris transfuga*. *J. Wildl. Dis.* **2012**, *48*, 517–519. [CrossRef]
18. Gutiérrez, Y. *Diagnostic Pathology of Parasitic Infections with Clinical Correlations*; Oxford University Press: Oxford, UK, 2000; p. 769.
19. Bugmyrin, S.V.; Spiridonov, S.E. First recond of natural *Baylisascaris transfuga* (Ascaridoidea, Nematoda) infection in wild rodents. *Parasitology* **2019**, *146*, 1714–1718. [CrossRef] [PubMed]
20. Abdelrasoul, K.; Fowler, M. Epidemiology of ascarid infection in captive carnivores. In Proceedings of the Annual Meeting of the American Association of Zoo Veterinarians, Denver, CO, USA, 7–11 October 1979; American Association of Zoo Veterinarians: Philadelphia, PA, USA, 1979; pp. 105–106.

21. Sato, H.; Matsuo, K.; Osanai, A.; Kamiya, H.; Akao, N.; Owaki, S.; Furuoka, H. Larva migrans by *Baylisascaris transfuga*: Fatal neurological diseases in Mongolian jirds, but not in mice. *J. Parasitol.* **2004**, *90*, 774–781. [CrossRef] [PubMed]
22. Gavin, P.J.; Kazacos, K.R.; Shulman, S.T. Baylisascariasis. *Clin. Microbiol. Rev.* **2005**, *18*, 703–718. [CrossRef] [PubMed]
23. Tiner, J.D. Fatalities in rodents caused by larval *Ascaris* in the central nervous system. *J. Mammal.* **1953**, *34*, 153–167. [CrossRef]
24. Wallach, J.D.; Boever, W.J. *Diseases of Exotic Animals Medical and Surgical Management*; WB Saunders CO: Philadelphia, PA, USA, 1983.
25. Crum, J.M.; Nettles, V.F.; Davidson, W.R. Studies on endoparasites of the black bear (*Ursus americanus*) in the southeastern United States. *J. Wildl. Dis.* **1978**, *14*, 178–186. [CrossRef] [PubMed]
26. Papini, R.; Renzoni, G.; Malloggi, M.; Casarosa, L. Visceral larva migrans in mice experimentally infected with *Baylisascaris transfuga* (Ascarididae: Nematoda). *Parasitologia* **1994**, *36*, 321–329.
27. King, J.M.; Black, H.C.; Hewitt, O.H. Pathology, parasitology and hematology of the black bear in New York. *N. Y. Fish Game J.* **1960**, *7*, 99–111.
28. Rogers, L.L. Parasites of black bears of the Lake Superior region. *J. Wildl. Dis.* **1975**, *11*, 189–192. [CrossRef]
29. Frechette, J.L.; Rau, M.E. Seasonal changes in the prevalance of ova of *Diphyllobothrium ursi* and *Baylisascaris transfuga* in the feces of the black bear (*Ursus americanus*). *J. Wildl. Dis.* **1978**, *14*, 342–344. [CrossRef]
30. Gau, R.J.; Kutz, S.; Elkin, B.T. Parasites in Grizzly Bears from the Central Canadian Arctic. *J. Wildl. Dis.* **1999**, *35*, 618–621. [CrossRef]
31. Testini, G.; Papini, R.; Lia, R.P.; Parisi, A.; Dantas-Torres, F.; Traversa, D.; Otranto, D. New insights into the morphology, molecular characterization and identification of *Baylisascaris transfuga* (Ascaridida, Ascarididae). *Vet. Parasitol.* **2011**, *175*, 97–102. [CrossRef] [PubMed]
32. Catalano, S.; Lejeune, M.; Tizzani, P.; Verocai, G.G.; Schwantje, H.; Nelson, C.; Duignan, P.J. Helminths of grizzly bears (*Ursus arctos*) and American black bears (*Ursus americanus*) in Alberta and British Columbia, Canada. *Can. J. Zool.* **2015**, *93*, 765–772. [CrossRef]
33. Bugmyrin, S.V.; Tirronen, K.F.; Panchenko, D.V.; Kopatz, A.; Hagen, S.B.; Eiken, H.G.; Kuznetsova, A.S. Helminths of brown bears (*Ursus arctos*) in the Kola Peninsula. *Parasitol. Res.* **2017**, *116*, 1755–1760. [CrossRef] [PubMed]
34. Štrkolcová, G.; Goldová, M.; Šnábel, V.; Špakulová, M.; Orosová, T.; Halán, M.; Mojžišová, J. A frequent roundworm *Baylisascaris transfuga* in over populated brown bears (*Ursus arctos*) in Slovakia: A problem worthy of attention. *Acta Parasitol.* **2018**, *63*, 167–174. [CrossRef]
35. Mituch, J. Helminth fauna of carnivores in Slovak and Czech Republics (In Slovak). *Folia Venatoria* **1972**, *2*, 161–171.
36. Goldova, M.; Ciberej, J.; Rigg, R. Medved hnedý (*Ursus arctos*) a parazitárne zoonózy. Brown bear (*Ursus arctos*) and parasitic zoonoses. *Folia Venatoria* **2003**, *33*, 123–127. (In Slovak)
37. Finnegan, S. Seasonal Dynamics in the Prevalence of *Baylisascaris transfuga* ova in the Faeces of the Brown Bear (*Ursus arctos*) in Slovakia. Master's Thesis, University of Veterinary Medicine and Pharmacy in Košice, Košice, Slovakia, 2009.
38. Major, P.; Molnár, L.; Štofík, J.; Goldová, M. Parasitofauna medved'a hnedého v NP Poloniny. Parasitofauna of the brown bear (*Ursus arctos*) in Poloniny National Park. In Proceedings of the Škola—Veda—prax I (School—Science—Practice), Košice, Slovakia, 24 September 2009; pp. 318–322. (In Slovak).
39. De Ambrogi, M.; Aghazadeh, M.; Hermosilla, C.; Huber, D.; Majnaric, D.; Reljic, S.; Riggins, J.E. Occurrence of *Baylisascaris transfuga* in wild populations of European brown bears (*Ursus arctos*) asidentified by a new PCR method. *Vet. Parasitol.* **2011**, *179*, 272–276. [CrossRef]
40. Orosová, T.; Goldová, M.; Ciberej, J.; Štrkolcová, G. Parasitofauna of brown bear (*Ursus arctos*) in the protected landscape area CHKO—Pol'ana. *Folia Veterinaria* **2016**, *60*, 20–24. [CrossRef]
41. Kresta, A.E.; Henke, S.E.; Pence, D.B. *Baylisascaris procyonis* in raccoons in Texas and its relationship to habitat characteristics. *J. Wildl. Dis.* **2010**, *46*, 843–853. [CrossRef]
42. Persson, I.L.; Wikan, S.; Swenson, J.E.; Mysterud, I. The diet of the brown bear *Ursus arctos* in the Pasvik Valley, northeastern Norway. *Wildl. Biol.* **2001**, *7*, 27–37. [CrossRef]

43. Coles, G.C.; Bauer, C.; Borgsteede, F.H.M.; Geerts, S.; Klei, T.R.; Taylor, M.A.; Waller, P.J. World Association for the Advancement of Veterinary Parasitology (W.A.A.V.P.) methods for the detection of anthelmintic resistance in nematodes of veterinary importance. *Vet. Parasitol.* **1992**, *44*, 35–44. [CrossRef]
44. Sprent, J.F.A. Notes on *Ascaris* and *Toxascaris*, with a definition of *Baylisascaris* gen. nov. *Parasitology* **1968**, *58*, 185–198. [CrossRef] [PubMed]
45. Kazakos, R.; Turek, J.J. Scanning electron microscopy of the eggs of *Baylisascaris procyonis*, *B. transfuga* and *Parascaris equorum* and their comparison with *Toxocara canis* and *Ascaris suum*. *Proc. Helm. Soc. Wash.* **1983**, *50*, 36–42.
46. Margolis, L.; Esch, G.W.; Holmes, J.C.; Kuris, A.M.; Schad, G.A. The use of eco-logical terms in parasitology (report of an ad hoc committee of the American Society of Parasitologists). *J. Parasitol.* **1982**, *68*, 131–133. [CrossRef]
47. Rausch, R.L. Notes on the black bear, *Ursus americanus*, Pallas, in Alaska, with particular reference to dentition and growth. *Z. Saugetierkd.* **1961**, *26*, 65–128.
48. Clark, J.D.; Loew, F.M.; Burns, K.F. The use of dichlorvos as anthelmintic in naturally parasitised bears. *JAVMA* **1969**, *155*, 1093–1097.
49. Choquette, L.P.E.; Gibson, G.G.; Pearson, A.M. Helminths of the grizzly bear, *Ursus actors*, in northern Canada. *Can. J. Zool.* **1969**, *47*, 167–170. [CrossRef]
50. Manville, M. Ecto- and endoparasites of the black bear in northern Wisconsin. *J. Wildl. Dis.* **1978**, *14*, 97–100. [CrossRef] [PubMed]
51. Reed, C.; Henke, S.E.; Kresta, A.E. Frequency of deposition and location of *Baylisascaris procyonis* eggs in raccoon feces. *J. Wildl. Dis.* **2012**, *48*, 190–194. [CrossRef] [PubMed]
52. Page, L.K.; Gehrt, S.D.; Titcombe, K.K.; Robinson, N.P. Measuring prevalence of raccoon roundworm (*Baylisascaris procyonis*): A comparison of common techniques. *Wildl. Soc. Bull.* **2005**, *33*, 1406–1412. [CrossRef]
53. Snyder, D.E.; Fitzgerald, P.R. Contaminative potential, egg prevalence, and intensity of Baylisascaris procyonis-infected raccoons (*Procyon lotor*) from Illinois, with a comparison to worm intensity. *Proc. Helminthol. Soc. Wash.* **1987**, *54*, 141–145.
54. Kazacos, K.R. *Baylisascaris Larva Migrans, Circular*; U.S. Geological Survey: Reston, VA, USA, 2016; p. 1412.
55. Hissa, R. Physiology of the European brown bear (*Ursus arctos arctos*). *Ann. Zool. Fennici* **1997**, *34*, 267–287.
56. Rigg, R. Ten years' experience of conservation and research work on large carnivores. Large carnivores: Management, research and public relation strategies of the protected areas. In Proceedings of the Alpine-Carpathian International Colloquium, Liptovský Ján, Slovakia, 2–4 July 2009.
57. Pelikán, V. Zaujímavosti z CHKO Muránska planina. Interesting observations from Muránska planina. *Spravodajca Chránených Uzemí Slovenska* **1983**, *2*, 94. (In Slovak)
58. Hell, P.; Slamečka, J. *Medveď v Slovenských Karpatoch a vo Svete [The Bear in the Slovak Carpathians and in the World]*; PaR Press: Bratislava, Slovakia, 1999; p. 150. (In Slovak)
59. Baláž, E. Ekológia medveďa hnedého (*Ursus arctos*) v Západných Tatrách a na Poľane [The Ecology of the Brown Bear (*Ursus arctos*) in the Western Tatras and in Poľana]. Master's Thesis, Technical University in Zvolen, Zvolen, Slovakia, 2002. (In Slovak).
60. Blizzard, E.L.; Davis, C.D.; Henke, S.; Long, D.B.; Hall, C.A.; Yabsley, M.J. Distribution, prevalence, and genetic characterization of *Baylisascaris procyonis* in selected areas of Georgia. *J. Parasitol.* **2010**, *96*, 1128–1133. [CrossRef]
61. Page, L.K.; Gehrt, S.D.; Cascione, A.; Kellner, K.F. The relationship between *Baylisascaris procyonis* prevalence and raccoon population structure. *J. Parasitol.* **2009**, *95*, 1314–1320. [CrossRef]
62. Kazacos, K.R.; Boyce, W.M. *Baylisascaris* larva migrans. *J. Am. Vet. Med. Assoc.* **1989**, *195*, 894–903.
63. Rigg, R.; Adamec, M. Status, ecology and management of the brown bear (*Ursus arctos*) in Slovakia. *Slovak Wildl. Soc.* **2007**, *6*, 128.

10

Changes in the Percentages of B- and T-Lymphocytes and Antibody Titres in Laying Hens Infested with *Dermanyssus gallinae*

Sylwia Koziatek-Sadłowska and Rajmund Sokół *

Department of Parasitology and Invasive Diseases, Faculty of Veterinary Medicine, University of Warmia and Mazury in Olsztyn, ul. Oczapowskiego 13, 10-719 Olsztyn, Poland; sylwia.koziatek@uwm.edu.pl

* Correspondence: rajmund.sokol@uwm.edu.pl.

Simple Summary: *Dermanyssus gallinae,* a hematophagous ectoparasite, adversely affects the health status of laying hens, leading to reduced egg production and significant economic losses in commercial poultry farms. The aim of this study was to determine the effect of *D. gallinae* on the immunological parameters (three lymphocyte subpopulations) and post-vaccination antibody titres (against most important avian pathogens) in layer hens during the egg production cycle. A total of 80 blood samples were collected at four time-points (B1–B4) from 10 Hy-Line Brown hens naturally infested with *D. gallinae*, which were randomly selected from a commercial layer farm. The infestation was monitored and treated twice with Biobeck PA 910 (active ingredient AI – silicon dioxide). The samples were collected before and after each treatment. The percentages of subpopulations of B cells and helper (Th) and cytotoxic (Tc) T cells were determined by flow cytometry. Antibody titres were determined by the immunoenzymatic method. The percentage of Th cells and post-vaccination anti-infectious bronchitis virus (anti-IBV) and anti-Newcastle disease virus (anti-NDV) antibodies decreased significantly at the second infestation peak when the number of parasites was twice higher than at the first infestation peak. There were non-significant correlations between the number of mites and antibody titres. These findings suggested that *D. gallinae* might inhibit humoral immune responses since the percentages of B cells and Th cells were negatively correlated with the number of mites. The percentage of Tc cells was positively correlated with the number of mites, which indicated that *D. gallinae* could stimulate cellular immune responses in infested laying hens. However, further research is needed to determine whether *D. gallinae* suppresses the production of vaccine-induced antibodies.

Abstract: (1) Background: *Dermanyssus gallinae*, a hematophagous ectoparasite, adversely affects the health status of laying hens, leading to reduced egg production and significant economic losses in commercial farms. The aim of this study was to determine the effect of *D. gallinae* on the development of post-vaccination immune responses in layer hens. (2) Methods: A total of 80 blood samples were collected at four time-points (B1–B4) from 10 Hy-Line Brown hens, randomly selected from a commercial layer farm. The flock was naturally infested with *D. gallinae* and treated twice with Biobeck PA 910 (AI silicon dioxide). The samples were collected before and after each treatment. The percentages of IgM+ B cells, CD3+/CD4+ T cells and CD3+/CD8a+ T cells were determined by flow cytometry; the titres of antibodies against avian encephalomyelitis, infectious bronchitis virus, Newcastle disease virus, *Ornithobacterium rhinotracheale*, reticuloendotheliosis virus and avian reovirus were determined by the immunoenzymatic method. (3) Results: The percentage of Th cells and post-vaccination anti-IBV and anti-NDV antibodies decreased significantly at the second infestation peak when the number of parasites was twice higher than at the first infestation peak. Non-significant negative correlations were found between the number of mites and the percentage of B cells (R = −0.845, $p > 0.05$) and between the number of mites and the percentage of Th cells (R = −0.522,

$p > 0.05$), and a significant positive correlation was noted between the number of mites and the percentage of Tc cells (R = −0.982, $p < 0.05$). There were non-significant correlations between the number of mites and antibody titres. (4) Conclusion: The present findings suggested that *D. gallinae* might inhibit immune responses since the percentages of B cells and Th cells were negatively correlated with the number of mites. The percentage of Tc cells was positively correlated with the number of mites, which indicated that *D. gallinae* could stimulate cellular immune responses in infested laying hens. However, further research is needed to determine whether *D. gallinae* suppresses the production of vaccine-induced antibodies.

Keywords: *D. gallinae*; hematophagous ectoparasite; poultry red mite; antibody titre; lymphocyte subpopulation

1. Introduction

Dermanyssus gallinae (De Geer, 1778) (*D. gallinae*), commonly known as poultry red mite (prm), is a temporary ectoparasite, feeding on the blood of wild and domestic birds [1–4]. It is currently the most serious mite pest in commercial caged layer hen farms [5–9]. Farm conditions favour mass occurrence and uncontrolled growth of the parasite. Such conditions include high, constant temperature, high relative air humidity, constant access to the host body and long production cycle (80 weeks) [8,10,11]. The parasite settles in numerous gaps in the poultry house construction and equipment where it goes through the development cycle of five life stages (egg, larva, protonymph, deutonymph and adults). It needs the host's blood for growth in the last three stages [1,12]. They feed briefly and return to their refugia [13,14]. This way of life makes it poorly accessible to acaricides [8,10,15]. Moreover, there have been increasing numbers of reports on the prm resistance to acaricides [16–18]. The implementation of enriched cages (in line with the EU Directive 1999.74/EC) has probably led to a significant and uncontrolled proliferation of *D. gallinae* [8,19]. Under heavy infestation, the welfare of the laying hens significantly decreases. Upon puncturing the skin of the host, the mite introduces toxic saliva that can cause itching and irritation, which leads to distress and, consequently, poor feed conversion, reduced egg production and increased bird mortality [10,20,21].

Birds in commercial flocks of laying hens are given preventive vaccination until the 20th week of their lives. Not only are they important from the economic perspective, but they ensure consumer safety. Vaccination effectiveness may be affected by feed, genetic, environmental, chemical and biological (bacteria and viruses) factors. According to the literature, hens, which are chronically exposed to *D. gallinae*, do not produce a strong immune response against this parasite. A non-significant correlation between serum IgY level and red mite population levels has been observed [22]. Another study has revealed that *D. gallinae* feeding stimulates Th1 and pro-inflammatory cytokines/chemokines, initially followed by their subsequent down-regulation [23]. There is also a theory that *D. gallinae* might adopt a feeding strategy of minimal host interference, while *D. gallinae* could determine host immune status by nymphal/larval survival rates [24]. Our recent studies revealed that *D. gallinae* infestation caused somatic and psychogenic stress in layer hens, which led to lower humoral immunity decrease of γ-globulin in the blood of hens infested by *D. gallinae* [25,26]. Therefore, the question may be formulated, whether the pressure (feeding) of *D. gallinae* may have an immunosuppressive effect and affect the development of post-vaccination immune responses in laying hens. There has been no scientific research on the subject. The research on *D. gallinae*, in an ectoparasite–host immunological relationship, mainly concerns vaccines against this parasite.

Therefore, the aim of this study was to determine the percentages of subpopulations of B IgM+ cells, T cells CD3+/CD4+ (Th) and T cells CD3+/CD8a+ (Tc) by flow cytometry and the titres of antibodies against AE (avian encephalomyelitis), IBV (infectious bronchitis virus), NDV (Newcastle disease virus), ORT (*Ornithobacterium rhinotracheale*), REV (reticuloendotheliosis virus) and REO (avian reovirus) using the immunoenzymatic method with ELISA tests (IDEXX, USA) in the peripheral blood of laying hens infested with *D. gallinae*, controlled with Biobeck PA 910 (active ingredient (AI) silicon dioxide).

2. Materials and Methods

2.1. Birds

Blood samples for analyses were collected from 10 randomly selected laying hens from an industrial laying hen farm naturally infested with *D. gallinae*. A flock of 56,400 hens of the Hy-Line Brown line was kept in battery cages for 54 weeks in conditions complying with the valid standards. Hens were fed with high-quality feed and watered *ad libitum* from automatic drinkers. The air temperature in the hen house was 20–22 °C, and the relative humidity (RH) was 40%–60%. The birds were given prophylactic vaccinations as per the standard programme: *Salmonella enteritidis*—6–10 days, and 70–74 days, *Staphylococcus gallinarum*—42–46 days and 16 weeks, *Mycoplasma gallisepticum*, *Mycoplasma synoviae*—56–60 days, infectious bronchitis virus (IBV) and Newcastle disease virus (NDV)—35–39 days and 13 weeks, Gumboro disease (IBD)—22–26 days and 30–34 days, avian encephalomyelitis (AE) and egg drop syndrome (EDS'76)—12–13 weeks. Day or week indicates the age range of the hen while vaccinated.

All procedures were conducted according to the prevailing national legislation on the use of animals in research. The experiment was carried out in compliance with the recommendations of the Local Ethics Committee for Animal Experimentation in Olsztyn (no. 59/2006).

2.2. Monitoring of the *Dermanyssus gallinae* Infestation

The infestation of *D. gallinae* was monitored in 2-week intervals. The parasites were caught with a system of traps fixed to the cages under the conveyor belt for egg collection, four at each of fixed selected places, on the second and the fourth row of cages [27]. The traps from each site were collected separately to a twist-type jar (0.9 L) and sent to the laboratory. The jars with their contents were cooled down for 30 min at a temperature of −20 °C to immobilise the parasites and count them. The deposit was poured onto a 2 × 2 cm chequered Petri dish, and the parasite life stages; (a) adults, (b) larvae + nymphs, (c) eggs were counted with a binocular magnifying glass (Olympus, Type SZ, magn. 40×, Tokyo, Japan). The infestation size was presented as the average number of each life stage (Figure 1).

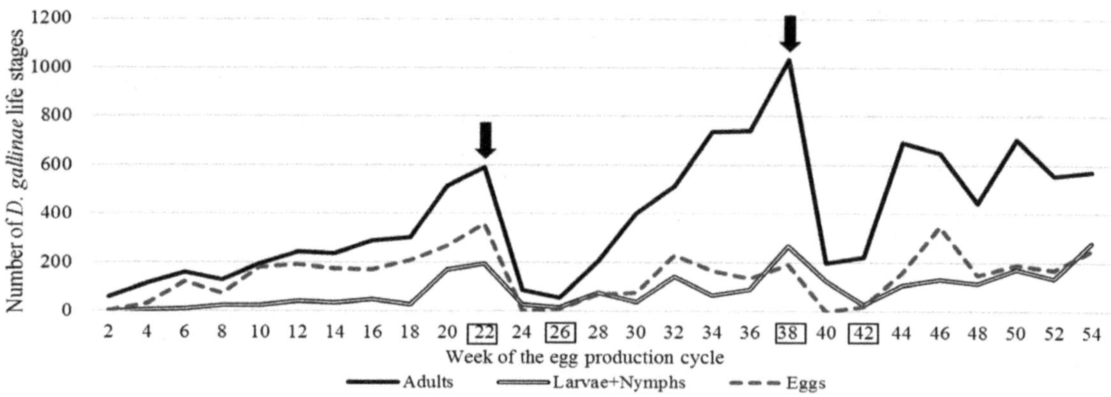

Figure 1. The size of the *Dermanyssus gallinae* population and its life stages following two applications of the acaricide product Biobeck PA 910 (AI silicon dioxide, Biologische Preparate, Brilon, Germany) during a 54-week production cycle. (Mite treatment MTI and MTII dates are marked by arrows, blood sampling B1–4 dates are marked by squares).

2.3. Controlling of the Dermanyssus gallinae Infestation

The infestation of *D. gallinae* was controlled with Biobeck PA 910 (AI silicon dioxide, Biologische Preparate, Brilon, Germany), which was applied in accordance with the manufacturer's guidelines at 1–2 g/hen by spraying onto the cages and hens with a device imparting static electricity to it. Two dates for mite treatment were established based on the results of ongoing monitoring of the number of different life stages. It was performed in the 22nd and 38th week of the production cycle. The first mite treatment (MTI) was performed after a rapid increase in the number of *D. gallinae* was observed—a nearly two-fold increase in the number of adults and eggs and a four-fold increase in the number of larvae + nymphs compared to week 16 (Figure 1). The second mite treatment (MTII) was performed after a two-fold increase, in the number of adults and larvae + nymphs, was recorded compared to week 32 (the number of eggs was similar).

2.4. Collection of the Blood Samples

Blood samples for cytometric and serological tests were collected at four time-points during the egg production cycle, from the wing vein of 10 randomly selected hens for each analysis. Blood samples were collected in the 22nd—B1 (before MTI), 26th—B2 (after MTI), 38th—B3 (before MTII), 42nd—B4 (after MTII) week of the production cycle. Hens were 40, 44, 56, 60 weeks old, respectively, in B1–B4. A total of 80 blood samples were tested (40 for each analysis). Hens were marked, and the blood was taken from the same hens each time.

2.5. Flow Cytometry Analysis

Blood samples in the amount of 1.5 mL were collected into test tubes with an anticoagulant EDTA-K2 (Sarstedt). Subsequently, blood was diluted 1:1 with PBS (phosphate-buffered saline) with 1% fetal calf serum (FCS). The blood samples were layered on 3 mL of Histopaque-1077 gradient (Sigma-Aldrich, Darmstadt, Germany) and centrifuged in 15 mL FALCON tubes at 400× g at the temperature of 25 °C for 30 min. After centrifuging, the layer of mononuclear cells was carefully collected into sterile tubes and washed twice with PBS with an addition of 1% FCS and subsequently suspended in 1 mL PBS. The cells were then counted by the chamber method. A total of 10^6 cells were collected from the suspension and transferred to cytometric tubes. Two microlitres of antibodies targeted at surface domains of the CD3 receptor (Mouse AntiChicken CD3-FITC clone CT-3, SouthernBiotech, Birmingham, AL, USA), CD4 receptor (Mouse AntiChicken CD4-FITC clone CT-4, SouthernBiotech, Birmingham, AL, USA) and CD8 receptor (Mouse AntiChicken CD8a-Cy5 clone 3-298, SouthernBiotech, Birmingham, AL, USA), T cells and immunoglobulin BCR (IgM^+) of B cells (Mouse AntiChickenIgM-SPRD clone M-1, SouthernBiotech, Birmingham, AL, USA) were added to each tube. The samples were incubated on ice for 30 min in darkness. Subsequently, the cells were washed twice in PBS, centrifuged at 250× *g* for 7 min at 4 °C, and the resulting cell pellets were suspended in 0.5 mL of fixing buffer (CellFIX, Becton Dickinson, Franklin Lakes, NJ, USA) and refrigerated. The samples were tested after 18 h with a flow cytometer FACSCanto II (Becton Dickinson, Franklin Lakes, NJ, USA). Immunophenotypic analysis of the lymphocytes was performed with a specialist software FlowJo (Tree Star, Inc., Ashland, OR, USA).

2.6. Serological Analysis (ELISA)

Blood samples were taken to sterile tubes and refrigerated for 1 h to separate the serum from morphotic elements. The blood was then centrifuged for 20 min at 4 °C at 1000× g. Portions of 1.5 mL of serum were transferred to microcentrifuge tubes. The titres of antibodies against AE (avian encephalomyelitis), IBV (infectious bronchitis virus), NDV (Newcastle disease virus), ORT (*Ornithobacterium rhinotracheale*), REO (avian reovirus) and REV (reticuloendotheliosis virus) were determined in accordance with the manufacturer's guidelines for commercial tests ELISA Pro Flok HEV Ab (Zoetis, Parsippany, NJ, USA). The absorbance was read out with a BioTek ELx800

(Winooski, VT, USA) plate reader. The data analysis and calculations were performed in the xCheck IDEXX (Westbrook, ME, USA) software environment.

2.7. Statistical Analysis

The results were analysed statistically by calculating mean values, standard error (SE) and coefficient of variation (CV%) for antibody titres. Differences between B1–B4 for lymphocyte subpopulations and antibody titres were analysed using repeated-measures ANOVA test or MANOVA test if the assumption of sphericity was violated (statistically significant Mauchly test). Tukey's post hoc test was used. The statistical significance was declared at $p < 0.05$. Pearson correlation coefficient test was used to determine the relationships between mite numbers and lymphocyte subpopulations and antibody titres.

3. Results

3.1. Development of the Dermanyssus gallinae Infestation

The mean number of different life stages of *D. gallinae* (adults, larvae + nymphs and eggs) in consecutive weeks of the production cycle of laying hens; dates of mite treatment (MTI and MTII); dates of blood sampling for assays (B1–B4) are shown in Figure 1. Two peaks in mite population (PI and PII, in the study called 'infestation peak') during the 54-week production cycle induced by mite treatment were recorded. The growth of the *D. gallinae* population was moderate until week 18. Subsequently, the growth rate increased. A two-fold increase in the number of adults, larvae + nymphs and eggs of *D. gallinae* was recorded in week 22 of the production cycle (592 adults, 194 larvae + nymphs and 357 eggs) compared to week 18. Mite treatment I (MTI) was performed, as a result of which the number of life stages of *D. gallinae* was reduced significantly (found: 56 adult forms, 16 larvae + nymphs and 10 eggs) in week 24 of the production cycle compared to week 22. The infestation remained at a low level for 2 weeks. Subsequently, it started to grow rapidly, starting with week 26. The reinfestation peak (PII) was observed in week 38 of the production cycle (found: 1034 adult forms, 268 larvae + nymphs and 191 eggs). The second mite treatment (MTII) was performed, which resulted in a statistically significant reduction in the number of individual life stages of *D. gallinae* in week 40 of the production cycle (found: 199 females, 124 larvae-nymphs and 1 egg). The effect persisted for the next 2 weeks. After that, the population started to regenerate, but statistically non-significant fluctuations of the numbers of individual life stages were observed. Adults in a number of 574, 282 larvae-nymphs and 251 eggs were observed in the 54th (final) week.

Each mite treatment procedure resulted in a reduction in the number of individual life stages for 2 weeks. After that time, the population re-grew, and the infestation development rate after the second mite treatment procedure was 2.4 times higher than the infestation development rate compared to MTI.

3.2. Changes in the Percentages of Lymphocytes Subpopulations

The percentages and changes in the populations of Th cells, Tc cells and B cells in laying hens infested with *D. gallinae* controlled with Biobeck PA 910 (AI silicon dioxide, Biologische Preparate, Brilon, Germany) are shown in Figure 2. The Th cells accounted for the highest portion of all the lymphocytes, followed by B cells and Tc cells in each assay (B1–4). There were 68.52% of Th cells of total lymphocytes at the infestation peak I (B1). The *D. gallinae* population decreased after Biobeck PA 910 (AI silicon dioxide, Biologische Preparate, Brilon, Germany) was applied (B2), and the percentage of the lymphocytes decreased non-significantly (61.25%), and the decrease was continued significantly at the infestation peak II (B3) (50.34%) compared to B1 ($p = 0.0002$) and B2 ($p = 0.018$). Subsequently, the percentage increased to 60.6% ($p = 0.028$) after another mite treatment compared to B3. The analysis of correlation revealed a non-significant negative correlation between mite number and B cells ($R = -0.845$, $p > 0.05$), a non-significant negative correlation between mite number and Th cells ($R = -0.522$, $p > 0.05$) and a significant positive correlation between mite number and Tc cells ($R = -0.982$, $p < 0.05$).

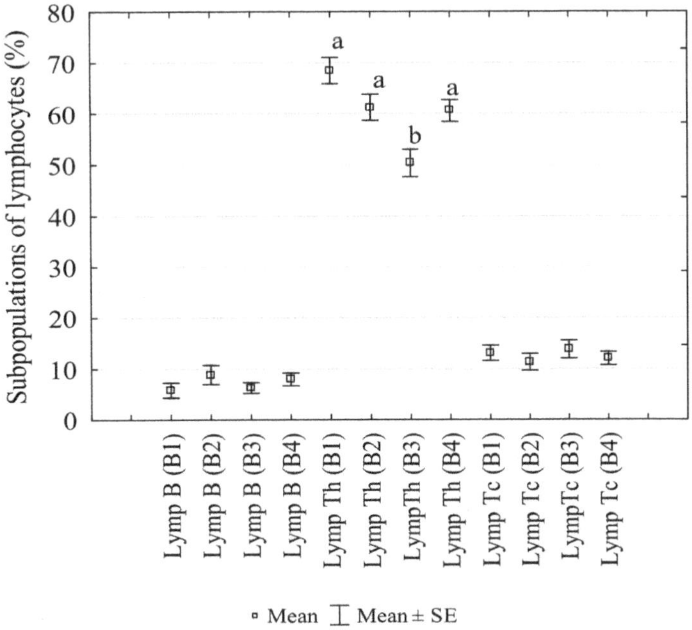

Figure 2. Changes in the percentages of B IgM+ cells (Lymp B), T CD3+CD4+ cells (Lymp Th) and T CD3+CD8a+ cells (Lymp Tc) in the peripheral blood of laying hens infested with *Dermanyssus gallinae*, controlled with Biobeck PA 910 (AI silicon dioxide, Biologische Preparate, Brilon, Germany). (B1–B4: blood sampling dates; a,b: different letters indicate statistical differences between groups).

3.3. The Changes in the Titres of Antibodies

The titres of antibodies against AE, IBV, NDV, REV, REO and ORT in laying hens infested with *D. gallinae*, controlled with Biobeck PA 910 (AI silicon dioxide, Biologische Preparate, Brilon, Germany), are shown in Figure 3. The study found a significant decrease in the titre of post-vaccination antibodies against IBV and NDV at the second infestation peak (B3) ($p = 0.014$ and $p = 0.001$, respectively). The titres of post-vaccination antibodies against AE did not change significantly during the study. However, a non-significant negative correlation was observed between mite numbers and AE titre ($R = -0.564$, $p > 0.05$). Antibodies against REO, REV and ORT were found despite the hens were not immunised earlier against those pathogens. The titres of antibodies against REO in subsequent weeks of the study were 7472, 8163, 2246, 1556. The titres of antibodies against REV were 121, 14, 19, 1. The titres of antibodies against ORT increased during the production cycle and were 402, 1904, 2921, 2150.

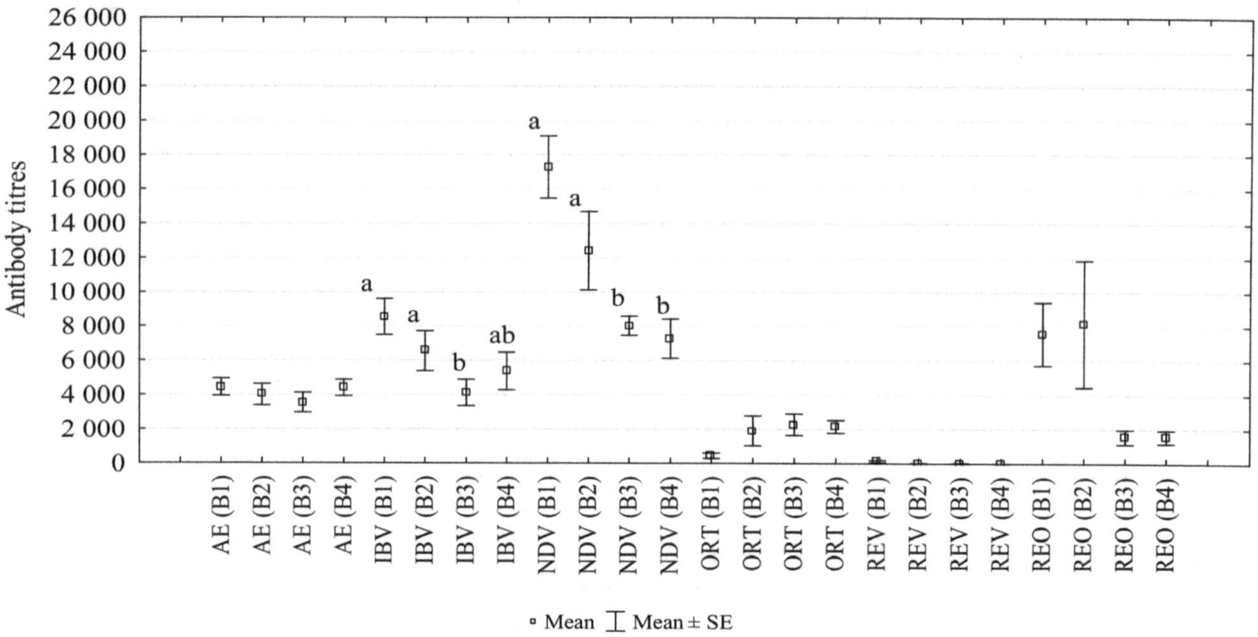

Figure 3. Changes in the titres of antibodies against AE (avian encephalomyelitis), IBV (infectious bronchitis virus), NDV (Newcastle disease virus), ORT (*Ornithobacterium rhinotracheale*), REV (reticuloendotheliosis virus) and REO (avian reovirus) in the peripheral blood of laying hens infested with *D. gallinae*, controlled with Biobeck. (B1–B4: blood sampling dates; a, ab, b: different letters indicate statistical differences between groups).

4. Discussion

This paper was the first report on the effect of *D. gallinae* infestation on a post-vaccination immune response in laying hens during the production cycle. Due to difficulties with access to the hen house free from the infestation of *D. gallinae*, we could not include a control group. Nevertheless, blood samples for cytometric and serological analyses were collected at the infestation peaks (on the day of mite treatment) and after the infestation subsided was recorded. Thus, we could observe the changes in the studied parameters under high and low mite pressure, which showed how *D. gallinae* might affect these parameters.

In the first infestation peak, no significant change in the percentages of B, Th or Tc cells or antibodies was observed. In the re-infestation of *D. gallinae* (infestation peak II), a significant decrease in the Th cells and IBV and NDV post-vaccination antibodies was observed.

Helper lymphocytes (Th) take part in the development of humoral response. They facilitate activation, proliferation and differentiation of B and Tc cells and have a CD4+ receptor on their surface. They also recognise antigens after they bind to class II of major histocompatibility complex (MHC) cells [28,29]. Our study showed a significant decrease in the percentage of these lymphocytes at the infestation peak II and a subsequent increase when the infestation subsided. These findings suggested that *D. gallinae* could inhibit the development of humoral immune response in infested laying hens.

Cytotoxic lymphocytes (Tc) play an important role in acquiring post-vaccine immunity. They are also called antigen-specific since they have a CD8+ receptor on their surface. A CD3+ receptor is present on the surface of most mature T cells and thymocytes. They are capable of destroying cells infected by a virus, cancer cells and of recognising proteins and glycoproteins (antigens) [28]. The percentage of these lymphocytes, as observed in this study, did not change significantly during the experiment. However, a strong positive correlation between mite numbers and those cells was reported. The percentage of these lymphocytes was seen to decrease during the periods of low *D. gallinae* infestation. These findings suggested that the parasite could stimulate the cellular immune response in infested laying hens, but the infestation was not sufficiently high to produce a significant effect.

B cells play a crucial role in the humoral immune response. They differentiate into memory cells and/or plasmatic cells, which produce antibodies specific to protein antigens in a complex process in which antigen-specific CD4+ helper cells take part [29,30]. Like Tc cells, the percentage of these lymphocytes, observed in this study, did not change significantly during the experiment. Only an increasing trend was observed for these lymphocytes during the period of low *D. gallinae* infestation. Despite the absence of statistical significance, these findings might suggest that *D. gallinae* could inhibit the post-vaccination humoral immune response. This was also testified to by a decrease in the post-vaccination antibody titre during the period of high *D. gallinae* infestation (Figure 3).

The titres of post-vaccination antibodies of AE, IBV, NDV changed during the cycle in a similar manner (Figure 3). They decreased with an increasing infestation (B1–B3), and their level increased after mite treatment (B4). A similar trend was observed in antibodies against REO, against which the hens were not immunised. On the other hand, antibodies against ORT showed an increasing trend in the B1–B3. The presence of antibodies against ORT in the blood of the hens under study, despite the absence of vaccination, indicated the occurrence of field infection. There was no correlation between mite numbers and antibody titres. Thus, there was insufficient evidence to support the hypothesis that *D. gallinae* has a negative effect on the production of post-vaccination antibodies in layer hens. Further study, including a larger sample size and negative control group, is required.

5. Conclusions

D. gallinae is currently considered to be the most bothersome ectoparasite in the commercial laying hen farms. Vaccines protect hens against pathogens, which is important from an economic perspective and consumer safety. Development of vaccine-induced immune responses might be affected by many factors. The role of *D. gallinae* as a potential immunosuppressor has been unknown. The present study was the first report in this area. The present findings suggested that *D. gallinae* might inhibit immune responses since the percentages of B cells and Th cells were negatively correlated with the number of mites. The percentage of Tc cells was positively correlated with the number of mites, which indicated that *D. gallinae* could stimulate cellular immune responses in infested laying hens. However, further research is needed to determine whether *D. gallinae* suppresses the production of vaccine-induced antibodies.

Author Contributions: Conceptualization, S.K.-S. and R.S.; methodology, S.K.-S. and R.S.; validation, R.S.; formal analysis, S.K.-S.; investigation, S.K.-S. and R.S.; resources, R.S.; data curation, R.S.; writing—original draft preparation, S.K.-S.; writing—review and editing, R.S.; visualization, S.K.-S.; supervision, R.S.; project administration, R.S.; funding acquisition, S.K.-S. and R.S. All authors have read and agreed to the published version of the manuscript.

Acknowledgments: Publication financially co-supported by the Minister of Science and Higher Education in the range of the program entitled "Regional Initiative of Excellence" for the years 2019–2022, Project No. 010/RID/2018/19, amount of funding PLN 12,000,000 PLN.

Abbreviations

AE	avian encephalomyelitis
ANOVA	analysis of variance
B1–B4	blood collection dates correspond to the assay groups
BCR	B-cell receptor
CD	cluster of differentiation
CV%	coefficient of variation
D. gallinae	Dermanyssus gallinae

FCS	fetal calf serum
IBV	infectious bronchitis virus
IGM	immunoglobulin M
Lymp Tc	lymphocytes T cells CD3+/CD8a+ (Tc)
Lymp B	lymphocytes B IgM+ cells
Lymp Th	lymphocytes T cells CD3+/CD4+ (Th)
MANOVA	multivariate analysis of variance
MHC	major histocompatibility complex
MTI-II	mite tratment dates
NDV	Newcastle disease virus
ORT	Ornithobacterium rhinotracheale
PBS	phosphate-buffered saline
PI-II	the peak in the mite population, in this study, referred to as infestation peak
prm	poultry red mite
REO	avian reovirus
REV	reticuloendotheliosis virus
RH	relative humidity
SE	standard error

References

1. Wood, H.P. The chicken mite: Its life history and habits. *US Dep. Agric.* **1917**, *553*, 1–14.
2. Chmielewski, W. Roztocze zamieszkujące gniazda wróbla domowego (Passer domesticus L). *Wiad Parazytol.* **1982**, *28*, 5–107.
3. Romaniuk, K.; Owczarzak-Podziemska, I. Występowanie saprobiontycznych i pasożytniczych roztoczy w ściółce ferm indyków. *Med. Weter.* **2002**, *58*, 298–299.
4. Roy, L.; Chauve, C. Historical review of the genus *Dermanyssus* Duges, 1834 (Acari: Mesostigmata: Dermanyssidae). *Parasite* **2007**, *14*, 87–100. [CrossRef]
5. Hoglund, J.; Nordenfors, H.; Uggla, A. Prevalence of the poultry red mite, *Dermanyssus gallinae*, in different types of production systems for egg layers in Sweden. *Poult. Sci.* **1995**, *74*, 1793–1798. [CrossRef] [PubMed]
6. Fiddes, M.D.; Le Gresley, S.; Parsons, D.G.; Epe, C.; Coles, G.C.; Stafford, K.A. Prevalence of the poultry red mite (*Dermanyssus gallinae*) in England. *Vet. Rec.* **2005**, *157*, 233–235. [CrossRef]
7. Van Emous, R.A. Wage war against the red mite! *Poult. Int.* **2005**, *44*, 26–33.
8. Sparagano, O.A.E.; Pavlicevic, A.; Murano, T.; Camarda, A.; Sahibi, H.; Kilpinen, O.; Mul, M.; Van Emous, R.A.; Le Bouguin, S.; Hoel, K.; et al. Prevalence and key figures for the poultry red mite *Dermanyssus gallinae* infections in poultry farm systems. *Exp. Appl. Acarol.* **2009**, *48*, 3–10. [CrossRef]
9. Sparagano, O.A.E.; George, D.R.; Harrington, D.W.; Giangaspero, A. Significance and control of the poultry red mite, *Dermanyssus gallinae*. *Ann. Rev. Entomol.* **2014**, *59*, 447–466. [CrossRef]
10. Chauve, C. The poultry red mite *Dermanyssus gallinae* (Dr Geer, 1778): Current situation and future prospects for control. *Vet. Parasitol.* **1998**, *79*, 239–245. [CrossRef]
11. Maurer, V.; Baumgartner, J. Temperature influence on life table statistics of the chicken mite *Dermanyssus gallinae* (Acari: Dermanyssidae). *Exp. Appl. Acarol.* **1992**, *15*, 27–40. [CrossRef] [PubMed]
12. Moss, W.W. The mite genus *Dermanyssus*: A survey, with description of *Dermanyssus trochilinis*, n. sp., and a revised key to the species (Acari: Mesostigmata: Dermanyssidae). *J. Med. Entomol.* **1978**, *14*, 627–640. [CrossRef]
13. Entrekin, D.L.; Oliver, J.H., Jr. Aggregation of the chicken mite, *Dermanyssus gallinae* (Acari: Dermanyssidae). *J. Med. Entomol.* **1982**, *1*, 671–678. [CrossRef] [PubMed]
14. Koenraadt, C.J.M.; Dicke, M. The role of volatiles in aggregation and host-seeking of the haematophagous poultry red mite *Dermanyssus gallinae* (Acari: Dermanyssidae). *Exp. Appl. Acarol.* **2010**, *50*, 191–199. [CrossRef]
15. Roy, L.; Chauve, C.; Buronfosse, T. Contrasted ecological repartition of the northern fowl mite *Ornithonyssus sylviarum* (Mesostigmata: Macronyssidae) and the chicken red mite *Dermanyssus gallinae* (Mesostigmata: Dermanyssidae). *Acarologia* **2010**, *50*, 207–219. [CrossRef]

16. Abdel-Ghaffar, F.; Semmler, M.; Al-Rasheid, K.; Mehlhorn, H. In vitro efficacy of ByeMite® and Mite-Stop® on developmental stages of the red chicken mite *Dermanyssus gallinae*. *Parasitol. Res.* **2009**, *105*, 1469–1471. [CrossRef]
17. Beugnet, F.; Chauve, C.; Gauthey, M.; Beert, L. Resistance of the red poultry mite to pyrethroids in France. *Vet. Rec.* **1997**, *140*, 577–579. [CrossRef]
18. Mul, M.; Van Niekerk, T.; Chirico, J.; Maurer, V.; Kilpinen, O.; Sparagano, O.A.E.; Thind, B.; Zoons, J.; Moore, D.; Bell, B.; et al. Control methods for *Dermanyssus gallinae* in systems for laying hens: Results of an international seminar. *Worlds Poult. Sci. J.* **2009**, *65*, 589–599. [CrossRef]
19. Chirico, J.; Tauson, R. Traps containing acaricides for the control of *Dermanyssus gallinae*. *Vet. Parasitol.* **2002**, *110*, 109–116. [CrossRef]
20. Cosoroaba, I. Massive *Dermanyssus gallinae* invasion in battery-husbandry raised fowls. *Rev. Med. Vet.* **2001**, *152*, 89–96.
21. Cencek, T. Prevalence of *Dermanyssus gallinae* in poultry farms in Silesia Region in Poland. *Bull. Vet. Inst. Pulawy.* **2003**, *47*, 465–469.
22. Arkle, S.; Guy, J.H.; Sparagano, O.A.E. Immunological effects and productivity variation of red mite (*Dermanyssus gallinae*) on laying hens—Implications for egg production and quality. *Worlds Poul. Sci. J.* **2006**, *62*, 249–257. [CrossRef]
23. Harrington, D.W.; Robinson, K.; Guy, J.; Sparagano, O.A.E. Characterization of the immunological response to *Dermanyssus gallinae* infestation in domestic fowl. *Transbound. Emerg. Diss.* **2010**, *57*, 107–110. [CrossRef] [PubMed]
24. Harrington, D.W.; Robinson, K.; Sparagano, O.A.E. Immune responses of the domestic fowl to *Dermanyssus gallinae* under laboratory conditions. *Parasitol. Res.* **2010**, *106*, 1425–1434. [CrossRef]
25. Kowalski, A.; Sokół, R. Influence of *Dermanyssus gallinae* (poultry red mite) invasion on the plasma levels of corticosterone, catecholamines and proteins in layer hens. *Pol. J. Vet. Sci.* **2009**, *12*, 231–235.
26. Sokół, R.; Koziatek-Sadłowska, S.; Michalczyk, M. The influence of *Dermanyssus gallinae* and different lighting regimens on selected blood proteins, corticosterone levels and egg production in layer hens. *Vet. Res. Commun.* **2019**, *43*, 31–36. [CrossRef]
27. Sokół, R.; Romaniuk, K. Przebieg i dynamika inwazji *Dermanyssus gallinae* w fermie kur niosek. *Med. Weter* **2007**, *63*, 484–486.
28. Arstila, T.P.; Vainio, O.; Lassila, O. Central role of CD4+ T cells in avian immune response. *Poult. Sci.* **1994**, *73*, 1019–1026. [CrossRef]
29. Chen, X.; Jensen, P.E. The role of B lymphocytes as antigen-presenting cells. *Arch. Immunol. Ther. Exp.* **2008**, *56*, 77–83. [CrossRef]
30. Parker, D.C. T cell-dependent B cell activation. *Ann. Rev. Immunol.* **1993**, *11*, 331–360. [CrossRef]

11

Ancylostoma ceylanicum: The Neglected Zoonotic Parasite of Community Dogs in Thailand and its Genetic Diversity among Asian Countries

Doolyawat Kladkempetch [1], Sahatchai Tangtrongsup [2,3] and Saruda Tiwananthagorn [4,5,*]

1 Master's Degree Program in Veterinary Science, Faculty of Veterinary Medicine, Chiang Mai University, Chiang Mai 50100, Thailand; doolyawat_kl@cmu.ac.th
2 Department of Companion Animal and Wildlife Clinic, Faculty of Veterinary Medicine, Chiang Mai University, Chiang Mai 50100, Thailand; sahatchai.t@cmu.ac.th
3 Research Center of Producing and Development of Products and Innovations for Animal Health and Production, Faculty of Veterinary Medicine, Chiang Mai University, Chiang Mai 50100, Thailand
4 Department of Veterinary Biosciences and Veterinary Public Health, Faculty of Veterinary Medicine, Chiang Mai University, Chiang Mai 50100, Thailand
5 Excellent Center in Veterinary Bioscience, Faculty of Veterinary Medicine, Chiang Mai University, Chiang Mai 50100, Thailand
* Correspondence: saruda.t@cmu.ac.th.

Simple Summary: Ancylostomiasis is a zoonotic disease caused by the *Ancylostoma* hookworm infection of dogs, cats, and other wildlife species and is frequently found in Asia and tropical regions. The present study had confirmed the species of hookworm in dogs and soil environments collected from temple communities. In addition, we investigated the association of hookworm-contaminated soil in temple areas to increase awareness and establish a regimen to prevent zoonotic hookworm transmission. Lastly, we analyzed the genetic diversity and evolution of hookworm in dogs and soil environments among Thai *A. ceylanicum* and other Asian populations and disclosed insight into their fundamental genetic relationship.

Abstract: *Ancylostoma ceylanicum* is a zoonotic helminth that is commonly found in domestic dogs and cats throughout Asia but is largely neglected in many countries. This study aimed to confirm the species of hookworm in dogs and soil environments and investigate the evolutionary analyses of *A. ceylanicum* among Thai and Asian populations. In a total of 299 dog fecal samples and 212 soil samples from 53 temples, the prevalence rates of hookworm infection by microscopic examination were 26.4% (79/299) and 10.4% (22/212) in dog and soil samples, respectively. A PCR-RFLP targeting the ITS region was then utilized to identify the hookworm species. In dogs, *A. ceylanicum* was the main hookworm species, and the rates of *A. ceylanicum* and *A. caninum* infections were 96.6% and 3.5%, respectively. The genetic characterization and diversity indices of the *A. ceylanicum cox1* gene among Thai and Asian populations were evaluated. Nine haplotypes were identified from Thai *A. ceylanicum*, in which the haplotype diversity and the nucleotide diversity were 0.4436 and 0.0036, respectively. The highest nucleotide diversity of Chinese *A. ceylanicum* populations suggested that it could be the ancestor of the populations. Pairwise fixation indices indicated that Thai *A. ceylanicum* was closely related to the Malaysian population, suggesting a gene flow between these populations. The temples with hookworm-positive dogs were associated with the presence of hookworm-contaminated soil, as these levels showed an approximately four-fold increase compared with those in temples with hookworm-negative dogs (OR = 4.38, 95% CI: 1.55–12.37). Interestingly, the genotypes of *A. ceylanicum* in the contaminating soil and infecting dogs were identical. Therefore, increased awareness and concern from the wider public communities with regard to the responsibility of temples and municipal offices to provide proper deworming programs to community dogs should be strongly endorsed to reduce the risk of the transmission of this zoonotic disease. In addition, parasitic examination and treatment should be strongly implemented before dogs are imported and exported worldwide.

Keywords: *Ancylostoma ceylanicum*; community dogs; ITS region; *cox1*; Thailand; population diversity

---

1. Introduction

Hookworms are soil-transmitted gastrointestinal nematodes of the Ancylostomatidae family that infect dogs, cats, and humans. These nematodes are endemic in tropical and subtropical regions of the world, including parts of China, Southeast Asia, Australia, and Africa [1–4]. Hookworms can infect the host by the fecal-oral route and through the skin penetration of the third-stage larvae [2]. Hookworm infection causes intestinal blood loss, anemia, malnutrition, and dermatitis [5]. Common species of hookworm infection in dogs include *Ancylostoma caninum*, *A. ceylanicum*, *A. braziliense*, and *Uncinaria stenocephala*, while *A. braziliense*, *A. tubaeforme*, *A. ceylanicum*, and *U. stenocephala* are commonly found in cats [6,7]. Recent studies have shown that ancylostomiasis in humans results from *Necator americanus*, *A. duodenale*, and *A. ceylanicum* [5,8,9]. Among *Ancylostoma* species, *A. ceylanicum* is the only species of animal hookworms known to produce patent infections in humans and is an important cause of zoonotic ancylostomiasis in Asia and Southeast Asia [9–14].

In general, the epidemiological study revealed that animal-derived *Ancylostoma* species are emerging due to human and animal interaction [15,16]. In Thailand, free-roaming community dogs have been widespread and come in close contact with people in some areas, such as temples and rural communities. The presence of hookworm larvae in soil reported by George et al. [5] confirmed that humans and dogs are at risk of infection from hookworm-contaminated soil. Additionally, a previous report in Malaysia from Ngui et al. [15] indicated that people who are not wearing shoes are at risk of hookworm infection from hookworm-contaminated soil. The opportunity for exposure to hookworm is high in children, farmers, and especially Buddhist monks, who do not wear shoes based on their practices and Buddhist tradition in Thai temples. Information regarding whether the soil in the area is contaminated with hookworm is, therefore, important for public health to promote awareness and establish a regimen to prevent zoonotic hookworm transmission.

The conventional method for hookworm diagnosis is coprological examination. However, this method cannot differentiate hookworm species due to the similar egg size and morphology. Morphological identification of adult hookworms is achievable, but the process is time-consuming and labor-intensive and requires personal skill [16]. Alternatively, molecular techniques have been developed for the identification of hookworms at the species level, such as polymerase chain reaction (PCR) assays and PCR with restriction fragment length polymorphism (PCR-RFLP) assays targeting the internal transcribed spacer (ITS) region [16]. The ITS region is a conserved region with a low mutation rate and has no intraspecific variation [17]. Thus, the ITS region is suitable as a genetic marker for hookworm species identification [18]. Recently, the cytochrome *c* oxidase subunit 1 (*cox1*) gene has been utilized to evaluate the evolution and relationship of hookworm species among the population [19,20], given its high intraspecific sequence variation from maternal inheritance and high evolutionary rates [21].

In Northern Thailand, a few reports have assessed the prevalence of hookworm infection in humans, domestic dogs, and cats. By microscopic examination, hookworm infection rates of approximately 21.3% in dogs and 13.9% in cats [22] and 12% in dogs and 4.5% in cats [23] have been reported in the lower northern region and in the Chiang Mai province of the upper northern region, respectively. The prevalence of hookworm infection in humans ranged from 0.6% to 13.4% [24,25]. However, the species of hookworm in Upper Northern Thailand have never been clarified. The present study, therefore, aimed to identify the species of hookworm in dogs and investigate the presence of hookworm contamination in the soil environment of community temples where there are high risks of communicable pathogen transmission. Furthermore, the genetic characteristics of *Ancylostoma* hookworm and the evolutionary genetic relationships among the Thai hookworm and the populations of neighboring Asian countries have been elucidated.

2. Materials and Methods

2.1. Study Area and Sample Size

The study area is located in the upper northern region of Thailand. Four provinces, including Chiang Mai (18°47′26″ N, 98°59′14″ E), Chiang Rai (20°01′05″ N, 99°40′22″ E), Lampang (18°17′21″ N, 99°29′26″ E), and Phayao (19°11′30″ N, 99°52′47″ E), were chosen and considered as high dog population density provinces (Figure 1). Sampling sites were 53 community temples that were chosen based on convenience and distribution from at least 3 districts in each province. The inclusion criteria for temple selection were (i) a human population density of more than 30 persons per sq. km. [26,27], (ii) no regular deworming program in dogs within 3 months, and (iii) ease of access and sample transportation to the laboratory. The sample size of 299 dog fecal samples for the detection of hookworm infection was calculated using the Win episcope 2.0 program [28] based on an estimated hookworm prevalence of 12.8% in dogs [29] and an error rate of 5% with a 95% level of confidence. The stratified sampling method was used to generate the number of samples per province based on dog population data [30].

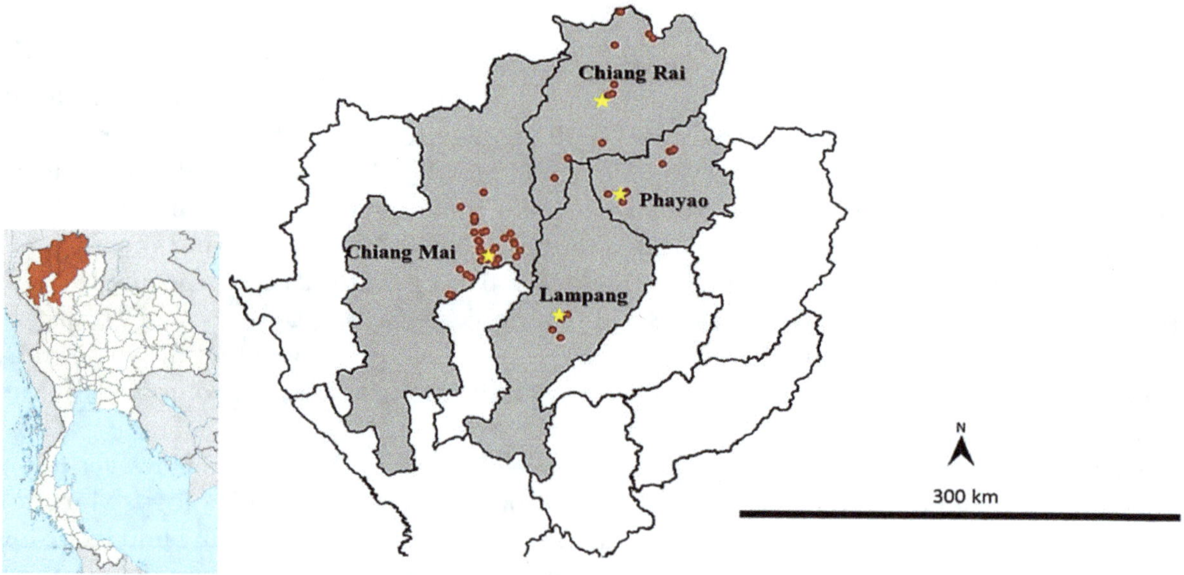

Figure 1. Map of the study areas in Thailand. The gray color indicates four study provinces, red dots indicate the location of sampling sites (temples), and stars indicate the capital city of each province.

All the owners signed an informed consent form, and the animal use was approved by the Ethics Committee of the Laboratory Animal Center, Faculty of Veterinary Medicine, Chiang Mai University (S41/2561), on 18 January 2019.

2.2. Sample Collection and Examination

2.2.1. Fecal and Soil Sample Collection

Samples were collected between June and September 2019. Two hundred and ninety-nine fecal samples were collected from the rectum of dogs or fresh fecal samples found on the ground. All the collected fresh feces were normal in appearance (medium to dark brown in color, soft to firm in texture) based on the WALTHAM fecal scoring system [31]. The dog ID, date of collection, temple name, district, province, cleaning housing program, and type of food were recorded. Soil environment samples were collected at the temple in the morning (08:00–10:00). For soil sample collection, the sites of sample collection were defined by 4 areas in each temple: (i) temple courtyard, (ii) dog dwelling area, (iii) human activity area (such as sand pagoda), and (iv) under the big tree. In the collection site that was not dirt ground, the soil sample for that site was obtained from the adjacent ground within a 2 m radius of the area. Soil samples were collected from moist areas within the selected sampling sites, and approximately 50 g (wet weight) was obtained by scraping the surface layer to gather a 0.09 square meter area using a metal spade. The soil samples were kept separately in a sealed plastic bag.

All the samples were stored on ice and transported to the Parasitology Laboratory, Faculty of Veterinary Medicine, Chiang Mai University. Samples were refrigerated at 4 °C upon arrival.

2.2.2. Microscopic Examinations of Fecal and Soil Samples

Fresh fecal samples were examined under a light microscope after simple floatation using zinc sulfate solution (specific gravity: 1.18) for the presence of eggs. The remainder of the fecal sample was stored at −20 °C until further molecular analysis. The Baermann technique was used to determine the presence of hookworm-like larvae in the soil samples [32]. Twenty grams of soil samples were primarily filtered through a tea strainer to remove any debris and then subjected to another filtration step using 2 sieve filters with pore sizes of 0.4 and 0.2 mm. The filtrated soil sample was cultured individually using tap water. Hookworm-like larvae containing sediments were stored at −20 °C until further molecular analysis could be carried out.

2.3. DNA Extraction

Genomic DNA (gDNA) samples from hookworm-positive samples were extracted using the NucleoSpin® DNA stool kit (Macherey-Nagel GmbH, Düren, Germany) according to the manufacturer's instructions. In the elution step, gDNA samples were eluted with 100 μL of elution buffer. The extracted DNA concentration and quality were determined using a spectrophotometer (Beckman Coulter DU® 730 Life Sciences, Pasadena, CA, USA) at wavelengths of 260 and 280 nm. All the gDNA samples were kept at −20 °C until the next step.

2.4. Molecular Analyses

2.4.1. Identification of Hookworm Species Using a Polymerase Chain Reaction-Restriction Fragment Length Polymorphism (PCR-RFLP) Assay Based on ITS Region

The PCR-RFLP assay, which was established by Traub et al. [16], was conducted to identify the species of hookworm in the positive dog fecal and soil samples. A forward primer RTGHF1 (5′-CGTGCTAGTCTTCAGGACTTTG-3′) and a reverse primer RTABCR1 (5′-CGGGAATTGCTATAAGCAAGTGC-3′) were used to amplify the 545-bp region of the internal transcribed spacer (ITS1, 5.8S, and ITS2). PCR amplification reactions were performed in a 25 μL reaction volume containing 10 ng of template gDNA (2–4 μL), 0.2 μM of each primer (0.5 μL of 10 μM), and 12.5 μL of 2× PCR Master Mix (KOD One™ PCR Mastermix; Toyobo, Japan). The thermocycling conditions were as follows: initial denaturation at 94 °C for 2 min, 45 cycles of amplification (94 °C for 30 s, 62 °C for 30 s, and 72 °C for 30 s), and a final extension at 72 °C for 5 min. The reaction was performed on a T100™ Thermal Cycler (Bio-Rad, Hercules, CA, USA). The amplified PCR products were digested with Hinf1 to differentiate *A. caninum* from *A. ceylanicum* and *U. stenocephala*. The digestions were performed at 37 °C for 16 h, using 1 unit of restriction enzyme and 1 μg of DNA (3–5 μL of PCR product) in a total reaction volume of 20 μL. The PCR products were analyzed using 2% agarose gels electrophoresis. Distilled water (DW) and the gDNA of *A. caninum* and *A. ceylanicum* were used as a negative and positive control, respectively.

2.4.2. PCR Assay and Nucleotide Analysis Based on *A. ceylanicum* and *A. caninum cox1* Gene

The mitochondrial *cox1* gene served as the target to assess the genetic characteristics and evolutionary analysis. The previously identified *A. ceylanicum*- and *A. caninum*-positive samples were successively subjected to PCR for the *cox1* gene using a set of primers described by Inpankaew et al. [33], including the forward primer AceyCOX1F (5′-GCTTTTGGTATTGTAAGACAG-3′) and the reverse primer AceyCOX1R (5′-CTAACAACATAATAAGTATCATG-3′), amplifying a 377-bp amplicon. The reactions were performed in a 50 μL reaction mixture volume, containing 10 ng of template gDNA (2–4 μL), 0.2 μM of each primer (1 μL of 10 μM), and 25 μL of 2× PCR Master Mix (KOD One™ PCR Mastermix; Toyobo, Japan). The PCR conditions were set as follows: initial denaturation at 94 °C for 2 min, 45 cycles of amplification (94 °C for 30 s, 55 °C for 30 s, and 68 °C for 45 s), and a final extension at 72 °C for 5 min. The reaction was performed using a T100™ Thermal Cycler (Bio-Rad, Hercules, CA, USA). The DW and gDNA of *A. caninum* and *A. ceylanicum* were used as negative and positive controls, respectively. The PCR products were purified using a NucleoSpin® PCR Clean-up Kit (Macherey-Nagel GmbH, Düren, Germany). Purified PCR products were submitted for fluorescent dye-terminator sequencing by Bio Basic, Inc. (Singapore, Singapore) in the sense and antisense directions using the PCR primer set described above. For nucleotide analysis, the *cox1* amplicons of 32 samples (29 *A. ceylanicum* samples from dogs, 2 *A. ceylanicum* samples from soil, and 1 *A. caninum* sample from dog) were selected based on the geographic distribution, covering all positive provinces.

2.5. Data Analyses

2.5.1. Prevalence of Hookworm Infection/Contamination

Positive fecal samples from the zinc sulfate flotation technique and positive soil samples from the Baermann technique were considered as positive for hookworm detection. The prevalence of hookworm infection in dogs and contamination in soil samples were estimated using the formula prevalence = (number of positives samples divided by the number of samples in dogs/soil examined) × 100. The association between hookworm-positive results and sampling areas was assessed using Fisher's exact test. The significance was defined as $p < 0.05$.

2.5.2. Phylogenetic Analysis

The *cox1* sequences were edited and manually aligned. The consensus sequences were generated using the BioEdit Sequence Alignment Editor [34] and then compared with the nucleotide sequences from GenBank using a Basic Local Alignment Search Tool (BLAST) analysis. Phylogenetic analysis was performed using MEGA X [35]. Multiple sequences were aligned using ClustalW (https://www.genome.jp/tools-bin/clustalw), and phylogenetic analysis was performed using a maximum likelihood (ML) method based on the Kimura 2-Parameter model. The consensus tree was obtained after a 1000-replication bootstrap analysis. The *cox1* sequences of *A. ceylanicum* from other areas of Thailand and other countries, including Malaysia, Cambodia, China, Japan, Papua New Guinea, Australia, and Tanzania, and *A. caninum* from Australia (NC012309) were used as reference sequences for tree construction (Table S1). In addition, the sequence of *A. duodenale* from China (accession number: NC003415) was used as an outgroup species.

2.5.3. Population Genetic Analysis

The DnaSP 6 program [36] was used for the haplotype analysis and calculations to determine the haplotype diversity (Hd), nucleotide diversity (π), and the number of variable sites (S). The gene flow among populations was analyzed by fixation index (F_{ST}) statistics using the Arlequin program Version 3.5 [37]. The gene flow of *A. ceylanicum* was analyzed using the reference sequences from Asian countries, including Thailand, China, Malaysia, and Cambodia (Table S2). The Network program [38] was used to generate a median-joining (MJ) network of *cox1* haplotypes and reference haplotypes and was subsequently drawn manually. The references haplotype and their frequency obtained from the NCBI database (https://www.ncbi.nlm.nih.gov/genbank/) are described above.

3. Results

3.1. Prevalence and Distribution of Hookworm Infection

A total of 299 fecal samples and 212 soil samples from 53 temples were examined microscopically, and the hookworm species were identified by PCR-RFLP targeting the ITS region. The prevalence rate of hookworm in dogs was 26.4% (79/299), as assessed by microscopic examination. PCR-RFLP successfully identified the species of hookworm in 58 samples, and the rates of *A. ceylanicum* and *A. caninum* infection were 96.55% (56/58) and 3.45% (2/58), respectively (Figure 1). On the other hand, the prevalence of hookworm-like larvae in soil was 10.38% (22/212), as assessed by microscopic examination (Table 1). However, PCR-RFLP only identified the species in 8 of 22 samples, and all the samples were identified as *A. ceylanicum* (Table 1).

Table 1. Summary of hookworm infection in dog fecal samples and soil samples in Thailand, as demonstrated by the microscopic results and subsequent PCR-RFLP targeting the ITS region.

Province	Fecal Samples									Soil Samples								
	Positive Microscopic			N_2	*A. ceylanicum*		*A. caninum*		n/a	Positive Microscopic			N_4	*A. ceylanicum*		*A. caninum*		n/a
	N_1	*n*	%		*n*	%	*n*	%	*n*	N_3	*n*	%		*n*	%	*n*	%	*n*
Chiang Mai	159	57	35.85 [a]	42	40	95.24	2	4.76	15	120	16	13.33	3	3	100	0	0	13
Chiang Rai	70	6	8.57 [b]	5	5	100	0	0	1	48	1	2.08	1	1	100	0	0	0
Lampang	20	9	45.00 [a]	5	5	100	0	0	4	16	3	18.75	2	2	100	0	0	1
Phayao	50	7	14.00 [b]	6	6	100	0	0	1	28	2	7.14	2	2	100	0	0	0
Total	299	79	26.42	58	56	96.55	2	3.45	21	212	22	10.38	8	8	100	0	0	14

N_1: total number of examined dog fecal samples assessed by microscopic examination; N_2: number of positive dog samples successfully assessed with PCR-RFLP; N_3: total number of examined soil samples by microscopic examination; N_4: number of positive soil samples successfully assessed with PCR-RFLP; n/a: species unidentified samples; superscripts (a,b) indicate test results of Chi-square on prevalence among four provinces (any measurements with shared superscript letters are not significantly different from each other at $p < 0.05$).

Considering the population, the temple-level prevalence of positive dogs and positive soils was 47.17% (25/53) and 26.42% (14/53), respectively (Table S3). A total of 10 temples were positive for hookworm both in dog and soil samples (Table S3). Although not statistically significant, the hookworm-positive results in dogs were speculated to be associated with the hookworm-positive results in the soil ($p = 0.06$). Regarding the different areas in each temple, we found that the soil from dog-dwelling areas had the highest rates of hookworm contamination (15.09%, 8/53), followed by the soil from human activity areas, such as sand pagoda (11.32%; 6/53); the areas under big trees (9.43%; 5/53); and the temple courtyard (5.66%, 3/53) (Table S4). However, the frequency of hookworm-contaminated soil in each sampling site in the temple exhibited no significant differences ($p > 0.05$; Fisher's exact).

3.2. Hookworm Species Confirmation and Genetic Characteristics of the *A. ceylanicum* Mitochondrial *cox1* Gene

The nucleotide BLAST of partial *cox1* sequences (315 bp) of 31 *A. ceylanicum* sequences exhibited a high identity (98.07–100%) with Thai *A. ceylanicum* (GenBank accession no. KF896595). An *A. caninum* sequence from a dog exhibited a 96.71% identity with *A. caninum* from Australia (GenBank accession no. AJ407962). The obtained *A. ceylanicum cox1* gene sequences from dog and soil isolates were classified into nine haplotypes, which were referred to as Acy-COX1-TH01 to Acy-COX1-TH09. The sequences of *A. ceylanicum* of dogs and soil were deposited in GenBank (DDBJ/EMBL/GenBank database accession no. LC533318-LC533327). The sequence of *A. caninum* was deposited as LC533328 (Table S5).

Genetic variation among nine haplotypes of Thai *A. ceylanicum*, as assessed by multiple alignment analysis, revealed 12 different variable sites, including 2 transversions and 10 transitions (Table 2).

Table 2. Multiple alignment of the partial *cox1* from 9 haplotypes of *A. ceylanicum* in this study.

Haplotype Name	Nucleotide Position on the *A. ceylanicum cox1* Gene											
	48	72	87	88	90	105	147	150	198	199	219	264
Acy-COX1-TH01	A	C	A	G	A	A	G	A	G	G	A	G
Acy-COX1-TH02	G	.	.	.	.	.	A	.	.	.	.	.
Acy-COX1-TH03	.	T	.	.	.	.	.	.	.	.	.	.
Acy-COX1-TH04	.	.	.	.	.	G	.	.	A	A	.	.
Acy-COX1-TH05	.	.	.	C	.	.	.	.	.	.	.	.
Acy-COX1-TH06	.	T	G	.	G	.	A	.	.	.	G	A
Acy-COX1-TH07	.	.	.	.	.	.	.	T	.	.	.	.
Acy-COX1-TH08	.	.	G	.	.	.	.	.	.	.	.	.
Acy-COX1-TH09	G	.	.	.	.	.	.	.	.	.	.	.

Dots indicated the matching of nucleotide position the *A. ceylanicum* sequence.

The distribution and frequencies of *A. ceylanicum* haplotypes in Upper Northern Thailand were analyzed and revealed that the Acy-COX1-TH01 haplotype was detected at the highest frequency at 74.2% (23/31 sequences). This haplotype was commonly observed in all four provinces and found in both fecal and soil samples. As displayed in Figure 2, the sequence of two soil isolates (Acy-COX1-TH01-soil) was close to Acy-COX1-TH01-dog. Six haplotypes are present in Chiang Mai (Acy-COX1-TH01 to TH06), 3 haplotypes are present in Lampang (Acy-COX1-TH01, TH08, and TH09), whereas only one or two haplotypes were observed in Chiang Rai (Acy-COX1-TH01 and TH07) and Phayao (Acy-COX1-TH01) provinces (Table S5). Regarding the relationship among the human and animal isolates, Thai Acy-COX1-TH01 was close to the sequences of *A. ceylanicum* from Malaysian people (MK792828), dog (MK792824), and cat (MK792825) that belong to the same haplotype MA02 (Figure 2 and Table S1). Similarly, Acy-COX1-TH03 was close to the sequences of *A. ceylanicum* from human (KC247737) and dog (KC247734) that belong to the haplotype Malaysian MA01. Regarding the relationship between *A. ceylanicum* and geographic distribution, a phylogenetic tree demonstrated that *A. ceylanicum* from Thailand and all reference countries, including Malaysia, Cambodia, China, Japan, Papua New Guinea, and one country from the African continent (Tanzania), were located in the same clade, with the exception of one human sequence in Australia (AJ407937) (Figure 2).

3.3. Population Analyses of the A. ceylanicum Mitochondrial cox1 Gene among Asian Countries

The haplotype network displayed a star-like pattern and exhibited a wide dispersal around the predominant haplotype Acy-COX1-TH01 (in this study). This haplotype was identical to haplotypes MA02 from Malaysia, CA01 from Cambodia, and CH01 haplotype from China (Figure 3). The second most abundant haplotype was Acy-COX1-TH03, which was placed in the same group as haplotype MA01 from Malaysia and haplotype CA03 from Cambodia. Acy-COX1-TH06 was the most distinct haplotype, which includes four nucleotide-substitutions and was delineated from the haplotype CA02 from Cambodia.

The genetic diversity of the Thai *A. ceylanicum* population has been analyzed and compared pairwise to the populations of Cambodia, Malaysia, and China. The Thai *A. ceylanicum cox1* population (32 sequences; 31 from this study and 1 sequence from Inpankaew et al. [33]) displayed the lowest genetic diversity—i.e., a haplotype diversity (Hd) of 0.4435 and a nucleotide diversity (π) of 0.0036 (Table 3).

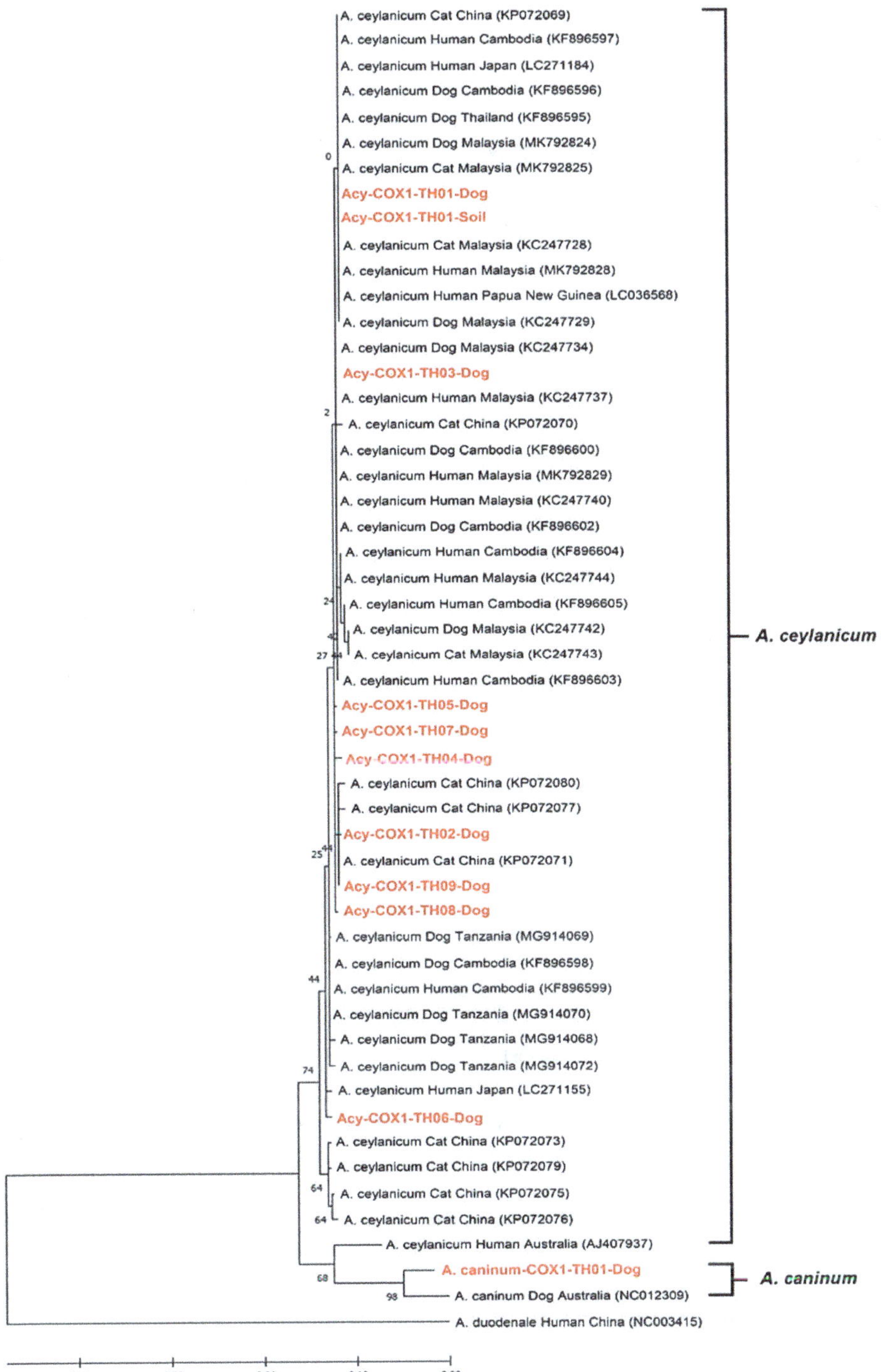

Figure 2. The evolutionary relationship of *A. ceylanicum* and *A. caninum* isolates from dogs and soil based on the 259-bp fragments of the mitochondrial cytochrome *c* oxidase subunit 1 (*cox1*) gene. The tree was constructed using a maximum likelihood method based on the Kimura 2-Parameter using the MEGA X software version 10.0.5. The number in each branch indicates the percentage of 1000 bootstrap replications. Sequences obtained from GenBank are indicated by their accession numbers.

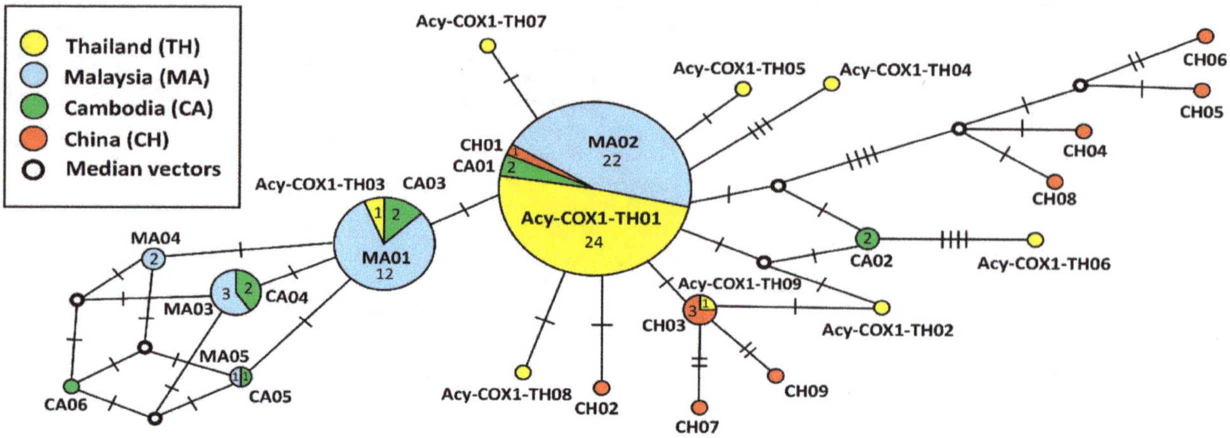

Figure 3. The haplotype network map of *A. ceylanicum* based on a fragment of the *cox1* gene from Thailand, Cambodia, China, and Malaysia. Circle size is scaled to frequencies of each haplotype. The hash marks indicate nucleotide substitutions among adjacent haplotypes.

Table 3. Summary of the genetic diversity of the 4 populations of *A. ceylanicum* based on the nucleotide sequences of the partial mitochondrial *cox1* gene.

Populations	N	Diversity			
		S	h	Hd ± SD	π ± SD
Thailand	32	11	9	0.4435 ± 0.1105	0.0036 ± 0.0028
Cambodia	10	6	6	0.9111 ± 0.0620	0.0088 ± 0.0059
Malaysia	40	4	5	0.6141 ± 0.0593	0.0043 ± 0.0006
China	12	17	9	0.9394 ± 0.0577	0.0201 ± 0.0118

N: numbers of *A. ceylanicum* sequences used; S: numbers of variable sites; h: numbers of haplotypes; Hd: haplotype diversity; SD: standard deviation; π: nucleotide diversity.

The highest haplotype diversity and nucleotide diversity were observed in the Chinese *A. ceylanicum* population (Hd = 0.9394; π = 0.0201), followed by the Cambodian and Malaysian populations. Pairwise (F_{ST}) indices between the Thai *A. ceylanicum* population and other reference populations were 0.2644, 0.2507, and 0.1526 for the Chinese, Cambodian, and Malaysian populations, respectively. In addition, the highest F_{ST} value of 0.3577 was observed between the Chinese and Malaysian populations. All the F_{ST} values were statistically significant (Table 4).

Table 4. The pairwise fixation index (F_{ST}) among four *A. ceylanicum* populations based on the partial mitochondrial *cox1* gene.

Populations	Thailand	Cambodia	Malaysia	China
Thailand	-			
Cambodia	0.2507	-		
Malaysia	0.1526	0.0999	-	
China	0.2644	0.1939	0.3577	-

All values were statistically significant ($p < 0.001$).

4. Discussion

The major hookworm species in the community dogs in Upper Northern Thailand was *A. ceylanicum*. We demonstrated an approximately 50% temple-level prevalence of hookworm infection in dogs, and these positive dogs were commonly living in the community temples and freely roaming in the surrounding communities. The prevalence of hookworm infection at the individual dog level in this study (26.4%) showed an approximately two-fold increase compared with previous studies in Chiang

Mai province (approximately 12%), as reported by Tiwananthagorn et al. (unpublished results) and Tangtrongsup et al. [23], and greater than that reported by Pumidonming et al. [22] in Lower Northern Thailand (21.3%). These differences are probably due to the different study areas and the inclusion criteria of no regular deworming program. The proportion of *A. ceylanicum* infection in dogs from our study in Upper Northern Thailand (96.6%) was higher than the previous report in the Lower Northern region, which reported a rate of 82.1% [22]. Recently, various studies have reported the rate of *A. ceylanicum* in hookworm infection in the bordering countries of Thailand: 94.4% of dogs in Cambodia, 52% of dogs in Malaysia [39], 77.8% of dogs in Laos [40], and 42.7% of dogs in China [7]. The failure of PCR amplification in some fecal and soil samples was noticed in the present study and was also noted in other studies. This failure could be due to the low intensity of infection, resulting in a reduced number of hookworm eggs, and some PCR inhibitors in the fecal and soil samples interfere with the amplification reaction [15,41]. Therefore, developing a more robust PCR assay to improve the diagnosis of hookworm infection is needed for the efficient control of this zoonosis.

The temples with hookworm-infected dogs are prone to have hookworm-contaminated soil. Here, we confirmed the presence of *A. ceylanicum* larvae in the soil. Moreover, the *A. ceylanicum* genotypes in dogs and soil were identical, suggesting the shedding of hookworm from dogs to the soil. The frequently detected areas in the positive temples included the dog's dwelling areas; human activity areas, such as the sand pagoda; and the areas under the big tree. These areas are the places that community people commonly access for the Buddhist rituals, ceremonies, commerce, and recreation. In addition, allowing dogs to roam freely with indiscriminate defecating areas in the Thai temples can lead to the widespread contamination of infective *A. ceylanicum* hookworm larvae in the environment and possible transmission to humans who occasionally go barefoot during these activities. As suggested in rural Malaysia, close contact with community dogs and cats was associated with *A. ceylanicum* hookworm infection in humans [42]. Previous reports worldwide have reported soil contaminated with hookworm in the public parks of Brazil and Malaysia [43,44], a tribal area of India [5], dog parks in Portugal [45], and organic farms in the Philippines [46]. Therefore, good hygienic practices of shoe-wearing and temple ground cleaning programs should be encouraged to reduce the risk of transmission [47]. In addition, reducing the number of free-roaming dog population size through a sterilization campaign or by sheltering free-roaming dogs should be implemented [48].

The molecular epidemiologic data, phylogenetic relationship, and population analysis obtained from the characterization of the *cox1* gene of *A. ceylanicum* hookworms strongly support the distribution of this parasite in the country, within the Asian continent, and possibly worldwide. A common haplotype of Thailand (Acy-COX1-TH01), which was observed in all four provinces of Upper Northern Thailand, suggested the circulation of *A. ceylanicum* in the region. Genetic differentiation analysis showed that Thai *A. ceylanicum* had the lowest haplotype diversity and nucleotide diversity, indicating minimal differences between haplotypes in Thailand. However, further studies in other regions of Thailand are necessary. The pairwise fixation index showed that Thai *A. ceylanicum* was mostly close to Malaysian *A. ceylanicum*, suggesting gene flow between these populations. In addition, the sharing haplotype of the *cox1* gene of *A. ceylanicum* among the countries (Acy-COX1-TH01 and MA02 and CA01 and CH01; or Acy-COX1-TH03 and MA01 and CA03) advocated the transmission and widespread geographic distribution among these countries [49]. The haplotype relationship between Malaysia and Cambodia populations revealed a very complex evolutionary pattern with some median vectors that indicated many lost or potential ancestors [50]. Interestingly, the Chinese *A. ceylanicum* exhibited the highest haplotype and nucleotide diversities, suggesting that the Chinese *A. ceylanicum* might be an ancestor of the populations in Asian countries. Our hypothesis is consistent with a previous study on the history of domestic dogs, in which China was the origin of the dog species [51]. Animals potentially migrated to accompany human colonization to other Asian countries and subsequently carried the parasites and allowed the parasites to colonize new habitats [51–53]. Hence, the transportation of companion animals should strictly follow the guidelines and regulations of each county to prevent the spreading of zoonotic hookworm.

Based on the phylogenetic tree, the sequences of *A. ceylanicum* from humans (MK792828-29), dogs (MK792824), and cats (MK792825) in Malaysia belong to the same haplotype MA02, confirming that transmission from dogs to humans has occurred. This species was also found in wildlife, such as Asian golden cat, leopard cat, civet, and wild canids [9,54,55]. The biological, epidemiological, and pathophysiological characteristics of *A. ceylanicum* in humans and other wildlife species in Thailand and their genetic diversity with isolates from companion animals deserve further investigation.

Integrated control programs intended for combining chemotherapeutic interventions by deworming programs with improvements in community hygiene and animal health programs will aid in curbing this potentially opportunistic zoonosis. For the deworming program of community dogs in Thailand, an oral dose of 10 mg/kg BW of pyrantel pamoate and the subcutaneous injection of 0.2–0.4 mg/kg BW ivermectin have been regularly administered for deworming; however, the efficacy of these regimens against *A. ceylanicum* in dogs remains unclear. Currently, many commercial drugs against *A. ceylanicum* infection in dogs have been tested at the laboratory level and exhibited greater than 99% efficacy within 3–7 days, including a combination of 15 mg/kg BW of febantel and 14.4 mg/kg BW of pyrantel embonate (Drontal® Plus, Bayer Animal health) [56], a spot-on of 2.5 mg/kg BW moxidectin (Advocate®, Bayer Animal health) [57], and 0.5 mg/kg BW milbemycin oxime (NexGard Spectra®, Boehringer Ingelheim) [58]. The clinical field assessment of the efficacy of anthelminthic agents against *A. ceylanicum* infection warrants further investigation.

5. Conclusions

In conclusion, this study provided the data, genetic characteristics, and evolutionary relationship of *A. ceylanicum* in Thailand and other Asian countries. We confirmed that *A. ceylanicum* was the predominant hookworm species in Northern Thailand, and the data fully supported the transmission dynamics from dogs to soil environments. Therefore, the awareness of *A. ceylanicum* transmission from dogs and soil in the temple should be raised. A proper schedule for the deworming of community dogs and the regular cleaning of the temple ground are suggested to reduce the risk of transmission of this zoonotic disease.

Author Contributions: Conceptualization, S.T. (Saruda Tiwananthagorn); methodology, D.K., S.T. (Sahatchai Tangtrongsup), and S.T. (Saruda Tiwananthagorn); software, D.K., S.T. (Sahatchai Tangtrongsup), and S.T. (Saruda Tiwananthagorn); validation, S.T. (Sahatchai Tangtrongsup), and S.T. (Saruda Tiwananthagorn); formal analysis, D.K., S.T. (Sahatchai Tangtrongsup), and S.T. (Saruda Tiwananthagorn); investigation, D.K. and S.T. (Saruda Tiwananthagorn); resources, D.K. and S.T. (Saruda Tiwananthagorn); data curation, D.K., S.T. (Sahatchai Tangtrongsup), and S.T. (Saruda Tiwananthagorn); writing—original draft preparation, D.K., S.T. (Sahatchai Tangtrongsup), and S.T. (Saruda Tiwananthagorn); writing—review and editing, S.T. (Sahatchai Tangtrongsup) and S.T. (Saruda Tiwananthagorn); visualization, S.T. (Saruda Tiwananthagorn); supervision, S.T. (Sahatchai Tangtrongsup) and S.T. (Saruda Tiwananthagorn); project administration, S.T. (Saruda Tiwananthagorn); funding acquisition, S.T. (Saruda Tiwananthagorn). All authors have read and agreed to the published version of the manuscript.

Acknowledgments: We would like to thank all the community dog owners for their valuable participation and the excellent assistance of Mrs. Duanghatai Sripakdee, Parasitological laboratory of Faculty of Veterinary Medicine, Chiang Mai University.

References

1. Liu, Y.; Shen, Y.; Zhang, T. Survey of the relationship between hookworm disease and socioeconomic factors. *Zhongguo Ji Sheng Chong Xue Yu Ji Sheng Chong Bing Za Zhi* **1999**, *17*, 399. [PubMed]
2. Bethony, J.; Brooker, S.; Albonico, M.; Geiger, S.M.; Loukas, A.; Diemert, D.; Hotez, P.J. Soil-transmitted helminth infections: Ascariasis, trichuriasis, and hookworm. *Lancet* **2006**, *367*, 1521–1532. [CrossRef]
3. Merino-Tejedor, A.; Nejsum, P.; Mkupasi, E.M.; Johansen, M.V.; Olsen, A. Molecular identification of zoonotic hookworm species in dog faeces from Tanzania. *J. Helminthol.* **2019**, *93*, 313–318. [CrossRef] [PubMed]
4. Gordon, C.A.; Kurscheid, J.; Jones, M.K.; Gray, D.J.; McManus, D.P. Soil-transmitted helminths in tropical Australia and Asia. *Trop. Med. Infect. Dis.* **2017**, *4*, 56. [CrossRef] [PubMed]
5. George, S.; Levecke, B.; Kattula, D.; Velusamy, V.; Roy, S.; Geldhof, P.; Sarkar, R.; Kang, G. Molecular identification of hookworm isolates in humans, dogs and soil in a tribal area in Tamil Nadu, India. *PLoS Negl. Trop. Dis.* **2016**, *10*, e0004891. [CrossRef]
6. Bowman, D.D.; Montgomery, S.P.; Zajac, A.M.; Eberhard, M.L.; Kazacos, K.R. Hookworms of dogs and cats as agents of cutaneous larva migrans. *Trends Parasitol.* **2010**, *26*, 162–167. [CrossRef] [PubMed]
7. Liu, Y.J.; Zheng, G.C.; Zhang, P.; Alsarakibi, M.; Zhang, X.H.; Li, Y.W.; Liu, T.; Ren, S.N.; Chen, Z.X.; Liu, Y.L.; et al. Molecular identification of hookworms in stray and shelter dogs from Guangzhou city, China using ITS sequences. *J. Helminthol.* **2015**, *89*, 196–202. [CrossRef]
8. Smout, F.A.; Skerratt, L.F.; Butler, J.R.A.; Johnson, C.N.; Congdon, B.C.; Thompson, R.C.A. The hookworm *Ancylostoma ceylanicum*: An emerging public health risk in Australian tropical rainforests and Indigenous communities. *One Health* **2017**, *3*, 66–69. [CrossRef]
9. Zibaei, M.; Nosrati, M.R.C.; Shadnoosh, F.; Houshmand, E.; Karami, M.F.; Rafsanjani, M.K.; Majidiani, H.; Ghaffarifar, F.; Cortes, H.C.E.; Dalvand, S.; et al. Insights into hookworm prevalence in Asia: A systematic review and meta-analysis. *Trans. R. Soc. Trop. Med. Hyg.* **2020**, *114*, 141–154. [CrossRef]
10. Palmer, C.S.; Traub, R.J.; Robertson, I.D.; Hobbs, R.P.; Elliot, A.; While, L.; Rees, R.; Thompson, R.C. The veterinary and public health significance of hookworm in dogs and cats in Australia and the status of *A. ceylanicum*. *Vet. Parasitol.* **2007**, *145*, 304–313. [CrossRef]
11. Traub, R.J. *Ancylostoma ceylanicum*, a re-emerging but neglected parasitic zoonosis. *Int. J. Parasitol.* **2013**, *43*, 1009–1015. [CrossRef] [PubMed]
12. Schar, F.; Inpankaew, T.; Traub, R.J.; Khieu, V.; Dalsgaard, A.; Chimnoi, W.; Chhoun, C.; Sok, D.; Marti, H.; Muth, S.; et al. The prevalence and diversity of intestinal parasitic infections in humans and domestic animals in a rural Cambodian village. *Parasitol. Int.* **2014**, *63*, 597–603. [CrossRef] [PubMed]
13. Kaya, D.; Yoshikawa, M.; Nakatani, T.; Tomo-Oka, F.; Fujimoto, Y.; Ishida, K.; Fujinaga, Y.; Aihara, Y.; Nagamatsu, S.; Matsuo, E.; et al. *Ancylostoma ceylanicum* hookworm infection in Japanese traveler who presented chronic diarrhea after return from Lao People's Democratic Republic. *Parasitol. Int.* **2016**, *65*, 737–740. [CrossRef] [PubMed]
14. Yoshikawa, M.; Ouji, Y.; Hirai, N.; Nakamura-Uchiyama, F.; Yamada, M.; Arizono, N.; Akamatsu, N.; Yoh, T.; Kaya, D.; Nakatani, T.; et al. *Ancylostoma ceylanicum*, novel etiological agent for traveler's diarrhea-report of four Japanese patients who returned from southeast Asia and Papua New Guinea. *Trop. Med. Health* **2018**, *46*, 6. [CrossRef] [PubMed]
15. Ngui, R.; Ching, L.S.; Kai, T.T.; Roslan, M.A.; Lim, Y.A. Molecular identification of human hookworm infections in economically disadvantaged communities in Peninsular Malaysia. *Am. J. Trop. Med. Hyg.* **2012**, *86*, 837–842. [CrossRef]
16. Traub, R.J.; Robertson, I.D.; Irwin, P.; Mencke, N.; Thompson, R.C. Application of a species-specific PCR-RFLP to identify *Ancylostoma* eggs directly from canine faeces. *Vet. Parasitol.* **2004**, *123*, 245–255. [CrossRef]
17. Romstad, A.; Gasser, R.B.; Nansen, P.; Polderman, A.M.; Chilton, N.B. *Necator americanus* (Nematoda: Ancylostomatidae) from Africa and Malaysia have different ITS-2 rDNA sequences. *Int. J. Parasitol.* **1998**, *28*, 611–615. [CrossRef]
18. Gasser, R.B.; Stewart, L.E.; Speare, R. Genetic markers in ribosomal DNA for hookworm identification. *Acta Trop.* **1996**, *62*, 15–21. [CrossRef]
19. Blouin, M.S. Molecular prospecting for cryptic species of nematodes: Mitochondrial DNA versus internal transcribed spacer. *Int. J. Parasitol.* **2002**, *32*, 527–531. [CrossRef]

20. Hu, M.; Chilton, N.B.; Gasser, R.B. The mitochondrial genomics of parasitic nematodes of socio-economic importance: Recent progress, and implications for population genetics and systematics. *Adv. Parasitol.* **2004**, *56*, 133–212. [CrossRef]
21. Avise, J.C.; Arnold, J.; Ball, R.M.; Bermingham, E.; Lamb, T.; Neigel, J.E.; Reeb, C.A.; Saunders, N.C. Intraspecific phylogeography: The mitochondrial DNA bridge between population genetics and systematics. *Annu. Rev. Ecol. Syst.* **1987**, *18*, 489–522. [CrossRef]
22. Pumidonming, W.; Salman, D.; Gronsang, D.; Abdelbaset, A.E.; Sangkaeo, K.; Kawazu, S.I.; Igarashi, M. Prevalence of gastrointestinal helminth parasites of zoonotic significance in dogs and cats in lower Northern Thailand. *J. Vet. Med. Sci.* **2017**, *78*, 1779–1784. [CrossRef]
23. Tangtrongsup, S.; Scorza, A.V.; Reif, J.S.; Ballweber, L.R.; Lappin, M.R.; Salman, M.D. Seasonal distributions and other risk factors for *Giardia duodenalis* and *Cryptosporidium* spp. infections in dogs and cats in Chiang Mai, Thailand. *Prev. Vet. Med.* **2020**, *174*, 104820. [CrossRef] [PubMed]
24. Piangjai, S.; Sukontason, K.; Sukontason, K.L. Intestinal parasitic infections in hill-tribe schoolchildren in Chiang Mai, northern Thailand. *Southeast Asian J. Trop. Med. Public Health* **2003**, *34* (Suppl. 2), 90–93.
25. Yanola, J.; Nachaiwieng, W.; Duangmano, S.; Prasannarong, M.; Somboon, P.; Pornprasert, S. Current prevalence of intestinal parasitic infections and their impact on hematological and nutritional status among Karen hill tribe children in Omkoi District, Chiang Mai Province, Thailand. *Acta Trop.* **2018**, *180*, 1–6. [CrossRef] [PubMed]
26. Energy Policy and Plannning Office, Ministry of Energy. The Provinces and Administrative Areas of Thailand. Available online: http://www.e-report.energy.go.th/area.html (accessed on 31 May 2019).
27. Royal Thai Government Gazette, The Secretariat of the Cabinet. Thailand Population. 2018. Available online: http://www.ratchakitcha.soc.go.th/DATA/PDF/2562/E/036/T_0032.PDF (accessed on 31 May 2019).
28. Thrusfield, M.; Ortega, C.; de Blas, I.; Noordhuizen, J.P.; Frankena, K. WIN EPISCOPE 2.0: Improved epidemiological software for veterinary medicine. *Vet. Rec.* **2001**, *148*, 567–572. [CrossRef] [PubMed]
29. Tiwananthagorn, S.; Chiang Mai University, Chiang Mai, Thailand. Unpublished Work. 2018.
30. Bureau of Disease Control and Veterinary Services, Department of Livestock Development. *Dog Population in Thailand*. 2016. Available online: http://dcontrol.dld.go.th/webnew/index.php/th/news-menu/2018-07-04-04-12-47/rabies/360-dogpop2016 (accessed on 31 May 2019).
31. Moxham, G. The WALTHAM faeces scoring system—A tool for veterinarians and pet owners: How does your pet rate? *Walth. Focus* **2001**, *11*, 24–25.
32. Gibbons, L.M.; Jones, A.; Khalil, L.F. *Manual for the 8th International Training Course on Identification of Helminth Parasites of Economic Importance*; CABI Institue of Parasitology, Wallingford: Oxon, UK, 1996.
33. Inpankaew, T.; Schar, F.; Dalsgaard, A.; Khieu, V.; Chimnoi, W.; Chhoun, C.; Sok, D.; Marti, H.; Muth, S.; Odermatt, P.; et al. High prevalence of *Ancylostoma ceylanicum* hookworm infections in humans, Cambodia, 2012. *Emerg. Infect. Dis.* **2014**, *20*, 976–982. [CrossRef]
34. Hall, T. BioEdit: A user-friendly biological sequence alignment editor and analysis program for Window 95/98/NT. *Nucleic Acids Symp. Ser.* **1996**, *41*, 95–98.
35. Kumar, S.; Stecher, G.; Li, M.; Knyaz, C.; Tamura, K. MEGA X: Molecular evolutionary genetics analysis across computing platforms. *Mol. Biol. Evol.* **2018**, *35*, 1547–1549. [CrossRef]
36. Rozas, J.; Ferrer-Mata, A.; Sanchez-DelBarrio, J.C.; Guirao-Rico, S.; Librado, P.; Ramos-Onsins, S.E.; Sanchez-Gracia, A. DnaSP 6: DNA sequence polymorphism analysis of large data sets. *Mol. Biol. Evol.* **2017**, *34*, 3299–3302. [CrossRef] [PubMed]
37. Excoffier, L.; Lischer, H.E. Arlequin suite ver 3.5: A new series of programs to perform population genetics analyses under Linux and Windows. *Mol. Ecol. Resour.* **2010**, *10*, 564–567. [CrossRef] [PubMed]
38. Bandelt, H.J.; Forster, P.; Rohl, A. Median-joining networks for inferring intraspecific phylogenies. *Mol. Biol. Evol.* **1999**, *16*, 37–48. [CrossRef] [PubMed]
39. Mahdy, M.A.; Lim, Y.A.; Ngui, R.; Siti Fatimah, M.R.; Choy, S.H.; Yap, N.J.; Al-Mekhlafi, H.M.; Ibrahim, J.; Surin, J. Prevalence and zoonotic potential of canine hookworms in Malaysia. *Parasit Vectors* **2012**, *5*, 88. [CrossRef]
40. Conlan, J.V.; Khamlome, B.; Vongxay, K.; Elliot, A.; Pallant, L.; Sripa, B.; Blacksell, S.D.; Fenwick, S.; Thompson, R.C. Soil-transmitted helminthiasis in Laos: A community-wide cross-sectional study of humans and dogs in a mass drug administration environment. *Am. J. Trop. Med. Hyg.* **2012**, *86*, 624–634. [CrossRef]

41. Schrader, C.; Schielke, A.; Ellerbroek, L.; Johne, R. PCR inhibitors—occurrence, properties and removal. *J. Appl. Microbiol.* **2012**, *113*, 1014–1026. [CrossRef]
42. Ngui, R.; Mahdy, M.A.; Chua, K.H.; Traub, R.; Lim, Y.A. Genetic characterization of the partial mitochondrial cytochrome oxidase *c* subunit I *(cox1)* gene of the zoonotic parasitic nematode, *Ancylostoma ceylanicum* from humans, dogs and cats. *Acta Trop.* **2013**, *128*, 154–157. [CrossRef]
43. Marques, J.P.; Guimaraes Cde, R.; Boas, A.V.; Carnauba, P.U.; Moraes, J. Contamination of public parks and squares from Guarulhos (Sao Paulo State, Brazil) by *Toxocara* spp. and *Ancylostoma* spp. *Rev. Inst. Med. Trop. Sao Paulo* **2012**, *54*, 267–271. [CrossRef]
44. Tun, S.; Ithoi, I.; Mahmud, R.; Samsudin, N.I.; Kek Heng, C.; Ling, L.Y. Detection of helminth eggs and identification of hookworm species in stray cats, dogs and soil from Klang Valley, Malaysia. *PLoS ONE* **2015**, *10*, e0142231. [CrossRef]
45. Ferreira, A.; Alho, A.M.; Otero, D.; Gomes, L.; Nijsse, R.; Overgaauw, P.A.M.; Madeira de Carvalho, L. Urban dog parks as sources of canine parasites: Contamination rates and pet owner behaviours in Lisbon, Portugal. *J. Env. Public Health* **2017**, *2017*, 5984086. [CrossRef]
46. Paller, V.G.V.; Babia-Abion, S. Soil-transmitted helminth (STH) eggs contaminating soils in selected organic and conventional farms in the Philippines. *Parasite Epidemiol. Control.* **2019**, *7*, e00119. [CrossRef]
47. Traub, R.J.; Inpankaew, T.; Sutthikornchai, C.; Sukthana, Y.; Thompson, R.C. PCR-based coprodiagnostic tools reveal dogs as reservoirs of zoonotic ancylostomiasis caused by *Ancylostoma ceylanicum* in temple communities in Bangkok. *Vet. Parasitol.* **2008**, *155*, 67–73. [CrossRef]
48. Smith, L.M.; Hartmann, S.; Munteanu, A.M.; Dalla Villa, P.; Quinnell, R.J.; Collins, L.M. The effectiveness of dog population management: A systematic review. *Animals* **2019**, *9*, 1020. [CrossRef] [PubMed]
49. Posada, D.; Crandall, K.A. Intraspecific gene genealogies: Trees grafting into networks. *Trends Ecol. Evol.* **2001**, *16*, 37–45. [CrossRef]
50. Guo, L.; Sun, B.; Sang, F.; Wang, W.; Lu, Z. Haplotype distribution and evolutionary pattern of miR-17 and miR-124 families based on population analysis. *PLoS ONE* **2009**, *4*, e7944. [CrossRef] [PubMed]
51. Wang, G.D.; Zhai, W.; Yang, H.C.; Wang, L.; Zhong, L.; Liu, Y.H.; Fan, R.X.; Yin, T.T.; Zhu, C.L.; Poyarkov, A.D.; et al. Out of southern East Asia: The natural history of domestic dogs across the world. *Cell Res.* **2016**, *26*, 21–33. [CrossRef] [PubMed]
52. Witt, K.E.; Judd, K.; Kitchen, A.; Grier, C.; Kohler, T.A.; Ortman, S.G.; Kemp, B.M.; Malhi, R.S. DNA analysis of ancient dogs of the Americas: Identifying possible founding haplotypes and reconstructing population histories. *J. Hum. Evol.* **2015**, *79*, 105–118. [CrossRef] [PubMed]
53. Loeurng, V.; Ichikawa-Seki, M.; Wannasan, A.; Sothyra, T.; Chaisowwong, W.; Tiwananthagorn, S. Genetic characterization of cambodian *Fasciola gigantica* and dispersal direction of the species in Asia. *Vet. Parasitol.* **2019**, *273*, 45–51. [CrossRef]
54. Biocca, E.; Chabaud, A. Redescription of *Seuratum mucronatum* (Nematoda-Cucullanidae). *Ann. Parasitol. Hum. Comp.* **1951**, *26*, 85–92. [CrossRef]
55. Smout, F.A.; Thompson, R.C.; Skerratt, L.F. First report of *Ancylostoma ceylanicum* in wild canids. *Int. J. Parasitol. Parasites Wildl.* **2013**, *2*, 173–177. [CrossRef]
56. Taweethavonsawat, P.; Chungpivat, S.; Satranarakun, P.; Traub, R.J.; Schaper, R. Efficacy of a combination product containing pyrantel, febantel and praziquantel (Drontal® Plus Flavour, Bayer Animal Health) against experimental infection with the hookworm *Ancylostoma ceylanicum* in dogs. *Parasitol. Res.* **2010**, *106*, 533–537. [CrossRef] [PubMed]
57. Taweethavonsawat, P.; Chungpivat, S.; Satranarakun, P.; Traub, R.J.; Schaper, R. Experimental infection with *Ancylostoma ceylanicum* in dogs and efficacy of a spot on combination containing imidacloprid 10% and moxidectin 2.5% (Advocate®/Advantage Multi, Bayer Animal Health). *Parasitol. Res.* **2010**, *106*, 1499–1502. [CrossRef] [PubMed]
58. Tielemans, E.; Lebon, W.; Dumont, P.; Taweethavonsawat, P.; Larsen, D.; Rehbein, S. Efficacy of afoxolaner plus milbemycin oxime chewable tablets (NexGard Spectra®, Merial) against adult *Ancylostoma ceylanicum* hookworm, in dogs. *Vet. Parasitol.* **2017**, *238*, 87–89. [CrossRef] [PubMed]

12

Antibacterial and Hemolytic Activity of *Crotalus triseriatus* and *Crotalus ravus* Venom

Adrian Zaragoza-Bastida [1], Saudy Consepcion Flores-Aguilar [2], Liliana Mireya Aguilar-Castro [2], Ana Lizet Morales-Ubaldo [1], Benjamín Valladares-Carranza [3], Lenin Rangel-López [1], Agustín Olmedo-Juárez [4], Carla E. Rosenfeld-Miranda [5] and Nallely Rivero-Pérez [1,*]

1 Universidad Autónoma del Estado de Hidalgo, Área Académica de Medicina Veterinaria y Zootecnia, Instituto de Ciencias Agropecuarias, Rancho Universitario Av. Universidad km 1, EX-Hda de Aquetzalpa, Tulancingo, Hidalgo 43600, Mexico; adrian_zaragoza@uaeh.edu.mx (A.Z.-B.); ubaldolizet8@gmail.com (A.L.M.-U.); ralolenin@gmail.com (L.R.-L.)

2 Universidad Autónoma del Estado de Hidalgo, Área Académica de Biología, Instituto de Ciencias Básicas e Ingeniería. Carretera Pachuca-Tulancingo S/N Int. 22 Colonia Carboneras, Mineral de la Reforma, Hidalgo 42180, Mexico; saudy.fa@gmail.com (S.C.F.-A.); profe_3192@uaeh.edu.mx (L.M.A.-C.)

3 Facultad de Medicina Veterinaria y Zootecnia Universidad Autónoma del Estado de México, El Cerrillo Piedras Blancas, Toluca 50295, Mexico; benvac2004@yahoo.com.mx

4 Centro Nacional de Investigación Disciplinaria en Salud Animal e Inocuidad (CENID SAI-INIFAP), Carretera Federal Cuernavaca-Cuautla No. 8534 / Col. Progreso, Jiutepec 62550, Morelos, Mexico; aolmedoj@gmail.com

5 Facultad de Ciencias Veterinarias, Universidad Austral de Chile, Isla Teja s/n, Casilla 567, Valdivia, Chile; crosenfe@uach.cl

* Correspondence: nallely_rivero@uaeh.edu.mx.

Simple Summary: Rattlesnakes (*Crotalus ravus* and *Crotalus triseriatus*) have some compounds that resemble polypeptides and proteins in their venoms which can be used in therapeutic treatment as antibacterial compounds. The aim of the present study is to evaluate the antibacterial and hemolytic activity of two rattlesnake venoms. The results of the present study indicate that the evaluated venoms have bactericidal activity against *Pseudomonas aeruginosa*, an important bacterium that affects animals and humans, thereby providing a new and efficient treatment alternative against this pathogenic bacterium.

Abstract: Rattlesnakes have venoms with a complex toxin mixture comprised of polypeptides and proteins. Previous studies have shown that some of these polypeptides are of high value for the development of new medical treatments. The aim of the present study is to evaluate, in vitro, the antibacterial and hemolytic activity of *Crotalus triseriatus* and *Crotalus ravus* venoms. A direct field search was conducted to obtain *Crotalus triseriatus* and *Crotalus ravus* venom samples. These were evaluated to determine their antibacterial activity against *Escherichia coli*, *Staphylococcus aureus* and *Pseudomonas aeruginosa* through the techniques of Minimum Inhibitory Concentration (MIC) and Minimum Bactericidal Concentration (MBC). Hemolytic activity was also determined. Antibacterial activity was determined for treatments (*Crotalus triseriatus* 2) CT2 and (*Crotalus ravus* 3) CR3, obtaining a Minimum Inhibitory Concentration of 50 µg/mL and a Minimum Bactericidal Concentration of 100 µg/mL against *Pseudomonas aeruginosa*. CT1 (*Crotalus triseriatus* 1), CT2, and CR3 presented hemolytic activity; on the other hand, *Crotalus ravus* 4 (CR4) did not show hemolytic activity. The results of the present study indicate for the first time that *Crotalus triseriatus* and *Crotalus ravus* venoms contain some bioactive compounds with bactericidal activity against *Pseudomonas aeruginosa* which could be used as alternative treatment in diseases caused by this pathogenic bacterium.

Keywords: *Crotalus ravus*; Crotalus triseriatus; venom; antibacterial activity; *Pseudomonas aeruginosa*; hemolytic activity

1. Introduction

Rattlesnakes are a species widely distributed through Mexico, occupying practically the whole territory. There exists a great variety of these species, among them, are *Crotalus triseriatus*, distributed in the States of Veracruz, Puebla, Tlaxcala, México, Morelos, and Michoacán and *Crotalus ravus*, which occupies the States of Morelos, México, Puebla, Tlaxcala, Guerrero, Oaxaca, and Hidalgo. These species are primarily recognized for their characteristic hemotoxic venoms [1–3].

Crotalid venoms are comprised mainly of enzymes that cause severe local inflammation, necrosis, hemorrhagic syndromes, and neurological manifestations. These responses would typically help rapid prey subjugation or capture, as well as serve as a defense mechanism [4].

Animal venoms, including that of snakes, are complex mixtures of bioactive compounds that contain large amounts of proteins, peptides, and small molecules that can be considered for use in a wide range of medical applications [5,6].

There are several examples in the development of treatments derived from snake venom compounds. One of the most widely known is Capoten®, a hypotensive agent, used for the treatment of congestive heart failure, diabetic nephropathy, and heart attacks. Another known example is Viprinex®, developed to treat acute strokes [7,8].

Aside from their qualities as potential therapeutic agents, venoms are currently considered as possible sources of molecules with antibacterial activity [9]. This, in fact, has a great impact on public health especially due to the increase of antibacterial resistant bacteria.

In 2017 the World Health Organization (WHO) compiled a list of antibiotic-resistant priority pathogens, among which, were the Gram-negative bacteria *Escherichia coli* and *Pseudomonas aeruginosa* bacteria resistant to carbapenems, and *Staphylococcus aureus* resistant to methicillin and vancomycin [10]. Due to the increased antibiotic resistance found in these pathogens, the aim of the present study was to evaluate, in vitro, the antibacterial and hemolytic response of *Crotalus triseriatus* and *Crotalus ravus* venoms on bacteria of public health importance.

2. Material and Methods

2.1. Field Sampling

Two field outings were carried out per month during each of the months of August, September, October and November 2018 in the state of Hidalgo, Mexico; covering the municipalities of Acatlán, Almoloya, Cuautepec de Hinojosa, Mineral del Chico, Mineral del Monte, Santiago Tulantepec, Singuilucan, Tula de Allende and Zacualtipán.

A direct search was conducted according to the methodology described by McDiarmid et al. in 2012. The rattlesnakes were trapped in accordance with the official norms for wildlife protection (NOM-059-SEMARNAT-2010) established by the government of Mexico and with a scientific collecting permit issued by General Directorate of Wildlife of the Secretariat of Environment and Natural Resources of Mexico (Office N° SGPA/SGVS/003613/18) [11,12].

2.2. Obtaining Venom Samples

Four samples were collected in the field, two of them belonging to the species *Crotalus triseriatus* (CT1 and CT2) and the remaining from the species *Crotalus ravus* (CR3 and CR4). A record of each individual was noted.

Once the samples were obtained, they were subjected to a lyophilization process and kept at −70 °C until further evaluation.

2.3. *Antibacterial Activity*

The venom's antibacterial activity was determined through the Minimum Inhibitory Concentration (MIC) and the Minimum Bactericidal Concentration (MBC) procedures, in accordance with the CLSI guidelines and with the standards published by Olmedo-Juárez et al., in 2019 and by Morales-Ubaldo et al., in 2020 [13–15].

Escherichia coli ATCC^{35218}, *Pseudomonas aeruginosa* ATCC^{9027}, and *Staphylococcus aureus* ATCC^{6538} strains were used to perform the evaluation. These samples were the same which were reactivated from cryopreservation in Müller–Hinton agar (BD Bioxon, Heidelberg, Germany) through simple strain technique to obtain isolated colonies. A Gram staining was performed to corroborate their morphology.

Once the purity was confirmed, one colony of each strain was inoculated in nutritive broth (BD Bioxon), and incubated under constant agitation at 70 rpm for 24 h at 37 °C. The bacterial cell suspension was adjusted to a 0.5 McFarland (Remel, R20421, Kansas, U.S.A.) standard (approximately 1.5×10^6 Colony Forming Units (CFU) per mL).

2.3.1. Minimal Inhibitory Concentration (MIC)

Micro-dilution was used to determine the MIC, evaluating different venom concentrations (100, 50, 25, 12.5, 6.25, 3.12, 1.56, 0.78 μg/mL).

In a sterile 96- well plate, 100 μL of each venom concentrations were added along with 10 μL of bacterial cell suspension previously adjusted to a 0.5 McFarland standard. The plates were incubated at 37 °C for 24 h at 70 rpm. Kanamycin (AppliChem 4K10421, Darmstadt, Germany) was used as a positive control (128 to 1 μg/mL) and nutritive broth as the negative control. Treatments were evaluated by triplicate.

After incubation 20 μL of a 0.04% (*w*/*v*) p-iodonitrotetrazolium (Sigma-Aldrich I8377, Missouri, U.S.A.) solution was added into each well and incubated for 30 min. The MIC was determined by the concentration at which the solution turned to a pinkish color.

2.3.2. Minimal Bactericidal Concentration (MBC)

After incubation and previous addition of p-iodonitrotetrazolium, 5 μL from each well was inoculated in Müller–Hinton agar (BD Bioxon) and incubated at 37 °C for 24 h. The MBC was considered as the lowest concentration where no visible growth of the bacteria was observed on the plates.

2.4. *Indirect Hemolytic Activity*

In accordance with the protocols described by Pirela et al., in 2006 with modifications, the venom's indirect hemolytic activity was evaluated [16]. A donor donkey blood sample was collected. The blood sample was stored in 10 mL sodium citrate (3.2%) tubes (DB Vacutainer) and in 3 mL EDTA (10.8 mg) tubes (BD Vacutainer).

Blood agar was used (Merck©, Darmstadt, Germany). To obtain plates with 8% blood concentration, 250 mL of agar base was prepared, and 20 mL of blood was added.

One hundred micrograms (100 μg) of each treatment were weighed out (lyophilized venom) and reconstituted in 1 mL of nutritive broth (BD Bioxon). Dilutions were made (100, 50, 25, 12.5, 6.25, 3.12 μg/mL) from this concentrated solution for further evaluation.

Four wells were made (6 mm diameter) on the plate's surface. Twenty micrograms (20 μL) were added of each concentrate to be evaluated. Treatments were performed by triplicate. Tween 80 at 100% (Sigma-Aldrich) and nutritive broth (BD Bioxon) were used as positive and negative controls, respectively. Plates were incubated for 24 h at 37 °C. Once the incubation period elapsed, hemolysis halos were measured (mm).

2.5. *Statistical Analysis.*

Obtained data were analyzed using two-way variance analysis (ANOVA) and a means comparison by Tukey at a significance level of 0.05% through Minitab 18 statistical package [17].

3. Results and Discussion

3.1. *Individuals Data*

A record of each individual was made with the following information: length, weight, age, and gender (Table 1). The characteristics of the rattlesnakes in the study coincided with those reported by Campbell and Lamar in 2004 [1], as seen in Figure 1.

Table 1. Individual data of trapped rattlesnakes in Hidalgo State.

Species	Species Characteristics	Individual Identification	Gender	Age	Length (cm)	Weight (g)
Crotalus triseriatus	Triangular head 8–10 rattles Postocular strip	CT1	Male	Adult	37	210
		CT2	Male	Adult	25	175
Crotalus ravus	Triangular head Thin rattle Symmetric scales in head	CR3	Male	Adult	25	180
		CR4	Male	Adult	25	175

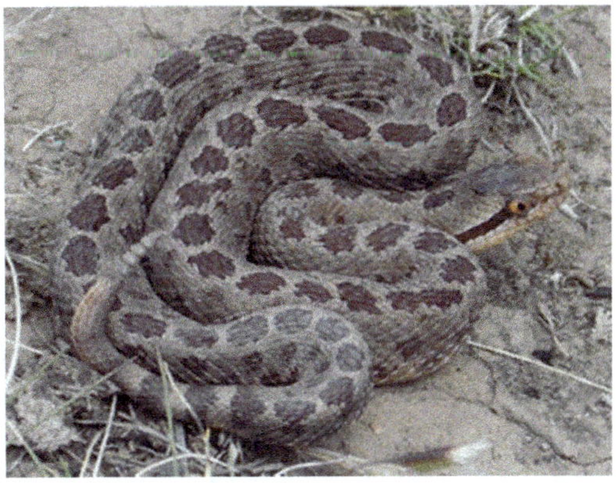

(**a**) *Crotalus triseriatus*

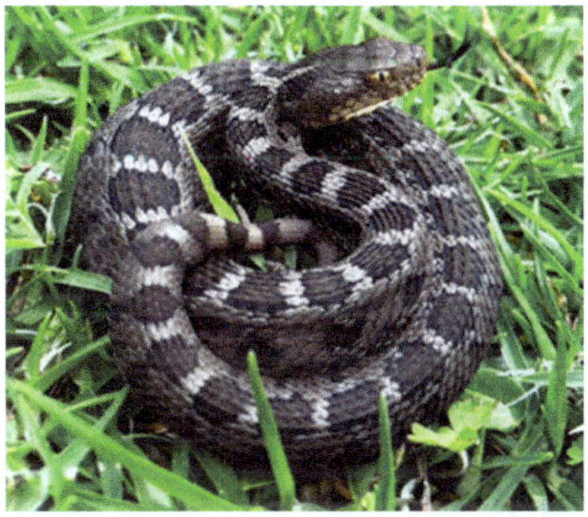

(**b**) *Crotalus ravus*

Figure 1. Captured species (**a**) *Crotalus triseriatus* and (**b**) *Crotalus ravus.*

3.2. *Antibacterial Activity*

A MIC of 50 µg/mL and an MBC of 100 µg /mL were determined as effective for treatments CT2 and CR3 over *P. aeruginosa* (Table 2, Figure 2). Nevertheless, antibacterial activity was not detected for *E. coli and S. aureus.*

Table 2. Minimal Inhibitory Concentration (MIC) and Minimal Bactericidal Concentration (MBC) of *Crotalus triseriatus and Crotalus ravus* venoms.

Evaluated Bacteria	Evaluated Treatments µg/mL (MIC/MBC)				Controls (MIC/MBC)	
	CT1	CT2	CR3	CR4	Nutritive Broth	Kanamycin (µg/mL)
E. coli	-	-	-	-	-	2/4
P. aeruginosa	-	$50^{a}/100^{A}$	$50^{a}/100^{A}$	-	-	$16^{b}/64^{B}$
S. aureus	-	-	-	-	-	1/4

CT1 *Crotalus triseriatus* 1, CT2 *Crotalus triseriatus* 2, CR3 *Crotalus ravus* 3, CR4 *Crotalus ravus* 4 ^{a,b} Different small letters indicate significant statistical differences between MIC ($p < 0.05$) ^{A,B} Different capital letters indicate significant statistical differences between MBC ($p < 0.05$)

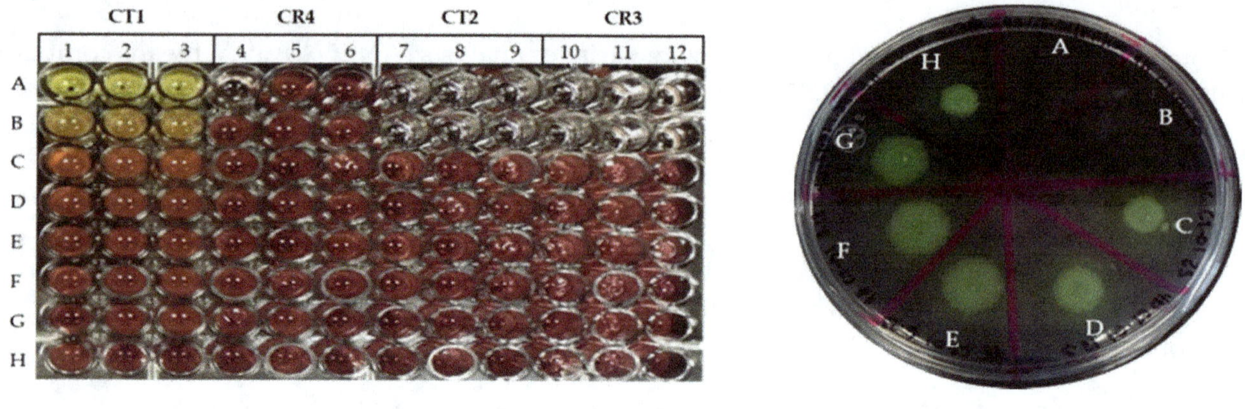

(**a**) MIC of venoms (**b**) MBC of CT2

Figure 2. Antibacterial activity of rattlesnake's venoms against *P. aeruginosa*: (**a**) columns 1–3, CT1 from 100 at 0.78 μg/mL, columns 4–6, CR4 from 100 at 0.78 μg/mL, columns 7–9, CT2 from 100 at 0.78 μg/mL, columns 10–12, CR3 from 100 at 0.78 μg/mL. The MIC value is read at the minimal concentration in which the color changes to pink; (**b**) Plate with *P. aeruginosa* + CT2 in Müller–Hinton agar; **A** CT2 to 100 μg/mL, **B** CT2 to 50 μg/mL, **C** CT2 to 25 μg/mL, **D** CT2 to 12.5 μg/mL, **E** CT2 to 6.25 μg/mL, **F** CT2 to 12.5 μg/mL, **G** CT2 to 6.25 μg/mL, **H** CT2 to 0.78 μg/mL. The MBC is read to the lowest concentration where no visible growth of the bacteria.

It was determined that the antibacterial response seen in treatments CT2 and CR3 were bactericidal, since the relation between MIC and MBC is less than 4, in accordance with González-Alamilla et al., in 2019 [18].

Boda et al., in 2019 evaluated the antibacterial activity of eleven crude venoms from different snake species including *Crotalus atrox* and *Crotalus polystictus* against *Staphylococcus aureus, Escherichia coli* and *Pseudomonas aeruginosa* among others, at varied concentrations of 500 to 1.95 μg/mL, determining a MIC and MBC of 125 and 500 μg/mL against *S. aureus* for *Crotalus atrox* and *Crotalus polystictus*, respectively. In the present study, antibacterial activity was not found for *S. aureus* and *E. coli* but was determined for *Pseudomonas aeruginosa*, obtaining a MIC of 50 and a MBC of 100 μg/mL for *C. triseriatus* and *C. ravus* (CT2 and CR3). According to Boda et al., 2019, the antibacterial activity of venoms from viperid species is probably due to their content of proteins with proteolytic activity [19].

Samy et al., in 2014, evaluated CaTx-II a toxin isolated from *Crotalus adamanteus* venom, determining a MIC of 7.8 μg/mL for *S. aureus* and 62.5 to 125 μg/mL for *P. aeruginosa*. Oguiura et al., in 2011, evaluated crotamine, a myotoxin from *Crotalus durissus* venom against different bacteria strains which included *E. coli, S. aureus*, and *P. aeruginosa*. They report a MIC of 100 μg/mL for *E. coli* and >200 μg/mL for the other two [20,21], a contrast with the results obtained in our present study since the antibacterial activity was not determined for *E. coli* or *S. aureus*. Since it was determined that a MIC of 50 μg/mL from *C. triseriatus* and *C. ravus* (CT2 and CR3) occurred in crude venom, the activity could be attributed to the presence of these bioactive compounds in the venom of the individuals used for this evaluation since both compounds were isolated from snake venom of the same genus (*Crotalus*).

Although the aim of the study did not include identifying the venom's active mechanism, it has been reported that phospholipase A_2 (CaTx-II) interacts with lipopolysaccharide (LPS), particularly with lipid A, a Gram-negative bacteria component, causing membrane permeabilization. Crotamine also has effects over some bacteria through membrane permeabilization, so it could be suggested that CT2 and CR3 treatments antibacterial activity is related to this mechanism [21,22].

In this respect, the efficiency of these compounds, specially phospholipase A_2 against antibiotic-resistant bacteria, holds promise for biotechnological applications, in this case, new medical treatment alternatives, however, it should be understood there are different antibacterial activity mechanisms from venom-based drugs [23,24].

In accordance with WHO, *P. aeruginosa* actually is in the critical priority group of the list of antibiotic-resistant pathogens. WHO has been expressing its interest by promoting the research and development of new antibiotics for this bacterium [10]. These results obtained herein show that CT2 and CR3 treatments demonstrated bactericidal activity against this pathogen showing its importance, since rattlesnake venoms or compounds thereof could be used to develop effective therapeutic agents to treat infections caused by *P. aeruginosa*.

3.3. Hemolytic Activity

With respect to the hemolysis produced, the generated halos showed significant statistical differences between them ($p < 0.05$) (Table 3). It was observed that CT1, CT2, and CR3 showed the highest hemolytic potential and there were no statistically significant differences between them at 100 μg/mL concentration compared with the other treatments (Figure 3).

Table 3. Hemolysis halos generated by *C. triseriatus* and *C. ravus* venoms.

Concentration (μg/mL)	Evaluated Treatments					
	CT1	CT2	CR3	CR4	Nutritive Broth	Tween 80
100	18.67 ± 1.53 ^{a,A,*}	17.00 ± 1.00 ^{a,A}	18.67 ± 1.15 ^{a,A,*}	0.0 ^{b}		
50	15.00 ± 0.0 ^{b,B}	12.33 ± 0.58 ^{c,B}	16.67 ± 0.58 ^{a,B}	0.0 ^{d}		
25	13.67 ± 0.58 ^{a,B,C}	13.67 ± 1.15 ^{a,B}	13.33 ± 0.58 ^{a,C}	0.0 ^{b}	0.00	20.33 ± 0.58 *
12.5	12.00 ± 1.00 ^{a,C}	10.00 ± 0.00 ^{a,b,C}	10.33 ± 0.58 ^{b,D}	0.0 ^{c}		
6.25	8.67 ± 0.58 ^{a,D}	8.33 ± 0.58 ^{a,C}	7.33 ± 0.58 ^{a,E}	0.0 ^{b}		
3.12	0.00 ± 0.00 ^{a,E}	0.00 ±0.00 ^{a,D}	0.00 ± 0.00 ^{a,F}	0.0 ^{a}		

^{a,b,c} Different letters indicate significant statistical differences between treatments ($p < 0.05$). ^{A,B,C} Different letters indicate significant statistical differences between concentrations ($p < 0.05$). * No statistical differences between treatments ($p > 0.05$). CT1 *Crotalus triseriatus* 1, CT2 *Crotalus triseriatus* 2, CR3 *Crotalus ravus* 3, and CR4 *Crotalus ravus* 4.

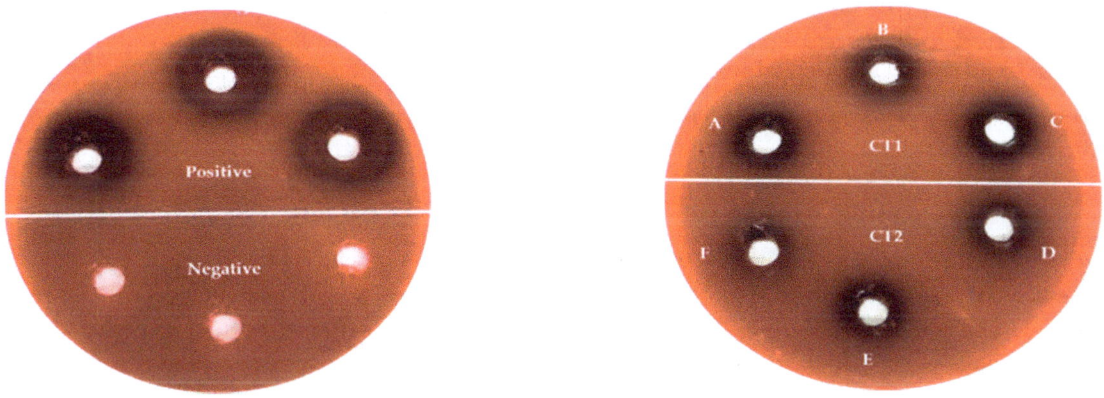

(**a**) Controls (**b**) Venoms

Figure 3. Indirect hemolytic activity of the rattlesnake's venoms: (**a**) hemolytic activity of controls, positive Tween 80, negative nutritive broth, (**b**) hemolytic activity of venoms **A**, **B**, **C** 100 μg/mL of CT1; **D**, **E**, **F** 100 μg/mL of CT2.

Macías-Rodríguez et al., in 2014 [25] evaluated the hemolytic activity of *Crotalus molossus* venom (*C. molossus molossus* and *C. molossus nigrescens*) at a 50 μg/mL concentration. In the present study, hemolytic halos were measured over different periods of time, (1, 2, 3, and 14 h). The results obtained showed that at 14 h halos generated measured 19.2 ± 1.5 and 17.00 ± 1.2 mm for *C. molossus molossus* and *C. m. molossus nigrescens*, respectively, whereas at the same concentration over a longer period of time (24 h) with the venoms of *C. triseriatus* and *C. ravus* generated smaller halos 15.00 ± 0.0 (CT1), 12.33 ± 0.58 (CT2), 16.67 ± 0.58 (CR3), and 0.00 ± 0.00 (CR4), showing the hemolytic potential of these species is lower.

On the other hand, Pirela et al., in 2006, determined that the indirect hemolytic dose of *Crotalus durissus cumanensis* venom to produce a 20 mm hemolytic halo was 379.51 ± 67.67 μg of venom [16]. In a similar study, Dos Santos et al. in 1993 obtained a dose of approximately 310 μg for the white venom and 350 μg for the yellow venom of *Crotalus durissus ruruima* to produce hemolytic halos of 20 mm [26]. With respect to *Crotalus triseriatus* and *Crotalus ravus* venoms, an average of 18.67 ± 1.53 mm was obtained at 100 μg/mL concentration of venom. Although there are no equivalent values in the measurements of hemolytic halos, the venom of *C.triseriatus* and *C. ravus* have close values in the measure of their halos in comparison with the other studies and in a lower venom concentration.

In accordance with Macías-Rodríguez et al., in 2014 [27], during the fall months, there exists a high proteomic concentration in rattlesnake venom. *C. ravus* and *C. triseriatus* were sampled in September and November, respectively, months which correspond to the autumn, while the individuals sampled by Pirela et al. in 2006 [16] were sampled in May, June, and July, months that have been shown to have decreased protein concentration. On the other hand, in 2010 Chippaux et al., [6] reported that the species *C. durissus durissus* and *C. durissus terrificus* have myotoxic and neurotoxic venoms compared to other species of the genus *Crotalus*, which mostly have hemotoxic and histologic venoms [28]. Therefore, due to this, in *C. triseriatus* and *C. ravus*, the highest concentration evaluated in this study (100 μg/mL) was enough to produce halos with measurements similar to those of the aforementioned study.

Treatment CR4, characterized by its transparent color, did not show hemolytic activity. This variation in color has been observed in other viperids. In the study carried out by Macías-Rodríguez et al., in 2014 [25], *C. molossus* presented a yellowish venom which turned out to be more hemolytic than *Crotalus tigris* venom, which was transparent in appearance, similar to *C. ravus* (CR4). Galán et al., in 2004 [29], reported that yellowish venoms have greater toxicity compared to white venoms. Lourenço et al., in 2013 [30], reported that the yellow coloration of the venom is due to the presence of crotamine, a myotoxin from rattlesnakes.

Snake venom complexity produces a source of bioactive molecules with different activities. The results obtained in this study confirm rattlesnake's crude venom contains compounds that could be used as therapeutic models, in this case, molecules with antibacterial activity. Although the venom cannot be used directly due to its high toxicity, some of its compounds will serve as prototypes for the development of new drugs.

4. Conclusions

Until today, there are no studies reporting on the antibacterial and hemolytic activity of the venoms of *C. triseriatus* and *C. ravus*. The results of the present study indicate that both rattlesnakes produce venoms rich in bioactive compounds with a bactericidal effect against *Pseudomonas aeruginosa*. These compounds could also serve as new antimicrobial drugs for the treatment of diseases caused by this bacterium; however, the isolation, identification, and evaluation of these molecules is necessary since it could present hemolytic activity.

Author Contributions: Conceptualization and Methodology, N.R.-P. and A.Z.-B.; Validation and Formal analysis, A.Z.-B., A.L.M.-U. and L.M.A.-C.; Investigation and Resources, N.R.-P., A.Z.-B. and L.R.-L.; Data curation, S.C.F.-A., C.E.R.-M. and A.O.-J.; Writing—original draft preparation, S.C.F.-A., A.L.M.-U and N.R.-P.; Writing—review and editing, A.Z.-B., B.V.-C., A.O.-J. and L.R.-L.; Supervision, N.R.-P., C.E.R.-M. and A.Z.-B.; Project administration, N.R.-P. and A.Z.-B.; Funding acquisition, N.R.-P., A.Z.-B. and L.M.A.-C. All authors have read and agreed to the published version of the manuscript.

Acknowledgments: The authors would like to acknowledge to the Universidad Autónoma del Estado de Hidalgo (UAEH) by for the support provided for carrying out the study in its facilities.

References

1. Campbell, J.A.; Lamar, W.W.; Brodie, E.D. *The Venomous Reptiles of the Western Hemisphere*; Cornell University Press: Ithaca, NY, USA, 2004; p. 528.
2. Mata-Silva, V.; Johnson, J.D.; Wilson, L.D.; García-Padilla, E. The herpetofauna of Oaxaca, Mexico: Composition, physiographic distribution, and conservation status. *Mesoam. Herpetol.* **2015**, *2*, 6–62.
3. Palacios-Aguilar, R.; Flores-Villela, O. An updated checklist of the herpetofauna from Guerrero, Mexico. *Zootaxa* **2018**, *4422*, 1–24. [CrossRef] [PubMed]
4. Chippaux, J. Snakebite in Africa: Current situation and urgent needs. In *Handbook of Venoms and Toxins of Reptiles*; CRC Press Inc.: London, UK, 2009; pp. 453–473.
5. Vetter, I.; Davis, J.L.; Rash, L.D.; Anangi, R.; Mobli, M.; Alewood, P.F.; Lewis, R.J.; King, G.F. Venomics: A new paradigm for natural products-based drug discovery. *Amino Acids* **2011**, *40*, 15–28. [CrossRef] [PubMed]
6. Prashanth, J.R.; Brust, A.; Jin, A.H.; Alewood, P.F.; Dutertre, S.; Lewis, R.J. Cone snail venomics: From novel biology to novel therapeutics. *Future Med. Chem.* **2014**, *6*, 1659–1675. [CrossRef]
7. Fox, J.W.; Serrano, S.M. Approaching the golden age of natural product pharmaceuticals from venom libraries: An overview of toxins and toxin-derivatives currently involved in therapeutic or diagnostic applications. *Curr. Pharm. Des.* **2007**, *13*, 2927–2934. [CrossRef] [PubMed]
8. Beeton, C. Targets and Therapeutic Properties. In *Handbook of Biologically Active Peptides*, 2nd ed.; Kastin, A.J., Ed.; Academic Press: Cambridge, MA, USA, 2013; pp. 473–482.
9. Vargas-Muñoz, L.J.; Estrada-Gomez, S.; Vásquez-Escobar, J. Toxinas de venenos de serpientes y escorpiones, una fuente natural de moléculas con actividad antimicrobiana. *Curare* **2015**, *2*. [CrossRef]
10. World Health Organization. WHO Publishes List of Bacteria for Which New Antibiotics are Urgently Needed. 2017. Available online: https://www.who.int/news-room/detail/27-02-2017-who-publishes-list-of-bacteria-for-which-new-antibiotics-are-urgently-needed (accessed on 15 December 2019).
11. McDiarmid, R.; Foster, M.; Guyer, C.; Gibbons, W.; Chernoff, N. *Reptile Biodiversity: Standard Methods for Inventory and Monitoring*; University of California Press: Berkely, CA, USA, 2012; p. 412.
12. SEMARNAT: Secretaría del Medio Ambiente y Recursos Naturales. México: Gobierno de México. 2016. Licencia de Colecta Científica con Propósitos de Enseñanza en Materia de vida Silvestre. Available online: https://www.gob.mx/tramites/ficha/licencia-de-colecta-cientifica-con-propositos-de-ensenanza-en-materia-de-vidasilvestre/SEMARNAT442 (accessed on 15 December 2019).
13. Clinical and Laboratory Standards Institute. *Methods for Dilution Antimicrobial Susceptibility Tests for Bacteria that Grow Aerobically (Approved Standards)*; CLSI document M7-A5; CLSI: Wayne, PA, USA, 2012.
14. Olmedo-Juárez, A.; Briones-Robles, T.I.; Zaragoza-Bastida, A.; Zamilpa, A.; Ojeda-Ramírez, D.; Mendoza-de Gives, P.; Olivares-Pérez, J.; Rivero-Perez, N. Antibacterial activity of compounds isolated from *Caesalpinia coriaria* (Jacq) Willd against important bacteria in public health. *Microb. Pathog.* **2019**, *136*, 103660. [CrossRef] [PubMed]
15. Morales-Ubaldo, A.; Hernández-Alvarado, J.; Valladares-Carranza, B.; Velázquez-Ordoñez, V.; Delgadillo-Ruiz, L.; Rosenfeld-Miranada, C.; Rivero-Pérez, N.; Zaragoza-Bastida, A. Actividad antibacteriana del extracto hidroalcohólico *Croton draco* sobre bacterias de importancia sanitaria. *Abanico Vet.* **2019**, *10*, 10. [CrossRef]
16. Pirela De las Salas, R.d.C.; López-Jonsthon, J.C.; Hernández Rangel, J.L. Caracterización toxinológica del veneno total de la serpiente de cascabel *Crotalus durissus cumanensis* (viperidae), presente en la localidad de Porshoure, Guajira Venezolana. *Rev. Cient.* **2006**, *16*, 232–238.
17. *Minitab 18 Statistical Software 2010*; Minitab, Inc.: State College, PA, USA, 2010; Available online: www.minitab.com (accessed on 15 November 2019).
18. González-Alamilla, E.N.; Gonzalez-Cortazar, M.; Valladares-Carranza, B.; Rivas-Jacobo, M.A.; Herrera-Corredor, C.A.; Ojeda-Ramírez, D.; Zaragoza-Bastida, A.; Rivero-Perez, N. Chemical Constituents of *Salix babylonica* L. and Their Antibacterial Activity Against Gram-Positive and Gram-Negative Animal Bacteria. *Molecules* **2019**, *24*, 2992. [CrossRef]
19. Boda, F.A.; Mare, A.; Szabó, Z.I.; Berta, L.; Curticapean, A.; Dogaru, M.; Man, A. Antibacterial activity of selected snake venoms on pathogenic bacterial strains. *Rev. Rom. Med. Lab.* **2019**, *27*, 305. [CrossRef]

20. Samy, R.P.; Kandasamy, M.; Gopalakrishnakone, P.; Stiles, B.G.; Rowan, E.G.; Becker, D.; Shanmugam, M.K.; Sethi, G.; Chow, V.T. Wound healing activity and mechanisms of action of an antibacterial protein from the venom of the eastern diamondback rattlesnake (Crotalus adamanteus). *PLoS ONE* **2014**, *9*, e80199-e. [CrossRef] [PubMed]
21. Oguiura, N.; Boni-Mitake, M.; Affonso, R.; Zhang, G. In vitro antibacterial and hemolytic activities of crotamine, a small basic myotoxin from rattlesnake Crotalus durissus. *J. Antibiot.* **2011**, *64*, 327–331. [CrossRef] [PubMed]
22. Santamaría, C.; Larios, S.; Angulo, Y.; Pizarro-Cerda, J.; Gorvel, J.P.; Moreno, E.; Lomonte, B. Antimicrobial activity of myotoxic phospholipases A2 from crotalid snake venoms and synthetic peptide variants derived from their C-terminal region. *Toxicon* **2005**, *45*, 807–815. [CrossRef] [PubMed]
23. Canhas, I.; Heneine, L.G.; Fraga, T.; Assis, D.; Borges, M.; Chartone-Souza, E.; Amaral Nascimento, A.M. Antibacterial activity of different types of snake venom from the Viperidae family against *Staphylococcus aureus*. *Acta Sci. Biol. Sci.* **2017**, *39*, 309. [CrossRef]
24. Bocian, A.; Hus, K. Antibacterial properties of snake venom components. *Chem. Pap.* **2019**. [CrossRef]
25. Macias-Rodríguez, E.; Martínez-Martínez, A.; Gatica-Colima, A.; Bojórquez-Rangel, G.; Plenge-Tellechea, L. Análisis comparativo de la actividad hemolítica entre las subespecies *Crotalus molossus* y *Crotalus molossus* nigrescens. *Revista Bio Ciencias* **2014**, *2*, 302–312.
26. Dos Santos, M.C.; Ferreira, L.C.L.; Da Silva, W.D.; Furtado, M.d.F.D. Caracterizacion de las actividades biologicas de los venenos 'amarillo' y 'blanco' de *Crotalus durissus ruruima* comparados con el veneno de *Crotalus durissus terrificus*. Poder neutralizante de los antivenenos frente a los venenos de *Crotalus durissus ruruim*. *Toxicon* **1993**, *31*, 1459–1469.
27. Macias-Rodríguez, E.; Díaz-Cárdenas, C.O.; Gatica-Colima, A.; Plenge, L. Variación estacional del contenido proteico y actividad de la PLA2 del veneno de *Crotalus molossus molossus* entre especímenes de origen silvestre y en cautiverio. *Acta Univ.* **2014**, *24*, 38–47. Available online: http://www.redalyc.org/articulo.oa?id=41630112002 (accessed on 15 December 2019).
28. De Roodt, A.R.; Estévez-Ramírez, J.; Paniagua-Solís, J.F.; Litwin, S.; Carvajal-Saucedo, A.; Dolab, J.A.; Robles–Ortiz, L.E.; Alagón, A. Toxicidad de venenos de serpientes de importancia médica en México. *Gac. Méd. Méx.* **2005**, *141*, 13–21.
29. Galán, J.A.; Sánchez, E.E.; Rodríguez-Acosta, A.; Pérez, J.C. Neutralization of venoms from two Southern Pacific Rattlesnakes (*Crotalus helleri*) with commercial antivenoms and endothermic animal sera. *Toxicon* **2004**, *43*, 791–799. [CrossRef] [PubMed]
30. Lourenço, A.; Zorzella-Creste, C.F.; Curtolo de Barros, L.; Delazari-dos Santos, L.; Pimenta, D.C.; Barraviera, B.; Ferreira, R.S., Jr. Individual venom profiling of *Crotalus durissus terrificus* specimens from a geographically limited region: Crotamine assessment and captivity evaluation on the biological activities. *Toxicon* **2013**, *69*, 75–81. [CrossRef] [PubMed]

13

Etiology, Epizootiology and Control of Maedi-Visna in Dairy Sheep

Aphrodite I. Kalogianni [1], Ioannis Bossis [1], Loukia V. Ekateriniadou [2] and Athanasios I. Gelasakis [1,*]

1 Laboratory of Anatomy and Physiology of Farm Animals, Department of Animal Science, Agricultural University of Athens (AUA), Iera Odos 75 str., 11855 Athens, Greece; afrokalo@aua.gr (A.I.K.); bossisi@aua.gr (I.B.)

2 Veterinary Research Institute, ELGO-Demeter, Thermi, 57001 Thessaloniki, Greece; ekateriniadou@vri.gr

* Correspondence: gelasakis@aua.gr

Simple Summary: Maedi-visna is a chronic viral disease of sheep with worldwide prevalence. It is caused by a small ruminant lentivirus. Its clinical manifestation includes primarily pneumonia and mastitis, and secondarily, arthritis and encephalitis. It causes substantial economic losses associated with involuntary culling or death of infected animals and reduced productivity, challenging the sustainability of dairy sheep farms. The extensive spread of the disease and the lack of treatment or vaccines render surveillance and prevention strategies indispensable. Currently, the major obstacles in controlling the disease are (i) the absence of an effective protocol for the early and definitive diagnosis of infected animals, utilizing appropriate, universally accepted serological and molecular techniques, (ii) the long interval between infection and seroconversion, and (iii) lack of understanding whether horizontal or vertical transmission are the most important route of infection. Therefore, the most appropriate measures for the control of the disease should include more frequent serological testing with available diagnostics and isolation or culling of seropositive animals, incorporation of artificial suckling, and strengthening of hygiene and biosecurity protocols.

Abstract: Maedi-visna (MV) in sheep is caused by maedi-visna virus (MVV), a small ruminant lentivirus (SRLV) that causes chronic infection and inflammatory lesions in infected animals. Pneumonia and mastitis are its predominant clinical manifestations, and the tissues infected by MVV are mainly the lungs, the mammary gland, the nervous system and the joints. MV has a worldwide distribution with distinct MVV transmission patterns depending on circulating strains and regionally applied control/eradication schemes. Nevertheless, the prevalence rate of MV universally increases. Currently, gaps in understanding the epizootiology of MV, the continuous mutation of existing and the emergence of new small ruminant lentiviruses (SRLVs) strains, lack of an effective detection protocol and the inefficiency of currently applied preventive measures render elimination of MV an unrealistic target. Therefore, modifications on the existing MV surveillance and control schemes on an evidentiary basis are necessary. Updated control schemes require the development of diagnostic protocols for the early and definitive diagnosis of MVV infections. The objectives of this review are to summarize the current knowledge in the epizootiology and control of MV in dairy sheep, to describe the research framework and to cover existing gaps in understanding future challenges regarding MV.

Keywords: maedi-visna virus; ovine progressive pneumonia; small ruminant lentivirus; dairy sheep

1. Introduction

Maedi-visna (MV) (also known as ovine progressive pneumonia, OPP) is an incurable viral disease of sheep with very long incubation period that leads to life-long infection [1]. It is caused by non-oncogenic exogenous retroviruses [2], namely, maedi-visna virus (MVV) and caprine arthritis-encephalitis virus (CAEV), both belonging to a subgroup of viruses known as small ruminant lentiviruses (SRLVs). These viruses are structurally identical, display similar pathogenicity, and have genetic variants/strains that can infect both sheep and goats [3,4]. Species-specific categorization of SRLVs is not always valid since cross-species transmission of certain genotypes is evident with the direction of transmission not being always apparent [4]. Clinical symptoms of SRLVs infections are strain-dependent. Most prevalent are symptoms associated with the respiratory tract, such as dyspnea and abdominal breathing due to chronic interstitial pneumonia. Symptoms associated with encephalitis include instability, paresis, and paralysis. Other clinical manifestations such as mastitis (indurated udder), arthritis (lameness), progressive weakness and, in some cases, death of infected animals may also occur [5]. The primary route of infection for newborn lambs is the consumption of colostrum and milk from infected ewes [3]. Horizontal transmission via respiratory secretions is also significant [4], whereas, vertical transmission (transplacental) [6] and transmission via semen during mating or artificial insemination are also possible [6], but their significance and extent has not been thoroughly investigated.

Recognizing the socio-economic impact of MV, the World Organization for Animal Health (OIE) has included it in the list of notifiable terrestrial and aquatic animal diseases, with significant impact on international trade of animals and their products [7]. In dairy sheep, economic losses associated with the disease are rather extensive. During the last 5 years, the situation seems to have worsened as accumulating evidence suggests an increase in prevalence of the disease especially in the European continent. The scarcity however of epizootiological data regarding inter- and intra-farm transmission of the disease is a major obstacle for the development and implementation of evidence-based disease-control and eradication programs [8]. In particular, in the case of dairy sheep, there is a considerable shortage of certified MVV-free sheep breeding stocks in the international market. This is an obvious drawback in newly established intensive sheep farms, where the interest to buy MVV-free breeding stocks with high productive potential is large. Hence, the need to establish MVV-free dairy sheep farms is now more urgent than ever and forms a major issue for the conservation and evolution of the dairy sheep sector worldwide.

As there is no treatment against MV and all efforts for the development of vaccines did not produce any satisfactory results [6], the control of the disease and the reduction of its prevalence have been achieved to some degree through controlled eradication programs aiming at diagnosis of the infected animals at an early stage. However, these programs are heterogeneous in terms of their planning and effectiveness, which highly depends on the number of participating farms, the regional prevalence of the disease, and the diagnostic methods applied to detect the infected animals [9]. It has now been recognized that early diagnosis of viral infection in MV is more complicated than originally thought and constitutes a major barrier for the effective eradication of the disease [10,11]. Most of the programs used for the control of the disease are based on serological tests to detect antibodies against the virus [12]. This way, only the seropositive animals are diagnosed and removed from the flock. However, many animals infected with the virus remain undiagnosed due to the late (from a few months to three years) seroconversion [13,14]. In the past, several papers have reviewed the status of MV in sheep industry [5,6,15–22]; nevertheless, the objectives of this review paper are to summarize and provide an integrated overview of the current knowledge regarding the epizootiology and control strategies of MV in dairy sheep, to describe the research framework and to cover existing gaps in understanding future challenges regarding MV.

2. Current State of the Art in Epizootiology of the Disease

MV was initially described in Iceland in 1939, possibly originating from the importation of live animals from Germany. Although clinical signs were apparent, the situation was likely underestimated or misdiagnosed for many years [5,15]. Eventually, it was transmitted among several countries through the trading of breeding stocks (e.g., Denmark in 1968, Canada in 1970, Hungary in 1972, France in 1976, Norway in 1979, and Finland in 1994) [15].

Nowadays, MV has a worldwide spread, with the exception of Iceland, New Zealand, and Australia which are considered MVV-free regions, but not CAEV-free [23]. Despite the scarcity of MV epizootiological data in the Mediterranean countries with developed dairy sheep sector (Spain, Italy, and Greece), field observations suggest increased seroprevalence [16]. Based on these observations and having recognized the significance of the disease, several European countries (e.g., France, Germany, Netherlands, Italy, Switzerland, and Spain) have applied eradication programs. However, the effectiveness of these programs in controlling the disease has been questionable [6].

The majority of SRLVs epizootiological studies worldwide (Table 1) is limited to primarily small-scale estimation of seroprevalence; nationwide monitoring and active surveillance schemes are scarce as they require a substantial funding which is not available in most cases.

Table 1. Epizootiological studies regarding small ruminant lentiviruses (SRLVs).

Region	Species	Seropositivity at Animal Level (%)	Seroprevalence at Flock Level (%)	Number of Flocks	Number of Animals	Reference
Spain (Aragon)	s	52.8	100.0	554	274,048	[9]
Spain (Northwestern)	s	25.0	53.0	78	15,155	[10]
Italy (Southern)	g	18.64	51.69	1060	4800	[24]
Greece	s	41.96	N/A	6	143	[25]
Belgium	s	9.0	17.0	87	555	[11]
	g	6.0	13.0	76	401	
Switzerland	s	9.0	N/A	241	5084	[12]
Poland (Central Eastern)	s	10.2	N/A	98	2925	[26]
Turkey (Central Anatolia)	s	9.3	N/A	N/A	279	[14]
	g	7.5			146	
Turkey (Instanbul)	s	15.3	N/A	4	542	[14]
Germany (Mecklenburg Western-Pomerania)	s	28.8	51.2	41	2229	[8]
Canada (Manitoba)	s	2.5	25.1	77	2207	[27]
China (Yunnan, Guizhou, Gansu, Ningxia, Shandong, Sichuan, Hunan, Guangdong, Chongqing, Guangxi, Jilin, Anhui)	s	4.6–50.0	N/A	24	672	[28]

s: sheep, g: goats, N/A: relative data is not available.

3. Etiology

There is a continuous effort for the identification and classification of SRLVs strains due to large genetic diversity of the isolated viruses [17,29]. To date, five strain groups, namely, A, B, C, D, and E with their subtypes have been identified in sheep and goats [1,18]. Group A consists of MVV strains and has 15 subtypes, group B consists of CAEV strains with 3 subtypes, whereas, the other three groups refer to strains which have been isolated from Norway (group C), Spain and Switzerland (group D), and Italy (group E) [18]. Some of the classical strains with known sequences are the K1514 (Iceland) and its neurovirulent clones KV1772-kv72/67 and LV1-1KS1, SA-OMVV (South Africa), EV1 (UK), and P1OLV (Portugal). Many of the fore-mentioned strains have been found to infect both sheep and goats (e.g., all the strains of groups B, C, and D as well as group A subtypes A1–A6, A9, and A11–A13). The subtype A15 has been isolated only from sheep and subtypes A7, A8, A10, A14, E1, and E2 only from goats. The classification of SRLVs, the species infected and the countries first reported are summarized in Table 2.

Table 2. Classification of SRLVs strains.

Group	Subtype	Strain	Origin Country	Species	Reference
A	A1	P1OLV	Portugal	s/g	[30]
		KV1772	Iceland	s/g	[31]
		LV1-1, KV1514	Iceland	s/g	[32,33]
		EV1	England	s/g	[34]
		SA-OMVV	South Africa	s/g	[35]
	A2	85/34	USA	s	[36]
	A3	697	Spain	s/g	[37]
	A4	SRLV-A4	Switzerland	s/g	[29]
	A5, A6, A9, A11-A13			s/g	[17,18]
	A7, A8, A10, A14			g	[17,18]
	A15			S	[17,18]
	A16 and A17		Poland	g	[38]
B	B1	FESC-752	Mexico	s/g	[39]
		CAEV-CO	USA	s/g	[40,41]
		GANSU	China	s/g	[42]
		SHANXI	China	s/g	[43]
	B2	S-496	Spain	s/g	[44]
	B3	Volttera and Fonni	Italy	s/g	[45]
	B4		Canada	g	[46]
C		1GA	Norway	s/g	[47,48]
D			Spain, Switzerland	s/g	[17,18]
E	E1	Rocaverano	Italy	g	[49,50]
	E2	Seui	Italy	g	[49,50]

s: sheep, g: goats.

Recently, phylogenetic analysis revealed a new strain (CRF01_ABSRLV) which was isolated from Canadian goats and possibly originating from the combination of A2 and B1 subtypes [51]. The mechanism for generation of retroviral recombined strains is complicated and not very well understood. However, it could be considered among possible explanations for the emergence of new SRLV strains [51,52].

4. Clinical Signs and Gross Pathology

In the majority of cases, virus replication is slow and the number of infected blood cells in the circulation is very low [53]. Therefore, the clinical disease is latent or progressive and in many cases, the clinical signs are not evident or characteristic of the disease at its early stages [3]. Immunosuppression of animals due to aging, co-existing of diseases and environmental stressors accelerates virus replication and clinical evidence of the disease becomes apparent. At the flock-level, serum detection of antibodies, the severity of clinical disease and the number of deaths/culled animals, can be affected by management practices and the co-existence of other diseases [18].

Clinical manifestation of SRLVs infection depends on the virus strain, the host immune response and the host genetic profile regarding resistance or susceptibility to the virus [54,55]. Lesions of SRLVs infection in tissues and organs are caused both by the immune response to the viral antigens and the viral replication itself [3]. The tissues mainly infected by MVV are located at the lungs, the mammary gland, the nervous system, and the joints [3,19]. Pneumonia and mastitis are the predominant clinical manifestations of MVV in sheep [3]. Less frequently, lesions such as lymphoid tissue hyperplasia may be apparent in kidneys, liver, and heart, indicating them as possible target organs [56,57]. Multiple-organ infection may be observed in the progression of the disease, but the severity of lesions varies among the affected organs [19].

Respiratory clinical signs include dyspnea and increased respiratory rate, caused by the characteristic lymphocytic interstitial pneumonia; at necropsy, the lungs appear discolored, enlarged, and diffusely firm with grey spots on the pleural surface and the mediastinal lymph nodes are often enlarged [19,23].

Symptoms from the nervous system include ataxia, paresis, weakness in hind limbs, incoordination or, in heavier cases, total paralysis, due to meningoencephalitis, astrocytosis, microgliosis, and focal secondary demyelination in the brain and the spinal cord [3,19].

In mammary gland, MVV can cause an indurative non-suppurative interstitial mastitis [3,19]. The udder is hard but not painful, with decreased milk production mainly noticed the first days postpartum, a situation usually described as "hard udder syndrome". The lymphocytic inflammatory pattern, caused by the replication of virus in macrophages and mammary gland epithelial cells, provokes the destruction of the acinar structure and the reduction of milk production [19].

Arthritis can also be the outcome of MVV infection, although it is less common in sheep [3,16,18,19]. The affected joints are usually the carpal and tarsal, but metatarsal, metacarpal and vertebral joints can also be affected [16,18,19]. Infiltration of the synovial membrane by mononuclear cells is followed by villous hypertrophy, angiogenesis, and finally fibrosis, mineralization, and necrosis of synovium and joint capsule [3]. In advanced arthritis cases, the cartilage is destructed and the articular capsule is fibrotic [18,19]. In the majority of cases, arthritis is progressive causing lameness and involuntary culling of the animal, whereas less often it may regress [3].

5. Transmission

The mechanisms and the significance of horizontal and vertical transmission of the MVV have not been fully clarified yet [3]. The major routes of transmission have been described; however, their significance and extent remain unclear. This information is critical for the efficient designation of the eradication protocols, especially in intensively reared dairy sheep.

The vertical transmission of MVV refers to the transmission of the virus from the ewe to the lamb during pregnancy (transplacental), at lambing or during suckling [6]. Opinions regarding transplacental transmission are controversial [15,58]. Seropositivity of 4- to 9-months old lambs derived by caesarean section, isolated after birth and not allowed to suckle seropositive dams support the transplacental transmission [59]. However, the possibility of horizontal transmission post-lambing, complicates the assessment of the significance of either transplacental or horizontal transmission [6,15]. Vertical transmission at lambing refers to the transmission of virus while the lamb passes through the ewe's genital tract and it is exposed to maternal body fluids and blood. The exact significance of this route of transmission remains unknown [6,58].

The most significant route of vertical transmission is considered to be the lactogenic, through the ingestion of colostrum and milk from infected dams [6]. MVV shows tropism to the epithelial cells of the mammary gland and the resident macrophages, where it can replicate [60]. It has been found that isolated lambs fed colostrum or milk from infected ewes seroconverted a few months later and some of them were diagnosed with clinical disease later in their adult life [15]. There is evidence that the lactogenic transmission is more significant in small ruminants than in primates due to the higher permeability of the digestive tract of small ruminants in the first 24 h post-lambing [61,62], allowing virions and infected cells to be absorbed by the lamb's intestine [62]. However, not all the subgroup variants of MVV are efficiently transmitted via the lactogenic route as the envelope varies among the different subgroups of the MVV determining some of its physicochemical properties and facilitating or not the lactogenic transmission [62].

Horizontal transmission of MVV includes the environmental, mechanical and iatrogenic routes and mainly refers to the transmission through respiratory secretions [63]. Lungs are the main target organ of MVV in the respiratory tract. In lungs, the virus infects monocytes, macrophages, and dendritic cells, and it can be horizontally transmitted via respiratory secretions containing these cells [3,15]. In severe cases, MVV causes the characteristic lesions of interstitial pneumonia. In general, the lower respiratory tract, constitutes the main route of infection [15,64]. This route of transmission is of major importance in intensive and permanently housed sheep in sheds with inadequate ventilation and high stocking density [19]. In general, many researchers support that the airborne transmission can be an equally significant route of transmission as the vertical transmission. For this reason, the segregation of newborn lambs or non-infected animals from the infected ones is of major importance for the control of MVV transmission [3,15,65]. The significance of transmission through contaminated barns, sheds, feeding and water equipment and pastures or reusable veterinary equipment has not been fully clarified [6,15]. The presence of the virus in the water and air from pens with infected animals [63] indicates that waterborne and airborne transmission in the farms cannot be disregarded. Infection of dairy sheep via the teat canal during milking has also been reported [15].

Sexual transmission of the MVV is theoretically possible but not yet confirmed. However, there is evidence of virus proliferation in the genitals of infected rams and the virus has been found in the semen of rams with leucocytospermia and rams positive for *Brucella ovis* [3,66]. In another study using real-time PCR, proviral DNA of SRLV was found in semen (intermittent shedding) and the genital tract of rams suggesting possible sexual transmission [67].

6. Risk Factors

There are several risk factors that influence transmission of MVV between and within flocks. These factors determine the likelihood of infection, the prevalence, the incidence rate and other epizootiological characteristics of the disease. Identification and mitigation of risk factors at the farm level is therefore crucial when establishing a MVV control/eradication program. Flock size/stocking density, intensity of the farming system [9–12,26,27], and age distribution [9–11] affect the likelihood of seropositivity at flock level, indicating the significant role of horizontal transmission in the epizootiology of MV [9]. For example, lower prevalence in extensively reared sheep can be attributed to the reduced stocking rates and limited direct contact between animals [68,69], conditions that reduce the exposure to MVV and the possibility of airborne transmission through respiratory droplets during exhalation, sneezing, and coughing [3,6]. In flocks where MV co-exists with pulmonary adenomatosis, the transmission is favored by the increased quantities of respiratory secretions produced by infected sheep [9,15]. In these cases, late removal of clinical cases of MV and non-isolation of seropositive animals are significant risk factors for the transmission and increased seroprevalence of the disease.

Inappropriate cleaning and disinfection of milking equipment [15,19], reuse of infected needles and surgical equipment, inadequate hygiene conditions inside the barn and grazing at common pasturelands are also potential risk factors for the horizontal transmission of MVV.

Importation of breeding stocks from flocks of unknown MVV-status is associated with increased seroprevalence of MV [10,27]. The remarkable absence of certified MVV-free flocks to produce breeding stocks and the use of seropositive rams for mating or artificial insemination are the main causes. Surprisingly, despite the lactogenic transmission of the virus through colostrum/milk during suckling, a reduced seroprevalence in the replacement stocks has been observed in flocks with increased suckling period [9]. This is possibly the result of a confounding effect of farming system; increased weaning age is mainly observed in semi-extensive and extensive systems, where horizontal transmission is limited. On the other hand, early weaning is mainly practiced in intensive systems where virus transmission is facilitated mostly due to the permanent housing, the increased stocking density and the inappropriate ventilation [9,10,70]. Nevertheless, the use of colostrum/milk from seropositive dams and natural suckling of newborn animals constitute major risk factors. Also, in mixed-species flocks (sheep and goats) the seroprevalence has been found to be higher, possibly due to cross-species transmission of several SRLVs strains [10,70].

There is evidence of genetic resistance/susceptibility against SRLVs [71]. Different alleles of the cellular *TMEM154* (*Transmembrane protein 154*) gene have been found to be associated with the occurrence of MV. Haplotypes carrying nucleotide sequences that code for the amino acid glutamate at position 35 are associated with increased susceptibility to MV, whereas haplotypes carrying nucleotide sequences that code for lysine at the same position are associated with resistance to MV [72–74]. Also, the haplotype responsible for the susceptibility seems to be dominant against the "resistant" haplotype [74]. Although there is indication for association between *TMEM154* mutations and control of MVV infection, there is no proven association for all the haplotypes [73]. Other genes associated with virus susceptibility are the *DPPA2* (*Developmental Pluripotency Associated* 2)/*DPPA4* (*Developmental Pluripotency Associated* 4), *SYTL3* (*Synaptotagmin-Like* 3), *CCR5* (*Chemokine receptor 5*), MHC (Major Histocompatability Complex), *TLR7, TLR8, TLR9* (*Toll-like receptors*) genes, and APOBEC3 (Apolipoprotein B mRNA-editing enzyme) proteins [75–77], whereas the zinc finger cluster, *C19orf42* (*Chromosome 19 Open Reading Frame 19*)/*TMEM38A* (*Transmembrane Protein 38A*) and *DLGAP1* (*Discs Large (Drosophila) Homolog-Associated Protein 1*) genes may be used in genetic selection programs to facilitate the control of the disease [78]. The tripartite motif-containing 5 (TRIM5) protein has been studied and has been proved to contribute to the restriction of MVV [79].

7. Diagnosis

Early and efficient diagnosis of MV is a critical parameter for the control and eradication of the disease. The diagnosis of SRLVs infections is based on the detection of antibodies against the virus proteins or the viral genome. Current control and eradication programs are based on serological tests (mainly enzyme-linked immunosorbent assays (ELISAs)) to detect antibodies against the virus [13]. Therefore, only the seropositive animals are considered infected and subsequently removed from the flock. This is a major drawback for the eradication of the disease as the immune response to the disease (seroconversion) requires a long period of time and thereby, many of the infected animals remain undiagnosed carriers of the virus [8,14]. The available assays for the detection of antibodies are the agar gel immunodiffusion (AGID) test, radioimmunoprecipitation assay (RIPA), Western blotting (WB) and ELISA, whereas, polymerase chain reaction (PCR) is used for the detection of proviral DNA as described below.

7.1. AGID Test

AGID test is commonly used as a diagnostic tool in MV control programs due to its simplicity. It is a highly specific diagnostic method but less sensitive than ELISA [6,19–21]. For this reason, it is supplementary used for the confirmation of the ELISA test [20].

7.2. RIPA

RIPA is as old as WB and both of them are considered as the reference standards. They have similar sensitivity and are mainly used as confirmatory assays [21,22]. RIPA is not frequently used due to its high cost and its difficult application.

7.3. WB

WB is a confirmatory laboratory test which has been used to detect antibodies in serum that recognize viral proteins. In general, WB is more sensitive than the ELISAs but more cumbersome and with lower throughput [6,21]. Cross-reactivity with non-specific cellular proteins is also a problem.

7.4. ELISA

ELISA is the most commonly used test in population screening and for the surveillance of SRLVs. It detects antiviral antibodies with satisfactory sensitivity and specificity, indicating the occurrence of infection and seroconversion at some point [6,20]. Seropositivity is not necessarily followed by clinical disease and a seronegative animal cannot be safely considered to be free of infection. In many cases, seroconversion requires several months even in early-infected animals (e.g., lambs infected via colostrum consumption) [17]. Except for this hurdle, the antigenic heterogeneity of SRLVs strains (especially among different subtypes, like the CAEV-like and the MVV-like) may limit the diagnostic performance of currently available ELISA [80]. Antibody titers present remarkable variations during an animal's life and in some cases, they are undetectable using an ELISA, which renders the test unreliable for a definitive diagnosis [17,21,22,81].

7.5. PCR

PCR can directly detect proviral DNA in fluids and tissues across the animal body (lungs, milk, peripheral blood, mammary gland, synovial membranes etc.). The most reliable cells for the detection of virus are the peripheral blood mononuclear cells [20,21]. The most significant advantage of PCR is its ability to detect infection before seroconversion. However, PCR is not a reference method and it is suggested to be combined with serological testing to overcome the problem of selective specificity associated with the lack of reliable universal primers [6,20,21]. PCR nested methods and Real-Time-PCR (RT-PCR) increase the sensitivity and specificity of the method, however, their use is less frequent [20,21,82].

8. Treatment–Vaccination

There is neither a treatment nor an effective vaccine against MV. In the past, there have been attempts for the development of attenuated and subunit vaccines but none of them proved to be effective in preventing viral infections [83–89]. The major obstacles for the development of an effective MV vaccine include the necessity for the induction of high antibody titers against the virus, the wide genetic variation of viral strains and its continuous mutations, the increased post-infection immunological reaction, the post-vaccination challenge on the immune system and the evidence that the production of SRLV-specific neutralizing antibodies, following vaccination with whole virus-, protein-, and live attenuated-vaccines, is not always protective and in some cases may favor persistent infection [3,54]. The last obstacle is correlated with the fact that the relationship of antibody production with the protection against the SRLVs infection is doubtful and the cellular immune response seems to be more critical [3,54]. Current research efforts for the development of an effective vaccine include pseudoviruses/viral particles, recombinant viruses carrying genes from MVV, and naked plasmids carrying MVV genes plus factors enhancing innate immune responses. However, the effectiveness of these alternative strategies has not been sufficiently validated and thus are considered inappropriate for commercial use [20,54].

9. Preventive and Eradication Measures

The preventive measures and management interventions that could aid in controlling or eradicating MV should be decided on case by case and include the following:

1. Annual, biannual, or more frequent blood sampling from the breeding stocks and serological and molecular testing for the diagnosis of the infected animals.

2. Post-lambing management primarily based on the application of artificial suckling and the use of colostrum and milk substitutes or pasteurized colostrum/milk. The management of colostrum involves the administration of bovine colostrum, commercial sheep colostrum or colostrum only from uninfected ewes or heat-treated colostrum (56 °C for 60 min) [6,20,90]. Artificial suckling should take place in an area isolated from adult animals, which has to be regularly cleaned and disinfected.

3. Immediate removal of animals with apparent clinical signs and positive laboratory diagnosis. The selective culling of these animals and their replacements with seronegative animals, or the grouping of animals according to their seroconversion status can be applied in areas with moderate seroprevalence [6,20,91]. The later strategy requires the spatial and managerial separation of seropositive and seronegative groups within the farm [20,91]. In flocks with high seroprevalence, the most efficient practice is the annual culling of the oldest and less productive seropositive animals and their exclusive replacement with seronegative breeding stocks. The selective culling of seropositive animals would not facilitate the rapid control of the disease, but can contribute to the reduction of seroprevalence and infection rate at flock-level, enhancing the potential of a more drastic elimination program in future time (i.e., culling of the remaining seropositive animals) [9,20].

4. Keeping the replacement animals, post-weaning, in separate housing facilities to avoid horizontal transmission of MVV through the contact with adult animals of the remaining flock.

5. Purchased animals should be from certified MVV-free farms. Imported animals need to remain on quarantine until the MV-status is determined using the most appropriate assays.

6. Regular cleaning and disinfection of facilities and equipment with appropriate disinfectants. The cleaning and disinfection schedule must include the barn (floor, walls, bedding), the milking machine, the feeders and the waterers.

7. Reduction of stocking density (sufficient area and volume) and adequate ventilation.

8. Implementation of general good hygiene practices. Use of disposable needles or sterilization of metal needles before their reuse is necessary. Similarly, the medical equipment should be sterilized after its use.

9. MV seronegative milking ewes should be grouped separately and machine-milked before the seropositive ones.

10. Grazing in communal pastures and sharing of infrastructures and equipment should be avoided when the MVV-status of the flocks is unknown.

11. Rams used either for mating or for semen collection need to be MVV-free [92]. Currently, attempts are being made to produce SRLVs-free breeding stocks via reproductive biotechnologies like artificial insemination and embryo transfer even from infected males and females, respectively. In the case of embryo transfer, this may be possible via the removal of cumulus oophorus cells [92].

12. Breeding for resistance could also be considered, but universally accepted resistant genotypes are yet to be developed [18].

The characterization of a flock as MVV-free demands two to five successive negative tests every 6 months, yearly or every 2 years (depending on the country). The trade of live animals is allowed when the animals have no clinical signs of MV, the adult animals are seronegative and MV has neither been clinically nor serologically diagnosed in the sheep flocks of origin during the last three years. Also, artificial insemination is allowed only using semen from seronegative rams. According to OIE, a country is considered MVV-free when <1.0% of herds are infected with 99.0% probability.

After the first implemented eradication program in Iceland, a lot of countries applied their own eradication programs (almost all the European countries and Canada) with variable results. The major obstacles for the successful implementation of eradication programs are (i) the possible refusal of farmers' participation [6,9], (ii) the breed variability, which, as previously mentioned associates with susceptibility and resistance against the disease, (iii) the genetic variability of the viral strains and the different epizootiological characteristics of the disease (virulence, transmission, seroconversion, seroprevalence at flock level, etc.) and (iv) the heterogeneous farming and herd health management systems. For this reason, the eradication program needs to be adjusted and optimized according to the fore-mentioned factors. An indicating classification of the flocks according to the observed seroprevalence could be: flocks with high (>70.0%), medium (40.0%–69.0%), low (10.0%–39.0%), very low (1.0%–9.0%) seroprevalence and the MVV-free flocks (<1.0%) [6,20].

The eradication measures when considered in a country-wide scale should include both species of small ruminants due to the fact that the cross transmission has been proven and is a significant risk factor in the spread of the virus [89]. Moreover, the existence of reference laboratories for the control of MV is of major importance [20]. These laboratories will be responsible for the surveillance of MV at national level and will coordinate all the efforts for the elimination of the disease [6].

Total replacement of seropositive flocks with breeding stocks from MVV-free flocks could be a sustainable option only in areas where the seroprevalence is very low and MVV-free flocks are available. Otherwise, there is a serious threat for significant monetary losses and restriction of genetic resources which may undermine the sustainability of the farms, particularly in areas with developed dairy sheep farming industry [20].

10. Conclusions and Future Challenges in Controlling MV

Epizootiological investigations regarding SRLVs infections are essential for the territorial mapping of virus distribution. The scarcity of detailed epizootiological data, in combination with the continuous mutations of SRLVs strains, render the creation of a universal, reliable and valid diagnostic protocol, and consequently the control of SRLVs, a rather complicated task.

For the early and definitive diagnosis of SRLVs infections, development of appropriate combinations of serological and molecular tests (ELISAs and PCR) on an evidential basis is suggested and forms a challenging research field in the future.

Determining the epizootiological traits of SRLVs infections and particularly the significance of the different routes of viral transmission will facilitate the decision-making process towards the determination of the most effective measures for the creation of MVV-free flocks. The global spread of SRLVs highlights the underestimation of the problem by the farmers and the insufficient implementation of the suggested preventive measures, which mainly focus on the lactogenic and airborne transmission of the disease, but may also be indicative of the failure in controlling the disease using these measures. Therefore, the significance of every other possible route of transmission (transplacental, sexual, and iatrogenic) needs to be carefully assessed and revised, and relevant preventive measures need to be integrated in the MV control protocols.

Exploitation of active surveillance programs and quantification of the consequences of SRLVs' infection on production [93], health and welfare traits are critical endeavors to determine the overall impact of the disease on the sustainability and resilience of the farms. For this reason, large-scale longitudinal and cohort studies are necessary to collect data for the determination of the most appropriate prediction models estimating the cost of the disease (production losses, involuntary culling/increased replacement rate, predisposition to other diseases and control measures), which remains unknown.

Breeding for resistance against SRLVs is an emerging research field. Specific genes have already been found to be associated with resistance or susceptibility to the disease and the discovery of additional genomic regions may increase the options for its control through marker-assisted selection (MAS) [76].

Despite the significant advances accomplished in SRLVs immunization studies, there are still important challenges to address, as vaccination against SRLVs may contribute to either controlling or enhancing MV [54]. Therefore, research efforts on the field of immunization have to be focused on the development of safe and effective vaccines, with the potential of universal application and mass production.

References

1. De Boer, G.F. Zwoegerziekte virus, the causative agent for progressive interstitial pneumonia (maedi) and meningo-leucoencephalitis (visna) in sheep. *Res. Vet. Sci.* **1975**, *18*, 15–25. [CrossRef]
2. Pálsson, P.A. Maedi-Visna. History and Clinical Description. In *Maedi-Visna and Related Diseases. Developments in Veterinary Virology*; Pétursson, G., Hoff-Jørgensen, R., Eds.; Kluwer Academic Publishers: Norwell, MA, USA, 1990; Volume 10, pp. 3–74. ISBN 978-1-4612-8892-3.
3. Blacklaws, B.A. Small ruminant lentiviruses: Immunopathogenesis of Visna-Maedi and caprine arthritis and encephalitis virus. *Comp. Immunol. Microbiol. Infect. Dis.* **2012**, *35*, 259–269. [CrossRef] [PubMed]
4. Leroux, C.; Cruz, J.C.; Mornex, J.F. SRLVs: A genetic continuum of lentiviral species in sheep and goats with cumulative evidence of cross species transmission. *Curr. HIV Res.* **2010**, *8*, 94–100. [CrossRef] [PubMed]
5. Straub, O.C. Maedi–Visna virus infection in sheep. History and present knowledge. *Comp. Immunol. Microbiol. Infect. Dis.* **2004**, *27*, 1–5. [CrossRef]

6. Peterhans, E.; Greenland, T.; Badiola, J.; Harkiss, G.; Bertoni, G.; Amorena, B.; Eliaszewicz, M.; Juste, R.A.; Kraβnig, R.; Lafont, J.P.; et al. Routes of transmission and consequences of small ruminant lentiviruses (SRLVs) infection and eradication schemes. *Vet. Res.* **2004**, *35*, 257–274. [CrossRef]
7. *Terrestial Animal Health Code*, 28th ed.; World Organization for Animal Health: Paris, France, 2019; Volume 2, ISBN 978-92-95108-86-8.
8. Hüttner, K.; Seelmann, M.; Feldhusen, F. Prevalence and risk factors for Maedi-Visna in sheep farms in Mecklenburg-Western-Pomerania. *Berl. Münch. Tierärztl.* **2010**, *123*, 463–467. [CrossRef]
9. Pérez, M.; Biescas, E.; de Andrés, X.; Leginagoikoa, I.; Salazar, E.; Berriatua, E.; Reina, R.; Bolea, R.; de Andrés, D.; Juste, R.A.; et al. Visna/Maedi virus serology in sheep: Survey, risk factors and implementation of a successful control programme in Aragón (Spain). *Vet. J.* **2010**, *186*, 221–225. [CrossRef]
10. Lago, N.; López, C.; Panadero, R.; Cienfuegos, J.; Pato, A.; Prieto, P.; Díaz, P.; Mourazos, N.; Fernández, G. Seroprevalence and risk factors associated with Visna/Maedi virus in semi-intensive lamb-producing flocks in northwestern Spain. *Prev. Vet. Med.* **2012**, *103*, 163–169. [CrossRef]
11. Michiels, R.; van Mael, E.; Quinet, C.; Welby, S.; Cay, A.B.; de Regge, N. Seroprevalence and risk factors related to small ruminant lentivirus infections in Belgian sheep and goats. *Prev. Vet. Med.* **2018**, *151*, 13–20. [CrossRef]
12. Schaller, P.; Vogt, H.R.; Strasser, M.; Nettleton, P.F.; Peterhans, E.; Zanoni, R. Seroprevalence of maedi-visna and border disease in Switzerland. *Schweiz. Arch. Tierh.* **2000**, *142*, 145–153.
13. Kaba, J.; Czopowicz, M.; Ganter, M.; Nowicki, M.; Witkowski, L.; Nowicka, D.; Szaluś-Jordanow, O. Risk factors associated with seropositivity to small ruminant lentiviruses in goat herds. *Res. Vet. Sci.* **2013**, *94*, 225–227. [CrossRef]
14. Azkur, A.K.; Aslan, M.E. Serological and Epidemiological Investigation of Bluetongue, Maedi-Visna and Caprine Arthritis-Encephalitis Viruses in Small Ruminant in Kirikkale District in Turkey. *Kafkas Univ. Vetr. Fak. Derg.* **2011**, *17*, 803–808. [CrossRef]
15. Blacklaws, B.A.; Berriatua, E.; Torsteinsdottir, S.; Watt, N.J.; de Andres, D.; Klein, D.; Harkiss, G.D. Transmission of small ruminant lentiviruses. *Vet. Microbiol.* **2004**, *101*, 199–208. [CrossRef] [PubMed]
16. Christodoulopoulos, G. Maedi–Visna: Clinical review and short reference on the disease status in Mediterranean countries. *Small Rumin. Res.* **2006**, *62*, 47–53. [CrossRef]
17. Ramírez, H.; Reina, R.; Amorena, B.; de Andrés, D.; Martínez, H.A. Small Ruminant Lentiviruses: Genetic Variability, Tropism and Diagnosis. *Viruses* **2013**, *5*, 1175–1207. [CrossRef] [PubMed]
18. Gomez-Lucia, E.; Barquero, N.; Domenech, A. Maedi-Visna virus: Current perspectives. *Vet. Med.* **2018**, *9*, 11–21. [CrossRef]
19. Minguijón, E.; Reina, R.; Pérez, M.; Polledo, L.; Villoria, M.; Ramírez, H.; Leginagoikoa, I.; Badiola, J.J.; García-Marín, J.F.; de Andrés, D.; et al. Small ruminant lentivirus infections and diseases. *Vet. Microbiol.* **2015**, *181*, 75–89. [CrossRef]
20. Reina, R.; Berriatua, E.; Lujan, L.; Juste, R.; Sanchez, A.; de Andres, D.; Amorena, B. Prevention strategies against small ruminant lentiviruses: An update. *Vet. J.* **2009**, *182*, 31–37. [CrossRef]
21. Herrmann-Hoesing, L.M. Diagnostic assays used to control small ruminant lentiviruses. *J. Vet. Diagn. Investig.* **2010**, *22*, 843–855. [CrossRef]
22. De Andres, D.; Klein, D.; Watt, N.J.; Berriatua, E.; Torsteinsdottir, S.; Blacklaws, B.A.; Harkiss, G.D. Diagnostic tests for small ruminant lentiviruses. *Vet. Microbiol.* **2005**, *107*, 49–62. [CrossRef]
23. López, A.; Martinson, S.A. *Respiratory System, Mediastinum, and Pleurae, In Pathologic Basis of Veterinary Disease*, 6th ed.; Zachary, J.F., Ed.; Mosby: St. Louis, MO, USA, 2017; pp. 471–560. ISBN 9780323357753.
24. Cirone, F.; Maggiolino, A.; Cirilli, M.; Sposato, A.; de Palo, P.; Ciappetta, G.; Pratelli, A. Small ruminant lentiviruses in goats in southern Italy: Serological evidence, risk factors and implementation of control programs. *Vet. Microbiol.* **2019**, *228*, 143–146. [CrossRef] [PubMed]
25. Karanikolaou, K.; Angelopoulou, K.; Papanastasopoulou, M.; Koumpati-Artopiou, M.; Papadopoulos, O.; Koptopoulos, G. Detection of small ruminant lentiviruses by PCR and serology tests in field samples of animals from Greece. *Small Rumin. Res.* **2005**, *58*, 181–187. [CrossRef]
26. Junkuszewa, A.; Dudko, P.; Bojar, W.; Olech, M.; Osinski, Z.; Gruszecki, T.M.; Kania, M.G.; Kuźmak, J.; Czerski, G. Risk factors associated with small ruminant lentivirus infection in eastern Poland sheep flocks. *Prev. Vet. Med.* **2016**, *127*, 44–49. [CrossRef] [PubMed]

27. Shuaib, M.; Green, C.; Rashid, M.; Duizer, G.; Whiting, T.L. Herd risk factors associated with sero-prevalence of Maedi-Visna in the Manitoba sheep population. *Can. Vet. J.* **2010**, *51*, 385–390.
28. Zhang, K.; He, J.; Liu, Y.; Shang, Y.; Liu, X. A Seroprevalence Survey of Maedi-Visna Among Twenty-Four Ovine Floks from Twelve Regions of China. *J. Integr. Agric.* **2013**, *12*, 2321–2323. [CrossRef]
29. Shah, C.; Boni, J.; Huder, J.B.; Vogt, H.R.; Muhlherr, J.; Zanoni, R.; Miserez, R.; Lutz, H.; Schüpbach, J. Phylogenetic analysis and reclassification of caprine and ovine lentiviruses based on 104 new isolates: Evidence for regular sheep-to-goat transmission and worldwide propagation through livestock trade. *Virology* **2004**, *319*, 12–26. [CrossRef]
30. Fevereiro, M.T.; Barros, S.S. Caracterização biológica e molecular de um lentivírus de ovino isolado em Portugal. *RPCV* **2004**, *99*, 27–39.
31. Andresson, O.S.; Elser, J.E.; Tobin, G.J.; Greenwood, J.D.; Gonda, M.A.; Georgsson, G.; Andrésdóttir, V.; Benediktsdóttir, E.; Carlsdóttir, H.M.; Mäntylä, E.O. Nucleotide sequence and biological properties of a pathogenic proviral molecular clone of neurovirulent visna virus. *Virology* **1993**, *193*, 89–105. [CrossRef]
32. Sonigo, P.; Alizon, M.; Staskus, K.; Klatzmann, D.; Cole, S.; Danos, O.; Retzel, E.; Tiollais, P.; Haase, A.; Wain-Hobson, S. Nucleotide sequence of the visna lentivirus: Relationship to the AIDS virus. *Cell* **1985**, *42*, 369–382. [CrossRef]
33. Staskus, K.A.; Retzel, E.F.; Lewis, E.D.; Silsby, J.L.; Sheila, C.S.T.; Rank, J.M.; Wietgrefe, S.W.; Haase, A.T.; Cook, R.; Fast, D.; et al. Isolation of replication-competent molecular clones of visna virus. *Virology* **1991**, *181*, 228–240. [CrossRef]
34. Sargan, D.R.; Bennet, I.D.; Cousens, C.; Roy, D.J.; Blacklaws, B.A.; Dalziel, R.G.; Watt, N.J.; Mc Connell, I. Nucleotide sequence of EV1, a British isolate of maedi-visna virus. *J. Gen. Virol.* **1991**, *72*, 1893–1903. [CrossRef] [PubMed]
35. Quérat, G.; Audoly, G.; Sonigo, P.; Vigne, R. Nucleotide sequence analysis of SA-OMVV, a visna-related ovine lentivirus: Phylogenetic history of lentiviruses. *Virology* **1990**, *175*, 434–447. [CrossRef]
36. Karr, B.M.; Chebloune, Y.; Leung, K.; Narayan, O. Genetic characterization of two phenotypically distinct North American ovine lentiviruses and their possible origin from caprine arthritis-encephalitis virus. *Virology* **1996**, *225*, 1–10. [CrossRef] [PubMed]
37. Glaria, I.; Reina, R.; Ramirez, H.; de Andres, X.; Crespo, H.; Jauregui, P.; Salazar, E.; Luján, L.; Pérez, M.M.; Benavides, J.; et al. Visna/Maedi virus genetic characterization and serological diagnosis of infection in sheep from a neurological outbreak. *Vet. Microbiol.* **2012**, *155*, 137–146. [CrossRef]
38. Olech, M.; Valas, S.; Kuźmak, J. Epidemiological survey in single-species flocks from Poland reveals expanded genetic and antigenic diversity of small ruminant lentiviruses. *PLoS ONE* **2018**, *13*, e0193892. [CrossRef]
39. Ramirez, H.; Glaria, I.; de Andres, X.; Martinez, H.A.; Hernandez, M.M.; Reina, R.; Iráizoz, E.; Crespo, H.; Berriatua, E.; Vázquez, J.; et al. Recombinant small ruminant lentivirus subtype B1 in goats and sheep of imported breeds in Mexico. *Vet. J.* **2011**, *190*, 169–172. [CrossRef]
40. Narayan, O.; Clements, J.E.; Strandberg, J.D.; Cork, L.C.; Griffin, D.E. Biological characterization of the virus causing leukoencephalitis and arthritis in goats. *J. Gen. Virol.* **1980**, *50*, 69–79. [CrossRef]
41. Saltarelli, M.; Querat, G.; Konings, D.A.; Vigne, R.; Clements, J.E. Nucleotide sequence and transcriptional analysis of molecular clones of CAEV which generate infectious virus. *Virology* **1990**, *179*, 347–364. [CrossRef]
42. Qu, J.; Guo, W.; Zhao, L.; Sheng, R.; Xiang, W. The gene cloning and sequence analysis of the whole genome of Caprine Arthritis Encephalitis virus (CAEV) GANSU strain. *Chin. J. Virol.* **2005**, *21*, 389–392.
43. Huang, J.; Sun, Y.; Liu, Y.; Xiao, H.; Zhuang, S. Development of a loop-mediated isothermal amplification method for rapid detection of caprine arthritis-encephalitis virus proviral DNA. *Arch. Virol.* **2012**, *157*, 1463–1469. [CrossRef]
44. Glaria, I.; Reina, R.; Crespo, H.; de Andres, X.; Ramirez, H.; Biescas, E.; Pérez, M.M.; Badiola, J.; Luján, L.; Amorena, B.; et al. Phylogenetic analysis of SRLV sequences from an arthritic sheep outbreak demonstrates the introduction of CAEV-like viruses among Spanish sheep. *Vet. Microbiol.* **2009**, *138*, 156–162. [CrossRef] [PubMed]
45. Bertolotti, L.; Mazzei, M.; Puggioni, G.; Carrozza, M.L.; Giudici, S.D.; Muz, D.; Juganaru, M.; Patta, C.; Tolari, F.; Rosati, S. Characterization of new small ruminant lentivirus subtype B3 suggests animal trade within the Mediterranean Basin. *J. Gen. Virol.* **2011**, *92*, 1923–1929. [CrossRef]

46. Santry, A.; de Jong, J.; Gold, A.C.; Walsh, S.R.; Menzies, P.I.; Wootton, S.K. Genetic characterization of small ruminant lentiviruses circulating in naturally infected sheep and goats in Ontario, Canada. *Virus Res.* **2013**, *175*, 30–44. [CrossRef] [PubMed]
47. Gjerset, B.; Jonassen, C.M.; Rimstad, E. Natural transmission and comparative analysis of small ruminant lentiviruses in the Norwegian sheep and goat populations. *Virus Res.* **2007**, *125*, 153–161. [CrossRef] [PubMed]
48. Gjerset, B.; Storset, A.K.; Rimstad, E. Genetic diversity of small-ruminant lentiviruses: Characterization of Norwegian isolates of Caprine arthritis encephalitis virus. *J. Gen. Virol.* **2006**, *87*, 573–580. [CrossRef]
49. Reina, R.; Grego, E.; Bertolotti, L.; de Meneghi, D.; Rosati, S. Genome analysis of small-ruminant lentivirus genotype E: A caprine lentivirus with natural deletions of the dUTPase subunit, vpr-like accessory gene, and 70-base-pair repeat of the U3 region. *J. Virol.* **2009**, *83*, 1152–1155. [CrossRef]
50. Reina, R.; Bertolotti, L.; Dei Giudici, S.; Puggioni, G.; Ponti, N.; Profiti, M.; Patta, C.; Rosati, S. Small Ruminant Lentivirus genotype E is widespread in Sarda Goat. *Vet. Microbiol.* **2010**, *144*, 24–31. [CrossRef]
51. L'Homme, Y.; Leboeuf, A.; Arsenault, J.; Fras, M. Identification and characterization of an emerging small ruminant lentivirus circulating recombinant form (CRF). *Virology* **2015**, *475*, 159–171. [CrossRef]
52. Pisoni, G.; Bertoni, G.; Puricelli, M.; Maccalli, M.; Moroni, P. Demonstration of coinfection with and recombination by caprine arthritis-encephalitis virus and maedi-visna virus in naturally infected goats. *J. Virol.* **2007**, *81*, 4948–4955. [CrossRef]
53. McNeilly, T.N.; Baker, A.; Brown, J.K.; Collie, D.; MacLachlan, G.; Rhind, S.M.; Harkiss, G.D. Role of Alveolar Macrophages in Respiratory Transmission of Visna/Maedi Virus. *J. Virol.* **2008**, *82*, 1526–1536. [CrossRef]
54. Reina, R.; de Andrés, D.; Amorena, B. Immunization against Small Ruminant Lentiviruses. *Viruses* **2013**, *5*, 1948–1963. [CrossRef] [PubMed]
55. Gayo, E.; Polledo, L.; Balseiro, A.; Martinez, C.P.; Garcia Iglesias, M.J.; Preziuso, S.; Rossi, G.; García Marín, J.F. Inflammatory Lesion Patterns in Target Organs of Visna/Maedi in Sheep and their Significance in the Pathogenesis and Diagnosis of the Infection. *J. Comp. Pathol.* **2018**, *159*, 49–56. [CrossRef] [PubMed]
56. Angelopoulou, K.; Brellou, G.D.; Vlemmas, I. Detection of Maedi-Visna Virus in the Kidneys of Naturally Infected Sheep. *J. Comp. Path.* **2006**, *134*, 329–335. [CrossRef] [PubMed]
57. Brellou, G.D.; Angelopoulou, K.; Poutahidis, T.; Vlemmas, I. Detection of Maedi-Visna Virus in the Liver and Heart of Naturally Infected Sheep. *J. Comp. Path.* **2007**, *136*, 27–35. [CrossRef]
58. Broughton-Neiswanger, L.E.; White, S.N.; Knowles, D.P.; Mousel, M.R.; Lewis, G.S.; Herndon, D.R.; Herrmann-Hoesing, L.M. Non-maternal transmission is the major mode of ovine lentivirus transmission in a ewe flock: A molecular epidemiology study. *Infect. Genet. Evol.* **2010**, *10*, 998–1007. [CrossRef]
59. Cutlip, R.C.; Lehmkuhl, H.D.; Jackson, T.A. Intrauterine transmission of ovine progressive pneumonia virus. Am. *J. Vet. Res.* **1981**, *42*, 1795–1797.
60. Bolea, R.; Monleón, E.; Carrasco, L.; Vargas, A.; de Andrés, D.; Amorena, B.; Badiola, J.J.; Luján, L. Maedi-visna virus infection of ovine mammary epithelial cells. *Vet. Res.* **2006**, *37*, 133–144. [CrossRef]
61. Preziuso, S.; Renzoni, G.; Allen, T.E.; Taccini, E.; Rossi, G.; DeMartini, J.C.; Braca, G. Colostral transmission of Maedi Visna virus: Sites of viral entry in lambs born from experimentally infected ewes. *Vet. Microbiol.* **2004**, *104*, 157–164. [CrossRef]
62. Pisoni, G.; Bertoni, G.; Manarolla, G.; Vogt, H.R.; Scaccabarozzi, L.; Locatelli, C.; Moroni, P. Genetic analysis of small ruminant lentiviruses following lactogenic transmission. *Virology* **2010**, *407*, 91–99. [CrossRef]
63. Radostits, O.M.; Gay, C.C.; Blood, D.C.; Hinchcliff, K.W. Ovine progressive pneumonia (Maedi, Maedi-Visna). In *Veterinary Medicine A Textbook of the Diseases of Cattle, Sheep, Pigs, Goats and Horses*, 9th ed., W.B. Saunders Company Ltd.: London, UK, 2000; pp. 1186–1189.
64. McNeilly, T.N.; Tennant, P.; Lujan, L.; Perez, M.; Harkiss, G.D. Differential infection efficiencies of peripheral lung and tracheal tissues in sheep infected with Visna/maedi virus via the respiratory tract. *J. Gen. Virol.* **2007**, *88*, 670–679. [CrossRef] [PubMed]
65. Villoria, M.; Leginagoikoa, I.; Luján, L.; Pérez, M.; Salazar, E.; Berriatua, E.; Juste, R.A.; Minguijón, E. Detection of small ruminant lentivirus in environmental samples of air and water. *Small Rumin. Res.* **2013**, *110*, 155–160. [CrossRef]
66. Preziuso, S.; Sanna, E.; Sanna, M.P.; Loddo, C.; Cerri, D.; Taccini, E.; Mariotti, F.; Braca, G.; Rossi, G.;

Renzoni, G. Association of maedi visna virus with Brucella ovis infectionin rams. *Eur. J. Histochem.* **2003**, *47*, 151–1588. [CrossRef] [PubMed]

67. Peterson, K.; Brinkhof, J.; Houwers, D.J.; Colenbrander, B.; Gadella, B.M. Presence of pro-lentiviral DNA in male sexual organs and ejaculates of small ruminants. *Theriogenology* **2008**, *69*, 433–442. [CrossRef] [PubMed]
68. Leginagoiko, I.; Daltabuit-Test, M.; Álvarez, V.; Arranz, J.; Juste, R.A.; Amorena, B.; de Andrés, D.; Luján, L.L.; Badiola, J.J.; Berriatua, E. Horizontal Maedi-Visna virus (MVV) infection in adult dairy-sheep raised under varying MVV-infection pressures investigated by ELISA and PCR. *Res. Vet. Sci.* **2006**, *80*, 235–241. [CrossRef]
69. Leginagoikoa, I.; Juste, R.A.; Barandika, J.; Amorena, B.; de Andrés, D.; Lujánc, L.; Badiola, J.; Beriattua, E. Extensive rearing hinders Maedi-Visna Virus (MVV) infection in sheep. *Vet. Res.* **2006**, *37*, 767–778. [CrossRef] [PubMed]
70. Alba, A.; Allepuz, A.; Serrano, E.; Casal, J. Seroprevalence and spatial distribution of Maedi–Visna virus and pestiviruses in Catalonia (Spain). *Small Rumin. Res.* **2008**, *78*, 80–86. [CrossRef]
71. Leginagoikoa, I.; Minguijon, E.; Juste, R.A.; Barandika, J.; Amorena, B.; de Andres, D.; Badiola, J.J.; Luján, L.; Berriatua, E. Effects of housing on the incidence of visna/maedi virus infection in sheep flocks. *Res. Vet. Sci.* **2010**, *88*, 415–421. [CrossRef]
72. Heaton, M.; Clawson, M.; Chitko-Mckown, C.; Leymaster, K.; Smith, T.; Harhay, G.P.; White, S.N.; Herrmann-Hoesing, L.M.; Mousel, M.R.; Lewis, G.S.; et al. Reduced Lentivirus Susceptibility in Sheep with TMEM154 Mutations. *PLoS Genet.* **2012**, *8*, e1002467. [CrossRef]
73. Alshanbari, F.A.; Mousel, M.R.; Reynolds, J.O.; Herrmann-Hoesing, L.M.; Highland, M.A.; Lewis, G.S.; White, N. Mutations in Ovis aries TMEM154 are associated with lower small ruminant lentivirus proviral concentration in one sheep flock. *Anim. Genet.* **2014**, *45*, 565–571. [CrossRef]
74. Leymaster, K.A.; Chitko-McKown, C.G.; Clawson, M.L.; Harhay, G.P.; Heaton, M.P. Effects of TMEM154 haplotypes 1 and 3 on susceptibility to ovine progressive pneumonia virus following natural exposure in sheep. *J. Anim. Sci.* **2013**, *91*, 5114–5121. [CrossRef]
75. Larruskain, A.; Jugo, B.M. Retroviral infections in sheep and goats: Small ruminant lentiviruses and host interaction. *Viruses* **2013**, *5*, 2043–2061. [CrossRef]
76. White, S.N.; Knowles, D.P. Expanding possibilities for intervention against small ruminant lentiviruses through genetic marker-assisted selective breeding. *Viruses* **2013**, *5*, 1466–1499. [CrossRef] [PubMed]
77. Stonos, N.; Wootton, S.K.; Karrow, N. Immunogenetics of small ruminant lentiviral infections. *Viruses* **2014**, *6*, 3311–3333. [CrossRef] [PubMed]
78. White, S.N.; Mousel, M.R.; Herrmann-Hoesing, L.M.; Reynolds, J.O.; Leymaster, K.A.; Neibergs, H.L.; Lewis, G.S.; Knowles, D.P. Genome-Wide Association Identifies Multiple Genomic Regions Associated with Susceptibility to and Control of Ovine Lentivirus. *PLoS ONE* **2012**, *7*, e47829. [CrossRef] [PubMed]
79. Jáuregui, P.; Crespo, H.; Glaria, I.; Luján, L.; Contreras, A.; Rosati, S.; de Andrés, D.; Amorena, B.; Towers, G.J.; Reina, R. Ovine TRIM5a Can Restrict Visna/Maedi Virus. *J. Virol.* **2012**, *86*, 9504–9509. [CrossRef]
80. Lacerenza, D.; Giammarioli, M.; Grego, E.; Marini, C.; Profiti, M.; Rutili, D.; Rosati, S. Antibody response in sheep experimentally infected with different small ruminant lentivirus genotypes. *Vet. Immunol. Immunopathol.* **2006**, *112*, 264–271. [CrossRef]
81. De Andrés, D.; Ramírez, H.; Bertolotti, L.; San Román, B.; Glaria, I.; Crespo, H.; Jáuregui, P.; Minguijón, E.; Juste, R.; Leginagoikoa, I.; et al. An insight into a combination of ELISA strategies to diagnose small ruminant lentivirus infections. *Vet. Immunol. Immunopathol.* **2013**, *152*, 277–288. [CrossRef]
82. Carrozza, M.L.; Mazzei, M.; Bandecchi, P.; Fraisier, C.; Pérez, M.; Suzan-Monti, M.; de Andrés, D.; Amorena, B.; Rosati, S.; Andrésdottir, V.; et al. Development and comparison of strain specific gag and pol real-time PCR assays for the detection of Visna/maedi virus. *J. Virol. Methods.* **2010**, *165*, 161–167. [CrossRef]
83. Cheevers, W.P.; Knowles, D.P.; McGuire, T.C.; Baszler, T.V.; Hullinger, G.A. Caprine arthritis–encephalitis lentivirus (CAEV) challenge of goats immunized with recombinant vaccinia virus expressing CAEV surface and transmembrane envelope glycoproteins. *Vet. Immunol. Immunopathol.* **1994**, *42*, 237–251. [CrossRef]
84. Petursson, G.; Matthiasdottir, S.; Svansson, V.; Andresdottir, V.; Georgsson, G.; Martin, A.H.; Agnarsdóttir, G.; Gísladóttir, E.; Arnadóttir, S.; Högnadóttir, S.; et al. Mucosal vaccination with an attenuated maedi-visna virus clone. *Vaccine* **2005**, *23*, 3223–3228. [CrossRef]
85. Gonzalez, B.; Reina, R.; Garcia, I.; Andres, S.; Glaria, I.; Alzueta, M.; Mora, M.I.; Jugo, B.M.; Arrieta-Aguirre, I.; de la Lastra, J.M.; et al. Mucosal immunization of sheep with a Maedi-Visna virus (MVV) env DNA vaccine protects against early MVV productive infection. *Vaccine* **2005**, *23*, 4342–4352. [CrossRef] [PubMed]

86. Torsteinsdottir, S.; Carlsdottir, H.M.; Svansson, V.; Matthiasdottir, S.; Martin, A.H.; Petursson, G. Vaccination of sheep with Maedi-visna virus gag gene and protein, beneficial or harmful? *Vaccine* **2007**, *25*, 6713–6720. [CrossRef] [PubMed]

87. de Andres, X.; Reina, R.; Ciriza, J.; Crespo, H.; Glaria, I.; Ramirez, H.; Grilló, M.J.; Pérez, M.M.; Andrésdóttir, V.; Rosati, S.; et al. Use of B7 costimulatory molecules as adjuvants in a prime-boost vaccination against Visna/Maedi ovine lentivirus. *Vaccine* **2009**, *27*, 591–600. [CrossRef]

88. Lin, Y.Z.; Shen, R.X.; Zhu, Z.Y.; Deng, X.L.; Cao, X.Z.; Wang, X.F.; Ma, J.; Jianga, C.G.; Zhao, L.P.; Lv, X.L.; et al. An attenuated EIAV vaccine strain induces significantly different immune responses from its pathogenic parental strain although with similar in vivo replication pattern. *Antiviral Res.* **2011**, *92*, 292–304. [CrossRef] [PubMed]

89. Brülisauer, F.; Vogt, H.; Perler, L.; Rüfenacht, J. Risk factors for the infection of Swiss goat herds with small ruminant lentivirus: A case-control study. *Vet. Rec.* **2005**, *157*, 229–233. [CrossRef] [PubMed]

90. Polledo, L.; González, J.; Fernández, C.; Miguélez, J.; Martínez-Fernández, B.; Morales, S.; Ferreras, M.C.; García Marín, J.F. Simple control strategy to reduce the level of Maedi-Visna infection in sheep flocks with high prevalence values (>90%). *Small Rumin. Res.* **2013**, *112*, 224–229. [CrossRef]

91. Pérez, M.; Munoz, J.A.; Biescas, E.; Salazar, E.; Bolea, R.; de Andrés, D.; Amorena, B.; Badiola, J.J.; Reina, R.; Luján, L. Successful Visna/maedi control in a highly infected ovine dairy flock using serologic segregation and management strategies. *Prev. Vet. Med.* **2013**, *112*, 423–427. [CrossRef]

92. Cortez-Romero, C.; Pellerin, J.L.; Ali-Al-Ahmad, M.Z.; Chebloune, Y.; Gallegos-Sánchez, J.; Lamara, A.; Pépin, M.; Fieni, F. The risk of small ruminant lentivirus (SRLV) transmission with reproductive biotechnologies: State-of-the-art review. *Theriogenology* **2013**, *79*, 1–9. [CrossRef]

93. Martínez-Navalón, B.; Peris, C.; Gómez, E.A.; Peris, B.; Roche, M.L.; Caballero, C.; Goyena, E.; Berriatua, E. Quantitative estimation of the impact of caprine arthritis encephalitis virus infection on milk production by dairy goats. *Vet. J.* **2013**, *197*, 311–317. [CrossRef]

14

Helminth Parasites among Rodents in the Middle East Countries

Md Mazharul Islam [1,2,*], Elmoubashar Farag [3,*], Mohammad Mahmudul Hassan [4], Devendra Bansal [3], Salah Al Awaidy [5], Abdinasir Abubakar [6], Hamad Al-Rumaihi [3] and Zilungile Mkhize-Kwitshana [7,8]

1 Department of Animal Resources, Ministry of Municipality and Environment, Doha, P.O. Box 35081, Qatar
2 School of Laboratory Medicine and Medical Sciences, College of Health Sciences, University of KwaZulu Natal, Durban 4000, South Africa
3 Ministry of Public Health, Doha, P.O. Box 42, Qatar; dbansal@moph.gov.qa (D.B.); halromaihi@moph.gov.qa (H.A.-R.)
4 Faculty of Veterinary Medicine, Chattogram Veterinary and Animal Sciences University, Khulshi, Chattogram 4225, Bangladesh; miladhasan@yahoo.com
5 Ministry of Health, P.O. Box 393, PC 113 Muscat, Oman; salah.awaidy@gmail.com
6 Infectious Hazard Preparedness (IHP) Unit, WHO Health Emergencies Department (WHE), World Health Organization, Regional Office for the Eastern Mediterranean, Cairo 11371, Egypt; abubakara@who.int
7 School of Life Sciences, College of Agriculture, Engineering & Science, University of KwaZulu Natal, Durban 40000, South Africa; mkhizekwitshanaz@ukzn.ac.za
8 South African Medical Research Council, Cape Town 7505, South Africa
* Correspondence: walidbdvet@gmail.com (M.M.I.); eabdfarag@moph.gov.qa (E.F.);

Simple Summary: The review was conducted to establish an overview of rodent helminths in the Middle East as well as their public health importance. Following a systematic search, 65 field research were identified, studied, and analyzed. The overall prevalence of cestodes, nematodes, and trematodes were 24.88%, 32.71%, and 10.17%, respectively. The review detected 21 species of cestodes, 56 nematodes, and 23 trematodes, from which 22 have zoonotic importance. *Capillaria hepatica*, *Hymenolepis diminuta*, *Hymenolepis nana*, and *Cysticercus fasciolaris* were the most frequent and widespread zoonotic helminths. The review identified that there is an information gap on rodent helminths at the humans-animal interface level in this region. Therefore, the public health importance of rodent-borne helminth parasites is not fully recognized. Countrywide detailed studies on rodent helminths, along with the impact on public health, should be conducted in this region.

Abstract: Rodents can be a source of zoonotic helminths in the Middle East and also in other parts of the world. The current systematic review aimed to provide baseline data on rodent helminths to recognize the threats of helminth parasites on public health in the Middle East region. Following a systematic search on PubMed, Scopus, and Web of Science, a total of 65 research studies on rodent cestodes, nematodes, and trematodes, which were conducted in the countries of the Middle East, were analyzed. The study identified 44 rodent species from which *Mus musculus*, *Rattus norvegicus*, and *Rattus rattus* were most common (63%) and recognized as the primary rodent hosts for helminth infestation in this region. Cestodes were the most frequently reported ($n = 50$), followed by nematodes (49), and trematodes (14). The random effect meta-analysis showed that the pooled prevalence of cestode (57.66%, 95% CI: 34.63–80.70, $I^2\% = 85.6$, $p < 0.001$) was higher in Saudi Arabia, followed by nematode (56.24%, 95% CI: 11.40–101.1, $I^2\% = 96.7$, $p < 0.001$) in Turkey, and trematode (15.83%, 95% CI: 6.25–25.1, $I^2\% = 98.5$, $p < 0.001$) in Egypt. According to the overall prevalence estimates of individual studies, nematodes were higher (32.71%, 95% CI: 24.89–40.54, $I^2\% = 98.6$, $p < 0.001$) followed by cestodes (24.88%, 95% CI: 19.99–29.77, $I^2\% = 94.9$, $p < 0.001$) and trematodes (10.17%,

95% CI: 6.7–13.65, $I^2\% = 98.3$, $p < 0.001$) in the rodents of the Middle East countries. The review detected 22 species of helminths, which have zoonotic importance. The most frequent helminths were *Capillaria hepatica*, *Hymenolepis diminuta*, *Hymenolepis nana*, and *Cysticercus fasciolaris*. There was no report of rodent-helminths from Bahrain, Jordan, Lebanon, Oman, United Arab Emirates, and Yemen. Furthermore, there is an information gap on rodent helminths at the humans-animal interface level in Middle East countries. Through the One Health approach and countrywide detailed studies on rodent-related helminths along with their impact on public health, the rodent control program should be conducted in this region.

Keywords: rodent; helminth; cestode; trematode; nematode; Middle East; meta-analysis

1. Introduction

Helminths are among the most diverse and geographically widespread groups of parasites that infect both humans and animals [1]. Although they are from different phyla or class (nematode, cestode, and trematode), the mode of transmission, infection, and pathogenesis, as well as host immune-responsiveness of these pathogens, follows a typical pattern. Approximately one-third of the world population is infected with one or more types of helminths. From amongst 300,000 species of helminths that typically infect vertebrates, 287 of them infect humans, from which 95% are either zoonoses or have evolved from animal parasites [2]. About 100 of the zoonotic helminths cause asymptomatic infection or mild symptoms in humans, while only a small percentage of them cause severe or even fatal infections [1]. In resource-poor countries, livestock is a source of food, production, income source, and deposit of wealth. Parasite infections in animals indirectly affect human health through financial hardship and malnutrition. Based on the burden of death, sickness, and treatment cost for both humans and animals for helminth infestation, the zoonotic parasites' socioeconomic burden was presented as high or low socioeconomic impact [3].

Rodents are significant sources of parasitic zoonosis in humans, serving as reservoirs and vectors of at least 70 zoonotic diseases, of which 16 are helminth parasites [4]. Consumption of uncooked/improperly cooked food contaminated with the infective larvae, eggs, or metacercariae is the primary source of humans infestation with helminth parasites [5,6]. When pilfering humans food, rodents pass stool or urine that contaminates said food, leading to transmission of zoonotic helminths from rodents to humans [7].

The Middle East is an intercontinental region with a total population of over 411 million [8] in 17 sovereign countries, including Bahrain, Cyprus, Egypt, Iran, Iraq, Israel, Jordan, Kuwait, Lebanon, Oman, Palestine, Qatar, Kingdom of Saudi Arabia (KSA), Syria, Turkey, United Arab Emirates (UAE), and Yemen. The majority of people in this region live in poverty [9], with the highest percentage being specific to Yemen, Syria, Egypt, Palestine, and Iraq [10,11]. Cultural diversity, weak economic policy, poor governance, rapid population growth, low educational structure, gender discrimination, underdeveloped infrastructure, and war and conflict have turned the region into a hot spot for many emerging and re-emerging diseases, including rodent-borne parasitic infections [9,12,13]. In the past, rodent-borne infections have led to multiple instances of a fatal epidemic, in part due to a lack of relevant information available on the subject, which makes it difficult to maintain public health sustainability [14,15].

Helminth infestations are mostly neglected diseases [16]. Therefore, the complete picture of zoonotic helminths is not well known in the Middle East area. Despite several studies being done on helminths in this region, no systematic review or meta-analysis was performed on rodent helminths, including zoonotic importance in the Middle East region. Our objective is to summarize baseline information on rodent helminths in this region using evidence-based records of the helminths detected in rodents in the Middle Eastern countries. The review also identifies the rodent helminths with public health importance in this region.

2. Materials and Methods

We followed PRISMA (Preferred Reporting Items for Systematic Reviews and Meta-Analysis) guidelines [17] to conduct the systematic review using a four-step approach: database search, evaluating relevant articles, data extraction, and summarizing. One author conducted the data search. Two authors were involved in critical evaluation and data extraction from the selected articles, while one author managed the compilation of said data. Afterward, two authors arranged the data and conducted the meta-analysis (Figure 1, Supplementary Table S1).

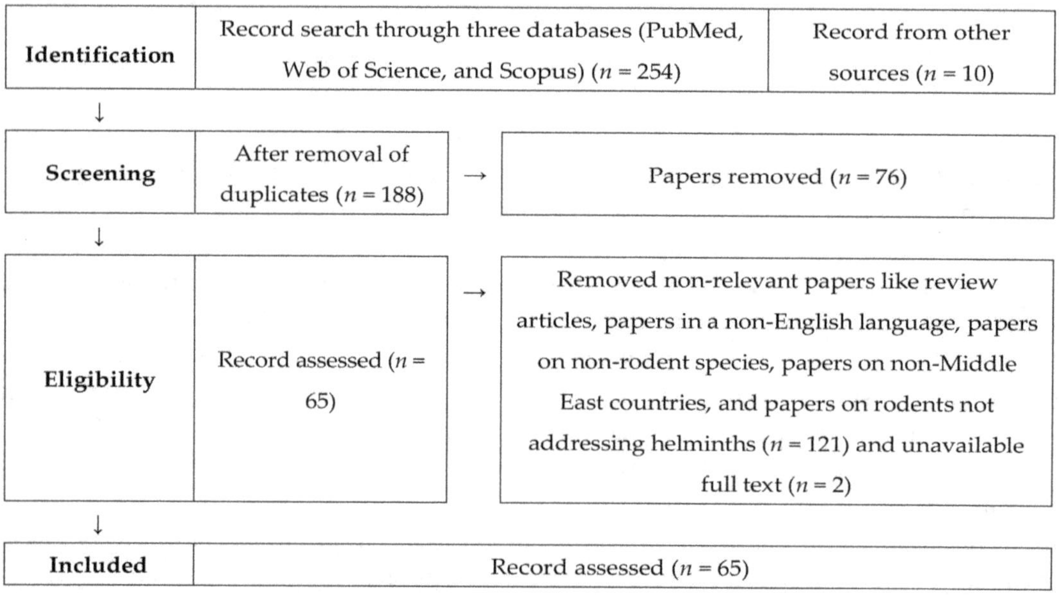

Figure 1. Systematic review PRISMA flow diagram describing the selection of published articles on rodent helminths in the Middle East and inclusion/exclusion process used in the study.

2.1. Search Strategy

A literature search on rodent helminth parasites in the Middle East was performed on 17 June 2019 through PubMed, Web of Science, and Scopus (Figure 1). The search included all the original research articles containing field evidence of helminth parasites (trematode, nematode, cestode) among rodents in the Middle East countries. The search did not have any date range of publication. The keywords included (Rodent OR Rat OR Jird OR Gerbil OR Vole OR Mouse OR Hamster OR Porcupine OR Squirrel OR Jerboa) AND (Endoparasite OR Helminth OR Cestode OR Trematode OR Nematode) AND (17 Middle East country names individually). Screening on the search was conducted as [Title/Abstract] in PubMed, [TITLE-ABS-KEY] in Scopus, and [Topic] in Web of Science.

2.2. Search of Relevant Articles

The data search results were processed using EndNote X9 (clarivate analytics, Philadelphia, PA, USA), which was also used to identify and exclude duplicate studies. Then we proceeded to peruse through the titles and abstracts to find the relevant articles. However, articles that were ambiguous regarding their relevance by their title and abstract were subjected to full-text analysis. Only documents published in English were considered for the review [18–82].

2.3. Data Extraction and Summarizing

Evidence-based field reports give a clear picture of any pathogen's availability, diversity, and dynamics in a locality [83,84]. We considered only the field reports containing rodent helminths for data abstraction. The extracted data included several variables such as country and location of sampling, season, year of sampling, rodent information (rodent species, sex, total rodent count, and the number of infected), helminth species and type, and possible associating factors of rodent infestation with helminth (Supplementary Table S2). The zoonotic rodent-borne helminths in this region were identified from the list of rodent helminths from this review with the support of published articles.

2.4. Data Analysis

The aggregated data was transcribed and stored in a Microsoft Excel spreadsheet, and then the data was forwarded to STATA/IC-13.0 (Stata Corp, 4905 Lakeway Drive, College Station, TX 77845, USA) for statistical analysis. Crude prevalence estimation was performed by dividing the total number of helminth-positive rodents with the total number of rodents sampled and expressed as a percentage. The crude estimate of prevalence was used throughout, the 95% confidence interval (CI), and the p-value were calculated on different types of helminths among the countries. Study variations among the studies were evaluated using the Chi-square (χ^2) test on Cochran's Q statistics (with p-value) followed by I^2 statistics to determine the study's degree of heterogeneity. Standard Error (SE) was calculated using a standard formula for proportion calculation. A random-effect meta-analysis model was applied using the "mean" command specifying random due to the study's high degree of heterogeneity ($I^2 > 75\%$). The output has been illustrated using a forest plot [85].

3. Results

3.1. Descriptive Analysis

The literature search returned 65 articles (Figure 1, Supplementary Table S2) published from 1969 to 2019. These articles were from 11 out of 17 Middle East countries, such as Cyprus, Egypt, Iran, Iraq, Israel, Kuwait, Palestine, Qatar, Saudi Arabia, Syria, and Turkey (Figure 2). No report on rodent helminths was available from Bahrain, Jordan, Lebanon, Oman, United Arab Emirates, and Yemen. Cestodes were the most frequently reported (50 articles) helminths in the Middle Eastern rodents, followed by nematodes (49), and trematodes (14).

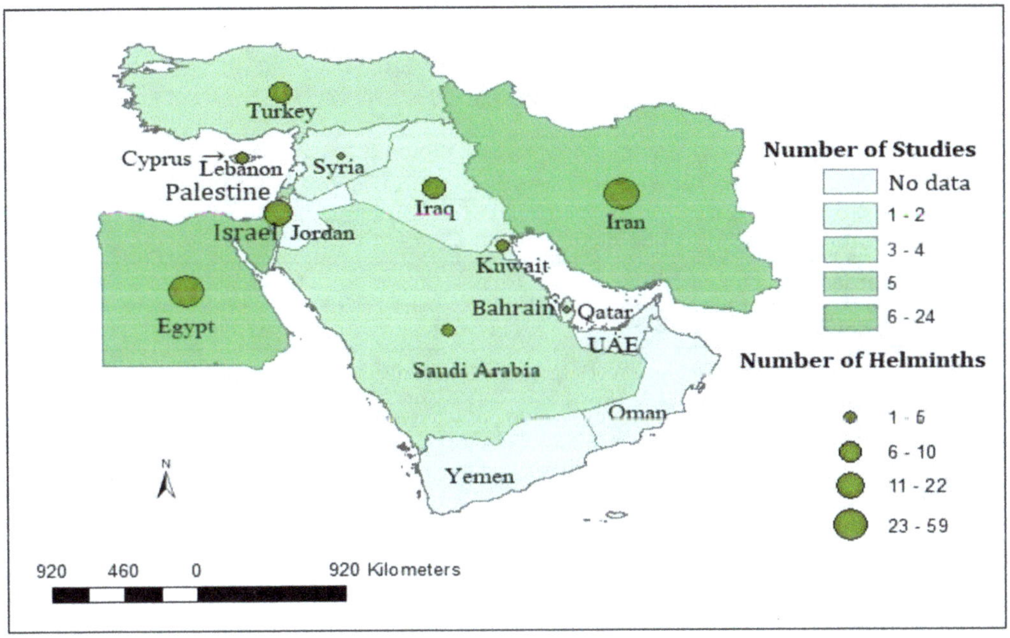

Figure 2. The map depicted the Middle East countries with the total number of studies and the number of helminths detected in rodents.

All 65 studies reported at least 9628 rodents (47% females and 53% males). A total of 44 rodent species from 6 families were listed (Supplementary Table S3). The analysis identified *Acomys dimidiatus, Jaculus jaculus, Meriones crassus, Mus musculus,* and *Rattus norvegicus, Rattus ratus* were widely distributed as these rodents were reported from where *Mus musculus* ($n = 1251$, 12.6%), *Rattus norvegicus* ($n = 3325$, 33.6%), and *Rattus rattus* ($n = 1694$, 17.1%) as the most common. Besides, three sub-species of *Rattus rattus*, such as *Rattus rattus alexandrines, Rattus rattus frugivorous,* and *Rattus rattus rattus*, are prevalent in the Middle East. Moreover, the review found some other rodents, which are important as zoonotic helminth carrier. These include *Acomys cahirinus, Acomys dimidiatus, Apodemus sylvaticus, Apodemus witherby, Arvicanthus niloticus, Calomyscus elburzensis, Cricetulus migratorius, Gerbillus cheesmani, Gerbillus gerbillus, Meriones libycus, Meriones persicus, Mesocricetus auratus, Microtus socialis, Microtus transcaspicus, Mus domesticus, Rhombomys opimus,* and *Tatera indica*. A total of 100 species of rodent helminths were identified. Based on the available data, the estimated pooled prevalence of the different types of parasites in rodents has been presented in Table 1. The random effect meta-analysis showed that the pooled prevalence of cestode ranged from 12.87% (95% CI: 5.17–20.57, $I^2\% = 80.6$, $p < 0.001$) in Turkey to 57.66% (95% CI: 34.63–80.70, $I^2\% = 85.6$, $p < 0.001$) in Saudi Arabia. The nematode prevalence was varying from 0.16% (95% CI: −0.15–0.47, $I^2\% = 0.0$) in Cyprus to 56.24% (95% CI: 11.40–101.1, $I^2\% = 96.7$, $p < 0.001$) in Turkey. Moreover, the prevalence of trematode ranged from 0.24% (95% CI: −0.11–0.59 $I^2\% = 0.0$, $p < 0.001$) in Iran to 15.83% (95% CI: 6.25–25.1, $I^2\% = 98.5$, $p < 0.001$) in Egypt.

Table 1. Estimated pooled prevalence of the rodent helminths in the Middle East countries.

Country	Parasite	Pooled Estimates (%)	95% CI	Heterogeneity Chi-Squared (χ^2)	$I^2\%$	*p*-Value
Cyprus	Nematode	0.160	−0.15–0.47	0.00	0	-
	Cestode	14.72	11.94–17.50	0.00	0	-
Egypt	Nematode	31.81	19.83–43.78	259.62	97.3	<0.001
	Cestode	27.49	23.72–31.26	17.18	70.9	<0.001
	Trematode	15.827	6.56–25.1	344.74	98.5	<0.001
Iran	Cestode	18.21	11.59–24.83	56.08	87.5	<0.001
	Nematode	33.93	16.52–51.35	154.53	96.8	<0.001
	Trematode	0.24	−0.11–0.59	0.19	0	<0.001
Palestine	Nematode	24.39	11.25–37.54	0.00	0	-
	Cestode	36.59	21.84–51.32	0.00	0	-
Qatar	Cestode	26.64	8.89–44.39	13.94	92.8	<0.001
Saudi Arabia	Cestode	57.66	34.63–80.70	6.74	85.6	<0.001
	Trematode	14.685	8.88–20.49	0.00	0	-
Turkey	Nematode	56.24	11.40–101.1	30.10	96.7	<0.001
	Cestode	12.87	5.17–20.57	10.34	80.6	<0.001

CI: confidence interval; I^2: inverse variance index; χ^2: Cochran's *Q* chi-square.

3.2. Rodent Cestodes in the Middle East Countries

Rodent cestodes information was available from all 11 Middle Eastern countries (Supplementary Table S3). A total of 21 rodent cestode species that belongs to 8 families have been reported in this review. Most of the cestodes were from Egypt and Iran (12 cestode species from each county). Out of 44 rodent species, *Mus musculus, Rattus norvegicus,* and *Rattus rattus* were frequently identified with the cestode infestation. Three species of cestodes have been frequently reported, viz: *Hymenolepis diminuta* (20 reports from 5 countries), *Hymenolepis nana* (30, 9), and *Cysticercus fasciolaris* (23, 4). Figure 3 shows the prevalence estimates from individual studies on cestodes in rodents of the Middle East countries, which ranged from 7.69 (95% CI: 2.22–13.17) to 68.57 (95% CI: 59.69–77.45) with an overall estimated prevalence 24.88 (95% CI: 19.99–29.77, $I^2\% = 94.9$, $p < 0.001$).

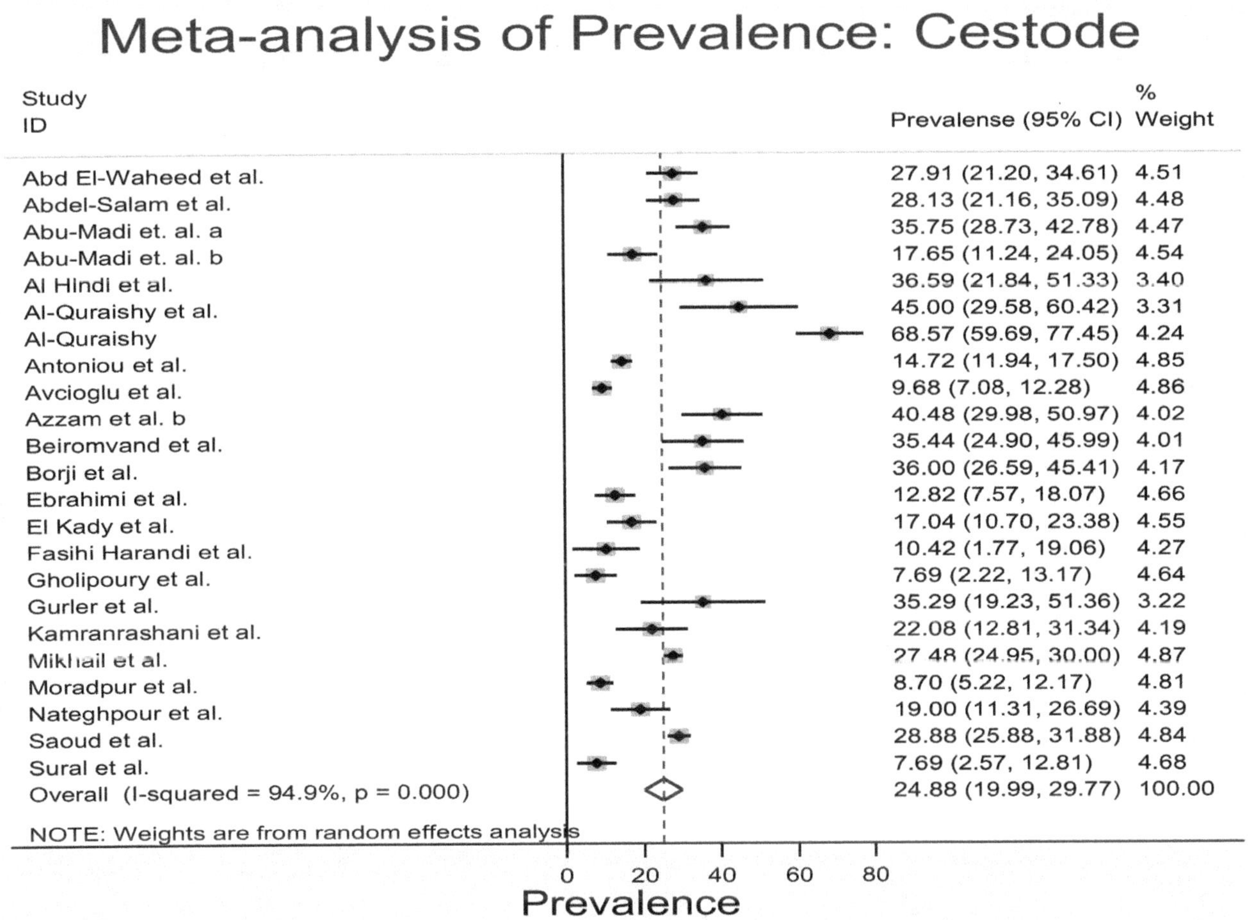

Figure 3. Forest plot of the prevalence estimates of cestode in rodents among the Middle East countries (the center dot representing point estimates whereas Gray Square representing the weight of each study to the meta-analysis).

3.3. Rodent Nematodes in the Middle East Countries

Rodent nematodes were studied in 8 countries in the Middle East, namely Cyprus, Egypt, Iran, Iraq, Israel, Kuwait, Palestine, and Turkey (Supplementary Table S3). Nematodes from 23 families represented the 56 nematode species in this region. Most of the rodent nematodes were reported from Egypt ($n = 24$) and Iran ($n = 31$) and the rodent species such as *Mus musculus*, *Rattus norvegicus*, *Rattus rattus*, *Meriones persicus*, *Acomys dimidiatus*, and *Tatera indica*. However, the nematodes, *Aspiculuris tetraptera*, *Capillaria hepatica*, *Syphacia obvelata*, *Streptopharagus kuntzi*, and *Trichuris muris* were most frequently reported and widely distributed. These nematodes were reported from three or more countries in the Middle East. Figure 4 shows the prevalence estimates from individual studies on nematodes in rodents of the Middle East countries, which ranged from 0.16 (95% CI: −0.15–0.47) to 79.41 (95% CI: 65.82–93.0) with an overall estimated prevalence of 32.71 (95% CI: 24.89–40.54, $I^2\% = 98.6$, $p < 0.001$).

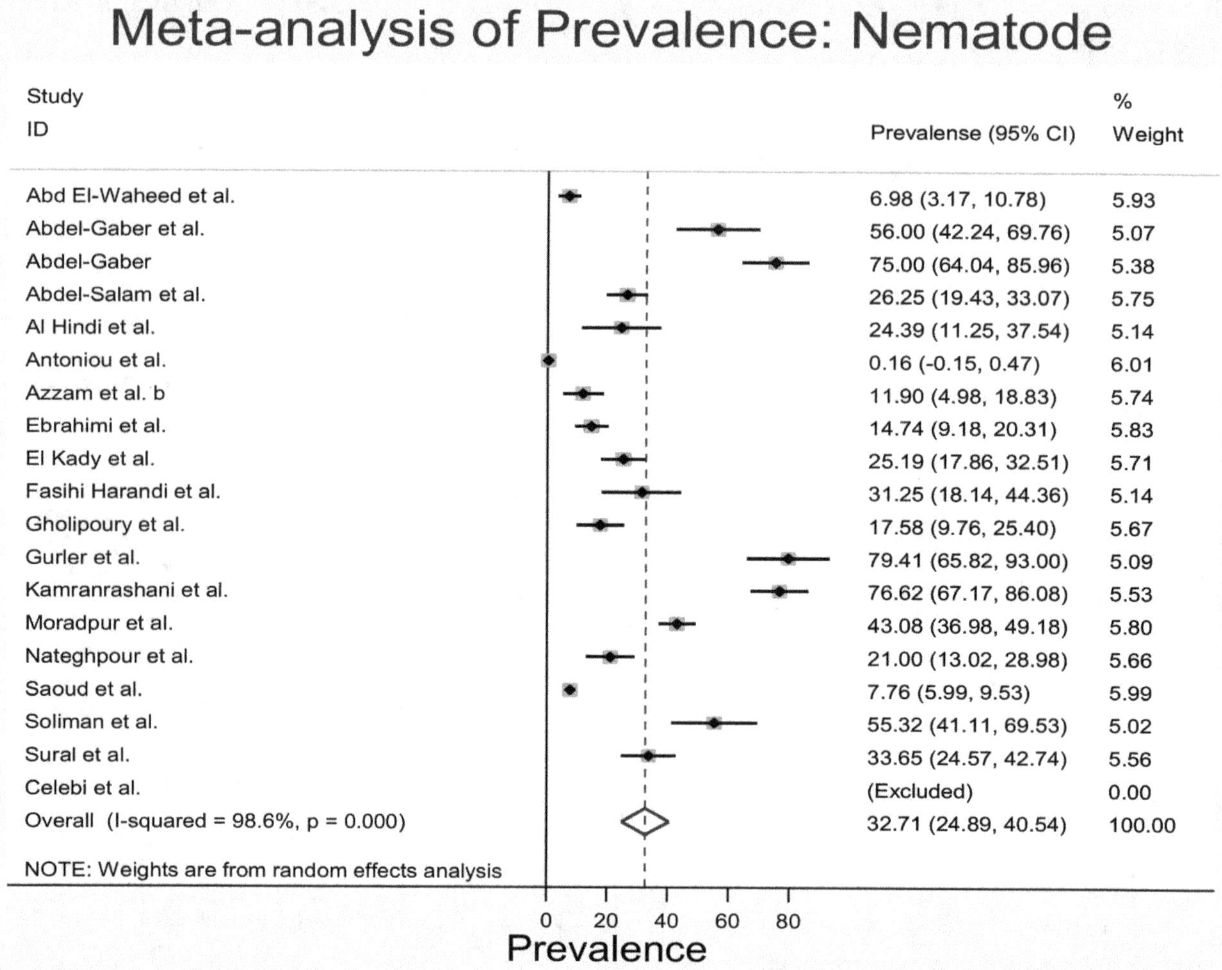

Figure 4. Forest plot of the prevalence estimates of nematode in rodents among the Middle East countries (the center dot representing point estimates whereas Gray Square representing the weight of each study to the meta-analysis).

3.4. Rodent Trematodes in the Middle East Countries

The reviewed studies reported rodent trematodes in Egypt, Iran, Israel, and Saudi Arabia (Supplementary Table S3). At least 23 trematode species from 11 families of trematodes were reported in the Middle Eastern rodents. Reports from Egypt ($n = 21$) were more descriptive of these trematodes. Moreover, *Fasciola* sp. was detected in Saudi Arabia, *Scaphiostomum* sp. in Israel, and *Notocotylus neyrai* and *Plagiorchis muris* were identified in Iran. The review found *Arvicanthus niloticus, Rattus norvegicus* and *Rattus rattus* are three rodent species important for trematode infestation. Figure 5 shows the prevalence estimates from individual studies on trematode in rodents of the Middle East countries, which ranged from 0.20 (95% CI: −0.19–0.59) to 36.90 (95% CI: 26.59–47.22) with an overall estimated prevalence of 10.17 (95% CI: 6.7–13.65, $I^2\% = 98.3$, $p < 0.001$).

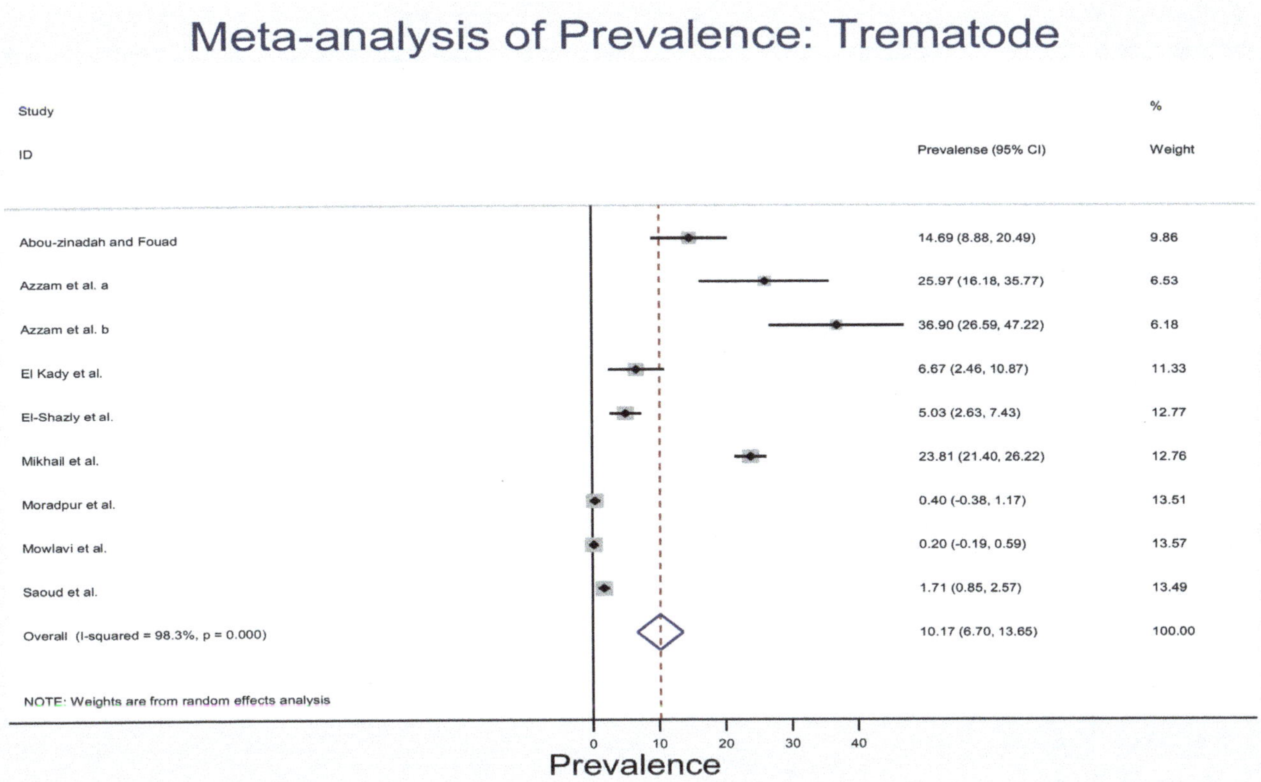

Figure 5. Forest plot of the prevalence estimates of trematode in rodents among the Middle East countries (the center dot representing point estimates, whereas Gray Square representing the weight of each study to the meta-analysis).

3.5. Zoonotic Importance of the Rodent Helminths in the Middle East Countries

Out of the 100 species of rodent helminths detected in this review, 22 species have zoonotic importance; 7 cestodes, 6 nematodes, and 9 trematodes. The zoonotic helminths, their hosts, and possible human infection sources have been illustrated in Table 2.

Table 2. Rodent-borne zoonotic helminths in the Middle East countries.

Parasites	Host	Source of Human Infection	Reference
	Rodent-borne zoonotic cestodes:		
Raillieitina celebensis and *R. demerariensis*.	DH: rodent; IH: ant and beetle	Ingestion of food contaminated with infected insects	[5,6]
Hymenolepis diminuta and *H. nana*	DH: rodent; IH: *H. diminuta*: flea and beetle. *H. nana* does not require IH.	Consumption contaminated food with rodent feces containing parasitic egg	[6,86,87]
Mesocestoides sp.	DH: dog and cat; 1st IH: ant and mite, 2nd IH: rodent, bird, amphibian, and reptile	Consumption of undercooked meat of amphibians and reptiles containing infective larva (tetrathyridium)	[5,6]
Taenia taeniaeformis	DH: cat; IH: rodent	There is a report that *Taenia taeniaformis* can infect humans	[88]
Echinococcus multilocularis	DH: dog, fox; IH: rat	Ingestion of embryonated eggs	[86]

Table 2. *Cont.*

Parasites	Host	Source of Human Infection	Reference
Rodent-borne zoonotic nematodes:			
Angiostrongylus cantonensis	DH: rat and mollusk; IH: snail, prawn, crab, and frog	Ingestion of uncooked IH or vegetables contaminated with infected larvae	[6]
Gongylonema pulchrum	DH: ruminant, pig, wild boar, non-human primate, carnivore, and rodent; IH: beetles and cockroaches	Ingestion of IH or drinking of water contaminated with infective larvae	[5,6]
Trichinella spp.	Pig, wild boar, and rodent	Ingestion of uncooked muscle with encysted larvae	[6]
Trichostrongylus spp.	Herbivorous animal	Consumption of food and water contaminated with animal feces containing infective larvae	[6]
Capillaria hepatica	Rat, carnivore, and humans	Consumption of food contaminated with feces containing embryonated eggs	[5]
Trichuris trichiura	Humans	Consumption of food contaminated with feces containing *Trichuris* egg.	[5]
Rodent-borne zoonotic trematodes:			
Echinochasmus sp., *Echinoparyphium recurvatum*, and *Echoinostoma* sp.	DH: humans, rat, duck 1st IH: snail, 2nd IH: snail, amphibian, bivalve, fish	Ingestion of uncooked fish containing metacercariae	[2,89]
Fasciola hepatica	DH: herbivore; IH: snail	Ingestion of metacercariae contaminated vegetable	[6,34]
Haplorchis *pumilio*, *Pygidiopsis genata*, *Stictodora tridactyla*, *Prosthodendrium* spp., and *Plagiorchis muris*	DH: dog, cat, rat, duck, humans; 1st IH: snail, 2nd IH: fish	Eating uncooked fish harboring viable metacercariae	[88,90]
Schistosoma mansoni	DH: Vertebrate animal; IH: snail	Penetrate the DH skin	[6,86]

Note: DH: Definite host, IH: Intermediate host.

4. Discussion

This study reviewed the literature published in English on helminths-infested rodents in the Middle East region. The majority of the studies (47 of 65) were from Iran and Egypt, most likely due to their long history of rodent-borne zoonotic disease (like murine typhus, plague, tularemia) epidemics, which resulted in millions of death [4,91–94]. Thus, this topic became a central focus of public health research in these countries. The present review found three commensal rodent species: *Mus musculus*, *Rattus norvegicus*, and *Rattus rattus* to be more common and carrying most of the zoonotic helminths within this region. Previous literature described that these species occupy different habitats with higher population density than the other species and pose considerable risk to public health [4]. Although rodent cestodes were most frequently reported ($n = 50$) helminth in this review, the meta-analysis detected the overall rodent nematode prevalence was highest (32.7%) compared to cestodes (24.88%) and trematodes (10.17%) prevalence. Out of the 22 zoonotic helminths detected in this review, *Capillaria hepatica*, *H. diminuta*, *H. nana*, and *C. fasciolaris* have been found as widespread distribution. Furthermore, some non-zoonotic helminths such as *Aspiculuris tetraptera*, *Syphacia obvelata*, *Streptopharagus kuntzi*, and *Trichuris muris* were reported from three or more countries in this region.

Rodents have several beneficiary activities in ecology, such as soil aeration and water absorption ability, biotic recovery, and insect control [4,95]. In this regard, the presence of healthy rodents is essential for ecology [96]. Helminths infestation in rodents affects their own health and can subsequently alter the rodent-environment ecology to a considerable degree. Moreover, rodent helminths are important for humans, livestock, and pet animal health. Hymenolepiais is a major zoonotic rodent cestode [6]. Fascioliasis is hazardous for livestock health as well as for humans [6,97]. The definite host of *Taenia taeniaeformis* is the cat, where a stage of this cestode lifecycle (the cystic form, *Cysticercus fasciolaris*) is completed in rodents. An increase of *Cysticercus fasciolaris* in rodents can increase the health risk of cats [98]. Thus, rodent helminths have an impact on the ecology as well as humans and animal health.

Rodent-borne zoonotic helminths incur significant socioeconomic losses, although the zoonotic helminths' socioeconomic burden can differ from species to species [3]. *Hymenolepis diminuta* and *Hymenolepis nana* are major zoonotic cestodes [3,99]. *Trichostrongylus* sp. and *Trichuris trichiura* are generally considered as major nematode threats [100]. The socioeconomic burden caused by *Angiostrongylus cantonensis, Gongylonema pulchrum, Trichinella* sp., and *Capillaria hepatica* are likely to be very low [3].

There is an information gap on rodent-borne zoonotic helminths in the Middle East countries. Some zoonotic cases of helminths infestation were reported in rodents by some countries in the Middle East, but none involved humans who might have been infected with the same helminths. Humans hymenolepiasis were reported in Bahrain [101], Cyprus [102], Jordan [103], Oman [104], Palestine [105], Qatar [106], and Yemen [107]. The *Hymenolepis nana* is a common zoonotic helminth transmitted from rodents to humans and the prevalence ranged from 0.15% to 12.2% in some Middle East countries with prevalence of specific countries such as Jordan (1.8%) [103], Oman (5.9%) [104], Palestine (1.0%) [105], Qatar (0.15%) [106], and Yemen (12.2%) [107]. Egg of *Hymenolepis diminuta* was detected from soil samples of school playgrounds of Jordan [108]. There is no report of rodent hymenolepiasis within these countries. *Echinococcus* spp. is a major helminth for human health, which was detected in rodents of Egypt, Iran, and Turkey. Human cases of alveolar hydatid cysts were reported from Iran, Kuwait, Saudi Arabia, and Turkey [109,110].

The rodent lungworm, *Angiostrongylus cantonensis*, causes eosinophilic meningomyelitis in humans, reported in Israel [111]. Gongylonema infection is reported in humans [112] and dromedaries [113] from Iran. *Trichinella* was a widespread parasite infecting humans and other mammals, although the former makes for a poor host for said organism [6]. There are reports of humans trichinellosis from Iran [114], Israel [115], Lebanon [116], and Turkey [117]. Human cases of trichostrongyliasis infestation were reported in Egypt [118], Iran [119], Israel [120], and Turkey [121]. Eggs of *Trichostrongylus* sp. were detected from soil samples of public places of Jordan [108] and Iraq [122]. Humans reports of *Trichuris trichiura* are available from Bahrain [123], Egypt [118], Israel [120], Jordan [103], Oman [104], Palestine [105], Qatar [124], Saudi Arabia [125], Turkey [126], and Yemen [107]. *Trichuris muris*, the rodent whipworm, does not have any zoonotic importance. Eggs of *Trichuris* were found in the soil of the public place of Iraq [122]. *Trichuris trichiura* is not a rodent specific nematode. The report of *Trichuris trichiura* in Iranian rodents [67] may be a case of accidental infestation.

Schistosoma and *Fasciola* are two major humans trematodes globally [3]. The high prevalence of *Fasciola* was recorded in Egypt, Iran, and Yemen [127]. Human cases of schistosomiasis were noted in Egypt [3], Iran [128], Israel [129], Jordan [103], Saudi Arabia [130], Turkey [131], and Yemen [3,132], whereas *Heterophyes heterophyes* were reported from Egypt and Saudi Arabia [133,134]. There are non-humans (fish, dogs, and cats) reports of *Pygidiopsis genata, Haplorchis pumilio, Haplorchis yokogawai*, and *Heterophyes heterophyes* from Egypt, Iran, Iraq, Israel, Palestine, Kuwait, Saudi Arabia, Turkey, UAE, and Yemen [135–138]. However, these rodent trematodes in the current review were mostly reported from Egypt and Iran.

Based on the meta-analysis, the overall prevalence of rodent trematodes was less than that of nematodes and cestodes in the Middle East, which had received more emphasis in other similar reports [110,127]. Efficient management of water resources are important factor for prevalence of trematode prevalence [139,140]. The presence of deserts means shortage of surface water in some of the countries of Arabian Peninsula such as Bahrain, Kuwait, Oman, Qatar, Saudi Arabia, and United Arab Emirates [141], which may be the cause of shortage of aquatic intermediate hosts of trematodes in these countries. Therefore, rodent trematodes are less reported in these countries. More research should be conducted to find rodent-borne trematodes in the countries of this region.

The reviewed articles in the current study described some of the factors that can influence the population of rodent-borne helminths within the Middle East, necessitating a need to develop a plan of action to control rodent helminths. The abundance of rodent-borne helminths depends on the host organism's prevalence and its distribution [29,44]. An increase in the rodent population may increase the risk of humans getting infected by rodent parasites [142]. Rodents who inhabit animal farms have easy access to animal feed, and thus, they can be considered a potential vector and reservoir of animal and zoonotic diseases where animals serve as hosts [26]. *Hymenolepis diminuta* in the rodent are linked with some insects as intermediate hosts, such as *Xenopsylla astia*, which has a clear seasonal pattern. In Qatar, a research found that rodents are more infested with *Hymenolepis diminuta* in summer due to the *X. astia* abundance [24]. Several studies reported that the prevalence of rodent helminths is increased with rodent age [23,24,35,51]. Rodent helminths infestation can change with rodent host species [48]. The nematode, *Syphacia obvelata*, was reported to be most abundant in *Mus musculus* [64].

Rodent population control is a primary way to control rodent zoonotic diseases [143,144]. The other contributing factors, such as rodent species, seasons of the year, intermediate host, rodent control management in the residential areas, and animal farms, should also be considered on rodent related zoonoses control. As most of the rodent-related zoonotic helminths are linked to herbivores and carnivores [5,6,86,88], it is vital to manage dogs, cats, and livestock animals to avoid the spread of helminth infestation. Thus, One Health practice comes as a practical approach to control rodent-borne helminth prevalence [145]. "One Health is a collaborative, multisectoral, and transdisciplinary approach - working at the local, regional, national, and global levels—with the goal of achieving optimal health outcomes recognizing the interconnection between people, animals, plants, and their shared environment" [146]. One Health practice by linking veterinary, medical, ecology, entomology, parasitology, zoology fields, and local people are essential for rodent helminths prevention and control.

5. Conclusions

Rodent helminths in the Middle Eastern countries have been documented, which also highlighted rodent-borne zoonotic helminths. *Rattus norvegicus*, *Rattus rattus*, and *Mus musculus* were the most frequently reported rodents and infected with helminth parasites. Out of the 22 rodent-related zoonotic helminths, *Capillaria hepatica*, *H. diminuta*, *H. nana*, and *C. fasciolaris* were most frequent in this region. The current study illustrates that there is an information gap on the availability, diversity, and dynamics of rodent helminths and their interaction between humans and animals in the Middle East. Thus, the public health importance of rodent-borne helminth parasites is not fully recognized. However, rodent control should be the primary concentration by a One Health approach to control the spread of these helminths at the humans-animal-environmental interface in the countries of this region. We also suggest countrywide and detailed studies be conducted on rodent-borne helminths along with their impact on public health in this region.

Author Contributions: Conceptualization, M.M.I., E.F. and Z.M.-K.; methodology, M.M.I., E.F. and M.M.H.; formal analysis, M.M.I. and M.M.H.; writing—original draft preparation, M.M.I., M.M.H. and Z.M.-K.; writing—review and editing, M.M.I., M.M.H., D.B., S.A.A., A.A., H.A.-R. and Z.M.-K.; visualization, D.B., E.F. and Z.M.-K.; supervision, Z.M.-K. All authors have read and agreed to the published version of the manuscript.

Acknowledgments: The authors acknowledge the Qatar National Library for providing some full-text articles and partially paying the publication fee.

References

1. Macpherson, C.N.L.; Craig, P.S. *Parasitic Helminths and Zoonoses in Africa*; Springer: Eindhoven, The Netherlands, 1991.
2. Bruschi, F. *Helminth Infections and Their Impact on Global Public Health*; Springer: Wien, Austria, 2014.
3. Torgerson, P.R.; Macpherson, C.N. The socioeconomic burden of parasitic zoonoses: Global trends. *Vet. Parasitol.* **2011**, *182*, 79–95. [CrossRef] [PubMed]
4. Rabiee, M.H.; Mahmoudi, A.; Siahsarvie, R.; Krystufek, B.; Mostafavi, E. Rodent-borne diseases and their public health importance in Iran. *PloS Negl. Trop. Dis.* **2018**, *12*. [CrossRef] [PubMed]
5. Centers for Disease Control and Prevention. DPDx A-Z Index. Available online: https://www.cdc.gov/dpdx/az.html (accessed on 5 September 2020).
6. Dhaliwal, B.B.S.; Juyal, P.D. *Parasitic Zoonoses*; Springer: New Delhi, India, 2013; pp. 1–135.
7. Meerburg, B.G.; Singleton, G.R.; Kijlstra, A. Rodent-borne diseases and their risks for public health. *Crit. Rev. Microbiol.* **2009**, *35*, 221–270. [CrossRef] [PubMed]
8. World Population Review. The Middle East Population. Available online: http://worldpopulationreview.com/continents/the-middle-east-population/ (accessed on 21 November 2019).
9. Dabrowski, M.; Wulf, L. Economic Development, Trade and Investment in the Eastern and Southern Mediterranean Region. *SSRN Electron. J.* **2013**, 10. [CrossRef]
10. The World Bank. GDP Growth; All Countries and Economies. Available online: https://data.worldbank.org/indicator/NY.GDP.MKTP.KD.ZG (accessed on 21 November 2019).
11. The World Bank. Palestine's Economic Update—October 2019. Available online: https://www.worldbank.org/en/country/westbankandgaza/publication/economic-update-october-2019 (accessed on 21 November 2019).
12. Buliva, E.; Elhakim, M.; Tran Minh, N.N.; Elkholy, A.; Mala, P.; Abubakar, A.; Malik, S.M.M.R. Emerging and Reemerging Diseases in the World Health Organization (WHO) Eastern Mediterranean Region-Progress, Challenges, and WHO Initiatives. *Front. Public Health* **2017**, *5*, 276. [CrossRef] [PubMed]
13. Stewart, F. Root causes of violent conflict in developing countries. *BMJ* **2002**, *324*, 342–345. [CrossRef]
14. Bannazadeh Baghi, H.; Alinezhad, F.; Kuzmin, I.; Rupprecht, C.E. A Perspective on Rabies in the Middle East-Beyond Neglect. *Vet. Sci.* **2018**, *5*, 67. [CrossRef]
15. Hashemi Shahraki, A.; Carniel, E.; Mostafavi, E. Plague in Iran: Its history and current status. *Epidemiol. Health* **2016**, *38*. [CrossRef]
16. World Health Organization. Neglected Tropical Diseases. Available online: https://www.who.int/neglected_diseases/diseases/en/ (accessed on 12 September 2020).
17. Moher, D.; Liberati, A.; Tetzlaff, J.; Altman, D.G. Preferred reporting items for systematic reviews and meta-analyses: The PRISMA statement. *PLoS Med.* **2009**, *6*. [CrossRef]
18. Abd el-Wahed, M.M.; Salem, G.H.; el-Assaly, T.M. The role of wild rats as a reservoir of some internal parasites in Qalyobia governorate. *J. Egypt. Soc. Parasitol.* **1999**, *29*, 495–503.
19. Abdel-Gaber, R.; Abdel-Ghaffar, F.; Al Quraishy, S.; Morsy, K.; Saleh, R.; Mehlhorn, H. Morphological Re-Description and 18 S rDNA Sequence Confirmation of the Pinworm *Aspiculuris tetraptera* (*Nematoda, Heteroxynematidae*) Infecting the Laboratory Mice Mus musculus. *J. Nematol.* **2018**, *50*, 117–132. [CrossRef] [PubMed]
20. Abdel-Gaber, R. Syphacia obvelata (*Nematode, Oxyuridae*) infecting laboratory mice *Mus musculus* (*Rodentia, Muridae*): Phylogeny and host-parasite relationship. *Parasitol. Res.* **2016**, *115*, 975–985. [CrossRef]
21. Abdel-Salam, F.A.; Galal, A.A.; Ali, M.K. The Role of Rodents as a Reservoir of Zoonotic Intestinal Parasites at Sohag Governorate, Egypt. *Assiut Vet. Med. J.* **1994**, *30*, 14.
22. Abou-Zinadah, N.Y.; Fouad, M.A. Anti-Fasciola antibodies among rodents and sheep in Jeddah, Saudi Arabia. *J. Egypt. Soc. Parasitol.* **2005**, *35*, 711–716. [PubMed]
23. Abu-Madi, M.A.; Behnke, J.M.; Mikhail, M.; Lewis, J.W.; Al-Kaabi, M.L. Parasite populations in the brown rat Rattus norvegicus from Doha, Qatar between years: The effect of host age, sex and density. *J. Helminthol.* **2005**, *79*, 105–111. [CrossRef]
24. Abu-Madi, M.A.; Lewis, J.W.; Mikhail, M.; El-Nagger, M.E.; Behnke, J.M. Monospecific helminth and arthropod infections in an urban population of brown rats from Doha, Qatar. *J. Helminthol.* **2001**, *75*, 313–320. [CrossRef]

25. Al Hindi, A.I.; Abu-Haddaf, E. Gastrointestinal parasites and ectoparasites biodiversity of *Rattus rattus* trapped from Khan Younis and Jabalia in Gaza strip, Palestine. *J. Egypt. Soc. Parasitol.* **2013**, *43*, 259–268. [CrossRef]
26. Allymehr, M.; Tavassoli, M.; Manoochehri, M.H.; Ardavan, D. Ectoparasites and Gastrointestinal Helminths of House Mice (*Mus musculus*) from Poultry Houses in Northwest Iran. *Comp. Parasitol.* **2012**, *79*, 283–287. [CrossRef]
27. Al-Quraishy, S.; Gewik, M.M.; Abdel-Baki, A.A. The intestinal cestode Hymenolepis diminuta as a lead sink for its rat host in the industrial areas of Riyadh, Saudi Arabia. *Saudi J. Biol. Sci.* **2014**, *21*, 387–390. [CrossRef] [PubMed]
28. Al-Qureishy, S. Lead concentrations in some organs of the rat *Meriones libycus* and its parasite Hymenolepis diminuta from Riyadh City, KSA. *J. Egypt. Soc. Parasitol.* **2008**, *38*, 351–358.
29. Antoniou, M.; Psaroulaki, A.; Toumazos, P.; Mazeris, A.; Ioannou, I.; Papaprodromou, M.; Georgiou, K.; Hristofi, N.; Patsias, A.; Loucaides, F.; et al. Rats as Indicators of the Presence and Dispersal of Pathogens in Cyprus: Ectoparasites, Parasitic Helminths, Enteric Bacteria, and Encephalomyocarditis Virus. *Vector Borne Zoonotic Dis.* **2010**, *10*, 867–873. [CrossRef]
30. Arzamani, K.; Salehi, M.; Mobedi, I.; Adinezade, A.; Hasanpour, H.; Alavinia, M.; Darvish, J.; Shirzadi, M.R.; Mohammadi, Z. Intestinal Helminths in Different Species of Rodents in North Khorasan Province, Northeast of Iran. *Iran. J. Parasitol.* **2017**, *12*, 267–273.
31. Ashour, A.A.; Lewis, J.W. Gongylonema aegypti n. sp. (Nematoda: Thelaziidae) from Egyptian rodents. *Syst. Parasitol.* **1986**, *8*, 199–206. [CrossRef]
32. Avcioglu, H.; Guven, E.; Balkaya, I.; Kirman, R.; Bia, M.M.; Gulbeyen, H.; Kurt, A.; Yaya, S.; Demirtas, S. First detection of *Echinococcus multilocularis* in rodent intermediate hosts in Turkey. *Parasitology* **2017**, *144*, 1821–1827. [CrossRef]
33. Azzam, K.M.; Abd El-Hady, E.A.; El-Abd, N. Survey of Natural Infection with Echinostoma liei in Aquatic Snails and Wild Rodents in Egypt. *Egypt. J. Biol. Pest. Control.* **2015**, *25*, 427–432.
34. Azzam, K.M.; El-Abd, N.M.; Abd El-Hady, E.A. Survey of endoparasites of different rodent species in Egypt. *Egypt. J. Biol. Pest. Control.* **2016**, *26*, 815–820.
35. Behnke, J.M.; Barnard, C.J.; Mason, N.; Harris, P.D.; Sherif, N.E.; Zalat, S.; Gilbert, F.S. Intestinal helminths of spiny mice (*Acomys cahirinus dimidiatus*) from St Katherine's Protectorate in the Sinai, Egypt. *J. Helminthol.* **2000**, *74*, 31–43. [CrossRef]
36. Behnke, J.M.; Harris, P.D.; Bajer, A.; Barnard, C.J.; Sherif, N.; Cliffe, L.; Hurst, J.; Lamb, M.; Rhodes, A.; James, M.; et al. Variation in the helminth community structure in spiny mice (*Acomys dimidiatus*) from four montane wadis in the St Katherine region of the Sinai Peninsula in Egypt. *Parasitology* **2004**, *129*, 379–398. [CrossRef]
37. Beiromvand, M.; Akhlaghi, L.; Fattahi Massom, S.H.; Meamar, A.R.; Darvish, J.; Razmjou, E. Molecular Identification of *Echinococcus multilocularis* Infection in Small Mammals from Northeast, Iran. *PLoS Negl. Trop. Dis.* **2013**, *7*. [CrossRef] [PubMed]
38. Borji, H.; Khoshnegah, J.; Razmi, G.; Amini, H.; Shariatzadeh, M. A survey on intestinal parasites of golden hamster (*Mesocricetus auratus*) in the northeast of Iran. *J. Parasit. Dis.* **2014**, *38*, 265–268. [CrossRef]
39. Celebi, B.; Taylan Ozkan, A.; Babur, C. *Capillaria Hhepatica* in mouse (*Apodemus flavicollis*) from Giresun Province of Turkey. *Turk. Parazitol. Derg.* **2014**, *38*, 208–210. [CrossRef]
40. Ebrahimi, M.; Sharifi, Y.; Nematollahi, A. Assessment of gastrointestinal helminths among house mice (*Mus musculus*) caught in the north-west of Iran, with a special view on zoonotic aspects. *Comp. Clin. Pathol.* **2016**, *25*, 1047–1051. [CrossRef]
41. El Gindy, M.S.; Morsy, T.A.; Bebars, M.A.; Sarwat, M.A.; Arafa, M.A.; Salama, M.M. Rodents as reservoir of zoonotic intestinal helminths in Suez Canal Zone with the possible immunological changes. *J. Egypt. Soc. Parasitol.* **1987**, *17*, 259–273.
42. El Kady, G.A.; Gheneam, Y.M.; Bahgat, I.M. Zoonotic helminthes of commensal rodents in Talkha Center, Dakahlia Governorate. *J. Egypt. Soc. Parasitol.* **2008**, *38*, 863–872.
43. El Shazly, A.M.; Morsy, T.A.; el Kady, G.A.; Ragheb, D.A.; Handousa, A.E.; Ahmed, M.M.; Younis, T.A.; Habib, K.S. The helminthic parasites of rodents in Dakahlia Governorate, with reference to their Egyptian helminth fauna. *J. Egypt. Soc. Parasitol.* **1994**, *24*, 413–428.

44. Elshazly, A.M.; Awad, S.I.; Azab, M.S.; Elsheikha, H.M.; Abdel-Gawad, A.G.; Khalil, H.H.; Morsy, T.A. Helminthes of synanthropic rodents (*Rodentia: Muridae*) from Dakahlia and Menoufia, Egypt. *J. Egypt. Soc. Parasitol.* **2008**, *38*, 727–740. [PubMed]
45. El-Shazly, A.M.; Romia, S.A.; el Ganayni, G.A.; Abou-Zakham, A.A.; Sabry, A.H.; Morsy, T.A. Antibodies against some zoonotic parasites in commensal rodents trapped from Dakahlia Governorate, Egypt. *J. Egypt. Soc. Parasitol.* **1991**, *21*, 169–177. [PubMed]
46. Fair, J.M.; Schmidt, G.D.; Wertheim, G. New species of Andrya and Paranoplocephala (*Cestoidea: Anoplocephalidae*) from voles and mole-rats in Israel and Syria. *J. Parasitol.* **1990**, *76*, 641–644. [CrossRef]
47. Fasihi Harandi, M.; Madjdzadeh, S.M.; Ahmadinejad, M. Helminth parasites of small mammals in Kerman province, southeastern Iran. *J. Parasit. Dis.* **2016**, *40*, 106–109. [CrossRef]
48. Garedaghi, Y.; Afshin Khaki, A. Prevalence of Gastrointestinal and Blood Parasites of Rodents in Tabriz, Iran, with Emphasis on Parasitic Zoonoses. *Crescent J. Med. Biol. Sci.* **2014**, *1*, 9–12.
49. Gholipoury, M.; Rezai, H.R.; Namroodi, S.; Arab Khazaeli, F. Zoonotic and Non-zoonotic Parasites of Wild Rodents in Turkman Sahra, Northeastern Iran. *Iran. J. Parasitol.* **2016**, *11*, 350–357.
50. Greenberg, Z. Helminths of mammals and birds of israel i. helminths of acomys spp. (*Rodentia, Murinae*). *Isr. J. Ecol. Evol.* **1969**, *18*, 25–38. [CrossRef]
51. Gurler, A.T.; Beyhan, Y.E.; Bolukbas, C.S.; Acici, M.; Umur, S. Gastro-intestinal helminths of wild rats (brown rat-*Rattus norvegicus*, Berkenhout 1769) in Samsun, Turkey. *Ank. Univ. Vet. Fak. Derg.* **2011**, *58*, 289–290. [CrossRef]
52. Haridy, F.M.; Morsy, T.A.; Ibrahim, B.B.; Abdel Gawad, A.G.; Mazyad, S.A. Rattus rattus: A new host for fascioliasis. *J. Egypt. Soc. Parasitol.* **2003**, *33*, 647–648. [PubMed]
53. Hasson, R.H. Zoonotic &Nonzoonotic Endoparasites of Rodents from Some Districts in Baghdad. *Diyala J. Pure Sci.* **2010**, *6*, 11.
54. Jones, A.; El-Azazy, O.M.E. *Coelomotrema aegyptiaca* sp, nov., an unusual prosthogonimid trematode from *Rattus norvegicus* (berkenhout) in Egypt. *J. Nat. Hist.* **1986**, *20*, 707–712. [CrossRef]
55. Kamranrashani, B.; Kia, E.; Mobedi, I.; Mohebali, M.; Zarei, Z.; Mowlavi, G.; Hajjaran, H.; Abai, M.; Sharifdini, M.; Kakooei, Z.; et al. Helminth Parasites of Rhombomys opimus from Golestan Province, Northeast Iran. *Iran. J. Parasitol.* **2013**, *8*, 78–84.
56. Khajeh, A.; Mohammadi, Z.; Darvish, J.; Razmi, G.R.; Ghorbani, F.; Mohammadi, A.; Mobedi, I.; Shahrokhi, A.R. A survey on endoparasites in wild rodents of the Jaz Murian depression and adjacent areas, southeast of Iran. *J. Parasit. Dis.* **2018**, *42*, 589–597. [CrossRef]
57. Khalil, L.F.; Hassounah, O.; Behbehani, K. Helminth parasites of rodents in Kuwait with the description of a new species *Abbreviata kuwaitensis* (*Nematoda: Physalopteridae*). *Syst. Parasitol.* **1979**, *1*, 67–73. [CrossRef]
58. Kia, E.B.; Homayouni, M.M.; Farahnak, A.; Mohebai, M.; Shojai, S. Study of Endoparasites of Rodents and their Zoonotic Importance In Ahvaz, South West Iran. *Iran. J. Public Health* **2001**, *30*, 4.
59. Kia, E.; Shahryary-Rad, E.; Mohebali, M.; Mahmoudi, M.; Mobedi, I.; Zahabiun, F.; Zarei, Z.; Miahipoor, A.; Mowlavi, G.; Akhavan, A.; et al. Endoparasites of rodents and their zoonotic importance in germi, dashte-mogan, ardabil province, Iran. *Iran. J. Parasitol.* **2010**, *5*, 15–20.
60. Meshkekar, M.; Sadraei, J.; Mahmoodzadeh, A.; Mobedi, I. Helminth Infections in *Rattus ratus* and *Rattus norvigicus* in Tehran, Iran. *Iran. J. Parasitol.* **2014**, *9*, 548–552.
61. Metwally, D.M.; Al-Enezy, H.A.; Al-Turaiki, I.M.; El-Khadragy, M.F.; Yehia, H.M.; Al-Otaibi, T.T. Gene-based molecular characterization of cox1 and pnad5 in Hymenolepis nana isolated from naturally infected mice and rats in Saudi Arabia. *Biosci. Rep.* **2019**, *39*. [CrossRef]
62. Mikhail, M.W.; Metwally, A.M.; Allam, K.A.; Mohamed, A.S. Rodents as reservoir host of intestinal helminthes in different Egyptian agroecosystems. *J. Egypt. Soc. Parasitol.* **2009**, *39*, 633–640.
63. Mirjalali, H.; Kia, E.B.; Kamranrashani, B.; Hajjaran, H.; Sharifdini, M. Molecular analysis of isolates of the cestode Rodentolepis nana from the great gerbil, Rhombomys opimus. *J. Helminthol.* **2016**, *90*, 252–255. [CrossRef]
64. Moradpour, N.; Borji, H.; Darvish, J.; Moshaverinia, A.; Mahmoudi, A. Rodents Helminth Parasites in Different Region of Iran. *Iran. J. Parasitol.* **2018**, *13*, 275–284.
65. Morsy, T.A.; Michael, S.A.; Bassili, W.R.; Saleh, M.S. Studies on rodents and their zoonotic parasites, particularly leishmania, in Ismailiya Governorate, A.R. Egypt. *J. Egypt. Soc. Parasitol.* **1982**, *12*, 565–585.

66. Mowlavi, G.; Mobedi, I.; Abedkhojasteh, H.; Sadjjadi, S.M.; Shahbazi, F.; Massoud, J. *Plagiorchis muris* (Tanabe, 1922) in *Rattus norvegicus* in Iran. *Iran. J. Parasitol.* **2013**, *8*, 486–490.
67. Nateghpour, M.; Motevalli-Haghi, A.; Akbarzadeh, K.; Akhavan, A.A.; Mohebali, M.; Mobedi, I.; Farivar, L. Endoparasites of wild rodents in Southeastern Iran. *J. Arthropod Borne Dis.* **2014**, *9*, 1–6.
68. Pakdel, N.; Naem, S.; Rezaei, F.; Chalehchaleh, A.A. A survey on helminthic infection in mice (*Mus musculus*) and rats (*Rattus norvegicus* and *Rattus rattus*) in Kermanshah, Iran. *Vet. Res. Forum Int. Q. J.* **2013**, *4*, 105–109.
69. Ranjbar, M.J.; Sarkari, B.; Mowlavi, G.R.; Seifollahi, Z.; Moshfe, A.; Abdolahi Khabisi, S.; Mobedi, I. Helminth Infections of Rodents and Their Zoonotic Importance in Boyer-Ahmad District, Southwestern Iran. *Iran. J. Parasitol.* **2017**, *12*, 572–579.
70. Sadighian, A.; Ghadirian, E.; Sadjadpour, E. Two new species of nematodes of lagomorphs and rodents from Iran. *J. Helminthol.* **1974**, *48*, 241–245. [CrossRef] [PubMed]
71. Saoud, M.F.; Ramadan, M.M.; Ashour, A.A.; Shahawy, A.A. On the helminth parasites of rodents in the Eastern Delta. I. General survey. *J. Egypt. Soc. Parasitol.* **1986**, *16*, 197–209.
72. Soliman, M.F.; Ibrahim, M.M.; Zalat, S.M. Gastrointestinal nematode community of spiny mice (Acomys dimidiatus) from St. Katherine, South Sinai, Egypt. *J. Parasit. Dis.* **2015**, *39*, 705–711. [CrossRef]
73. Sures, B.; Scheible, T.; Bashtar, A.R.; Taraschewski, H. Lead concentrations in *Hymenolepis diminuta* adults and *Taenia taeniaeformis* larvae compared to their rat hosts (*Rattus norvegicus*) sampled from the city of Cairo, Egypt. *Parasitology* **2003**, *127*, 483–487. [CrossRef] [PubMed]
74. Sursal, N.; Gokpinar, S.; Yildiz, K. Prevalence of intestinal parasites in hamsters and rabbits in some pet shops of Turkey. *Turk. Parazitol. Derg.* **2014**, *38*, 102–105. [CrossRef]
75. Wanas, M.Q.; Shehata, K.K.; Rashed, A.A. Larval occurrence of *Hydatigera taeniaeformis* Batsch (1786) (*Cestoda: Taeniidae*) in the liver of wild rodents in Egypt. *J. Egypt. Soc. Parasitol.* **1993**, *23*, 381–388.
76. Mohamed; Wanas, Q.A.; Shehata, K.K.; Rashed, A.A. Studies on the nematode parasites from Egyptian rodents. I. Spirurid nematodes. *J. Egypt. Soc. Parasitol.* **1994**, *23*, 851–863.
77. Wertheim, G.; Chabaud, A.G. Helminths of birds and mammals of Israel. VIII.—Skrjabinocapillaria rodentium n. sp. (*Nematoda Capillariidae*) from gerbillid and murid rodents. *Ann. De Parasitol. Hum. Comp.* **1979**, *54*, 65–68. [CrossRef]
78. Wertheim, G.; Giladi, M. Helminths of birds and mammals of Israel. VII.—*Pneumospirura rodentium* n. sp. (*Pneumospiruridae-Thelazioidea*). *Ann. Parasitol. Hum. Comp.* **1977**, *52*, 643–646. [CrossRef] [PubMed]
79. Wertheim, G. Helminths of Birds and Mammals from Israel: III. Helminths from Chromosomal Forms of the Mole-Rat, Spalax ehrenbergi. *J. Helminthol.* **1971**, *45*, 161–169. [CrossRef]
80. Yousefi, A.; Eslami, A.; Mobedi, I.; Rahbari, S.; Ronaghi, H. Helminth Infections of House Mouse (*Mus musulus*) and Wood Mouse (*Apodemus sylvaticus*) from the Suburban Areas of Hamadan City, Western Iran. *Iran. J. Parasitol.* **2014**, *9*, 511–518.
81. Yousif, F.; Ibrahim, A. The first record of *Angiostrongylus cantonensis* from Egypt. *Z. Parasitenkdunde* **1978**, *56*, 73–80. [CrossRef] [PubMed]
82. Zarei, Z.; Mohebali, M.; Heidari, Z.; Davoodi, J.; Shabestari, A.; Haghi, A.M.; Khanaliha, K.; Kia, E.B. Helminth infections of meriones persicus (Persian jird), *Mus musculus* (house mice) and cricetulus migratorius (grey ham-ster): A cross-sectional study in Meshkin-Shahr district, north-west Iran. *Iran. J. Parasitol.* **2016**, *11*, 213–220.
83. Nijsten, T.; Stern, R.S. How Epidemiology Has Contributed to a Better Understanding of Skin Disease. *J. Investig. Dermatol.* **2012**, *132*, 994–1002. [CrossRef] [PubMed]
84. Neta, G.; Brownson, R.C.; Chambers, D.A. Opportunities for Epidemiologists in Implementation Science: A Primer. *Am. J. Epidemiol.* **2018**, *187*, 899–910. [CrossRef]
85. Higgins, J.P.; Thompson, S.G. Quantifying heterogeneity in a meta-analysis. *Stat. Med.* **2002**, *21*, 1539–1558. [CrossRef]
86. Chatterjee, K.D. *Parasitology: Protozoology and Helminthology in Relation to Clinical Medicine: With Two Hundred Fourteen Illustrations*; CBS Publishers & Distributors: New Delhi, India, 2012.
87. Gárate, I.; Jimenez, P.; Flores, K.; Espinoza, B. Xenopsylla cheopis record as natural intermediate host of Hymenolepis diminuta in Lima, Peru. *Rev. Peru. Biol.* **2011**, *18*, 249–252. [CrossRef]
88. Stěrba, J.; Barus, V. First record of Strobilocercus fasciolaris (*Taenidae-larvae*) in man. *Folia Parasitol.* **1976**, *23*, 221–226.

89. Toledo, R.; Esteban, J.G. An update on human echinostomiasis. *Trans. R. Soc. Trop. Med. Hyg.* **2016**, *110*, 37–45. [CrossRef]
90. Boyce, K. Transmission Ecology of Gastrointestinal Trematodes of Small Mammals, Malham Tarn, North Yorkshire, UK. Ph.D. Thesis, University of Salford, Salford, UK, July 2013.
91. Loftis, A.D.; Reeves, W.K.; Szumlas, D.E.; Abbassy, M.M.; Helmy, I.M.; Moriarity, J.R.; Dasch, G.A. Surveillance of Egyptian fleas for agents of public health significance: Anaplasma, bartonella, coxiella, ehrlichia, rickettsia, and Yersinia pestis. *Am. J. Trop. Med. Hyg.* **2006**, *75*, 41–48. [CrossRef]
92. Trevisanato, S.I. The 'Hittite plague', an epidemic of tularemia and the first record of biological warfare. *Med. Hypotheses* **2007**, *69*, 1371–1374. [CrossRef] [PubMed]
93. Bishara, J.; Hershkovitz, D.; Yagupsky, P.; Lazarovitch, T.; Boldur, I.; Kra-Oz, T.; Pitlik, S. Murine typhus among Arabs and Jews in Israel 1991–2001. *Eur. J. Epidemiol.* **2004**, *19*, 1123–1126. [CrossRef] [PubMed]
94. Rosenthal, T.; Michaeli, D. Murine typhus and spotted fever in Israel in the seventies. *Infection* **1977**, *5*, 82–84. [CrossRef] [PubMed]
95. Khaghani, R. The economic and health impact of rodent in urban zone and harbours and their control methods. *Ann. Mil. Health Sci. Res.* **2007**, *4*, 1071–1078.
96. Morand, S.; Bordes, F. Parasite diversity of disease-bearing rodents of Southeast Asia: Habitat determinants and effects on sexual size dimorphism and life-traits. *Front. Ecol. Evol.* **2015**, *3*. [CrossRef]
97. Radostits, O.M.; Done, S.H. *Veterinary Medicine: A Textbook of the Diseases of Cattle, Sheep, Pigs, Goats, and Horses*; Elsevier Saunders: Philadelphia, PA, USA, 2007.
98. Rodan, I.; Sparkes, A.H. Chapter 8-Preventive Health Care for Cats. In *The Cat, Little, S.E., Ed.*; W.B. Saunders: Saint Louis, MO, USA, 2012; pp. 151–180. [CrossRef]
99. Dorny, P.; Praet, N.; Deckers, N.; Gabriel, S. Emerging food-borne parasites. *Vet. Parasitol.* **2009**, *163*, 196–206. [CrossRef]
100. Youn, H. Review of zoonotic parasites in medical and veterinary fields in the Republic of Korea. *Korean J. Parasitol.* **2009**, *47*, S133–S141. [CrossRef]
101. Amin, O.M. Pathogenic micro-organisms and helminths in sewage products, Arabian Gulf, country of Bahrain. *Am. J. Public Health* **1988**, *78*, 314–315. [CrossRef]
102. Berger, S. *Infectious Diseases of Cyprus*; Incorporated Gideon e-book series; Global Infectious Diseases and Epidemiology Network Informatics: Winconsin, WI, USA, 2019.
103. Al-Lahham, A.B.; Abu-Saud, M.; Shehabi, A.A. Prevalence of Salmonella, Shigella and intestinal parasites in food handlers in Irbid, Jordan. *J. Diarrhoeal Dis Res.* **1990**, *8*, 160–162.
104. Patel, P.K.; Khandekar, R. Intestinal parasitic infections among school children of the Dhahira Region of Oman. *Saudi Med. J.* **2006**, *27*, 627–632.
105. Astal, Z. Epidemiological survey of the prevalence of parasites among children in Khan Younis governorate, Palestine. *Parasitol. Res.* **2004**, *94*, 449–451. [CrossRef]
106. Abu-Madi, M.A.; Behnke, J.M.; Boughattas, S.; Al-Thani, A.; Doiphode, S.H.; Deshmukh, A. Helminth infections among long-term-residents and settled immigrants in Qatar in the decade from 2005 to 2014: Temporal trends and varying prevalence among subjects from different regional origins. *Parasites Vectors* **2016**, *9*, 153. [CrossRef]
107. Alharbi, R.A.; Alwajeeh, T.S.; Assabri, A.M.; Almalki, S.S.R.; Alruwetei, A.; Azazy, A.A. Intestinal parasitoses and schistosome infections among students with special reference to praziquantel efficacy in patients with schistosomosis in Hajjah governorate, Yemen. *Ann. Parasitol.* **2019**, *65*, 217–223. [CrossRef]
108. Abo-Shehada, M.N. Prevalence of Toxocara ova in some schools and public grounds in northern and central Jordan. *Ann. Trop Med. Parasitol.* **1989**, *83*, 73–75. [CrossRef]
109. Geramizadeh, B.; Baghernezhad, M. Hepatic Alveolar Hydatid Cyst: A Brief Review of Published Cases from Iran in the Last 20 Years. *Hepat Mon.* **2016**, *16*. [CrossRef]
110. Al-Aboody, M.S.; Omar, M.A.; Alsayeqh, A.F. Epizootiology of zoonotic parasites in Middle East: A comprehensive review. *Ann. Parasitol.* **2020**, *66*, 125–133. [CrossRef] [PubMed]
111. Fellner, A.; Hellmann, M.A.; Kolianov, V.; Bishara, J. A non-travel related case of Angiostrongylus cantonensis eosinophilic meningomyelitis acquired in Israel. *J. Neurol. Sci.* **2016**, *370*, 241–243. [CrossRef]
112. Molavi, G.H.; Massoud, J.; Gutierrez, Y. Human Gongylonema infection in Iran. *J. Helminthol.* **2006**, *80*, 425–428. [CrossRef]

113. Mirzayans, A.; Halim, R. Parasitic infection of Camelus dromedarius from Iran. *Bull. Soc. Pathol Exot. Fil.* **1980**, *73*, 442–445.
114. Moazeni, M.; Khamesipour, F.; Anyona, D.N.; Dida, G.O. Epidemiology of taeniosis, cysticercosis and trichinellosis in Iran: A systematic review. *Zoonoses Public Health* **2019**, *66*, 140–154. [CrossRef]
115. Eisenman, A.; Einat, R. A family outbreak of trichinosis acquired in Israel. *Harefuah* **1992**, *122*, 702–704, 751. [PubMed]
116. Haim, M.; Efrat, M.; Wilson, M.; Schantz, P.M.; Cohen, D.; Shemer, J. An outbreak of Trichinella spiralis infection in southern Lebanon. *Epidemiol. Infect.* **1997**, *119*, 357–362. [CrossRef]
117. Turk, M.; Kaptan, F.; Turker, N.; Korkmaz, M.; El, S.; Ozkaya, D.; Ural, S.; Vardar, I.; Alkan, M.Z.; Coskun, N.A.; et al. Clinical and laboratory aspects of a trichinellosis outbreak in Izmir, Turkey. *Parasite* **2006**, *13*, 65–70. [CrossRef]
118. El Shazly, A.M.; Awad, S.E.; Sultan, D.M.; Sadek, G.S.; Khalil, H.H.; Morsy, T.A. Intestinal parasites in Dakahlia governorate, with different techniques in diagnosing protozoa. *J. Egypt. Soc. Parasitol.* **2006**, *36*, 1023–1034.
119. Ghanbarzadeh, L.; Saraei, M.; Kia, E.B.; Amini, F.; Sharifdini, M. Clinical and haematological characteristics of human trichostrongyliasis. *J. Helminthol.* **2019**, *93*, 149–153. [CrossRef]
120. Greenberg, Z.; Giladi, L.; Bashary, A.; Zahavi, H. Prevalence of intestinal parasites among Thais in Israel. *Harefuah* **1994**, *126*, 507–509, 563.
121. Akdemir, C.; Helvaci, R. Evaluation of parasitology laboratory results of a group of people older than 15 years of age in Kutahya. *Turk. Parazit. Derg.* **2007**, *31*, 129–132.
122. Nooraldeen, K. Contamination of public squares and parks with parasites in Erbil city, Iraq. *Ann. Agric. Environ. Med.* **2015**, *22*, 418–420. [CrossRef]
123. Mukhtar, A. Intestinal parasites in the state of Bahrain. *Indian J. Pathol. Microbiol.* **1995**, *38*, 341–344. [PubMed]
124. Abu-Madi, M.A.; Behnke, J.M.; Ismail, A. Patterns of infection with intestinal parasites in Qatar among food handlers and housemaids from different geographical regions of origin. *Acta Trop.* **2008**, *106*, 213–220. [CrossRef]
125. Amer, O.S.O.; Al-Malki, E.S.; Waly, M.I.; AlAgeel, A.; Lubbad, M.Y. Prevalence of Intestinal Parasitic Infections among Patients of King Fahd Medical City in Riyadh Region, Saudi Arabia: A 5-Year Retrospective Study. *J. Parasitol. Res.* **2018**, *2018*. [CrossRef] [PubMed]
126. Yentur Doni, N.; Yildiz Zeyrek, F.; Simsek, Z.; Gurses, G.; Sahin, I. Risk Factors and Relationship between Intestinal Parasites and the Growth Retardation and Psychomotor Development Delays of Children in Sanliurfa, Turkey. *Turk. Parazitol. Derg.* **2015**, *39*, 270–276. [CrossRef]
127. Hotez, P.J.; Savioli, L.; Fenwick, A. Neglected tropical diseases of the Middle East and North Africa: Review of their prevalence, distribution, and opportunities for control. *PLoS Negl. Trop. Dis.* **2012**, *6*. [CrossRef]
128. Rollinson, D.; Knopp, S.; Levitz, S.; Stothard, J.R.; Tchuem Tchuente, L.A.; Garba, A.; Mohammed, K.A.; Schur, N.; Person, B.; Colley, D.G.; et al. Time to set the agenda for schistosomiasis elimination. *Acta Trop.* **2013**, *128*, 423–440. [CrossRef]
129. Hornstein, L.; Lederer, G.; Schechter, J.; Greenberg, Z.; Boem, R.; Bilguray, B.; Giladi, L.; Hamburger, J. Persistent Schistosoma mansoni infection in Yemeni immigrants to Israel. *Isr. J. Med. Sci.* **1990**, *26*, 386–389. [PubMed]
130. Taha, H.A.; Soliman, M.I.; Banjar, S.A. Intestinal parasitic infections among expatriate workers in Al-Madina Al-Munawarah, Kingdom of Saudi Arabia. *Trop Biomed.* **2013**, *30*, 78–88.
131. Kiremit, M.C.; Cakir, A.; Arslan, F.; Ormeci, T.; Erkurt, B.; Albayrak, S. The bladder carcinoma secondary to schistosoma mansoni infection: A case report with review of the literature. *Int. J. Surg. Case. Rep.* **2015**, *13*, 76–78. [CrossRef]
132. Al-Mekhlafi, A.M.; Abdul-Ghani, R.; Al-Eryani, S.M.; Saif-Ali, R.; Mahdy, M.A. School-based prevalence of intestinal parasitic infections and associated risk factors in rural communities of Sana'a, Yemen. *Acta Trop.* **2016**, *163*, 135–141. [CrossRef]
133. El-Shazly, A.M.; el-Nahas, H.A.; Soliman, M.; Sultan, D.M.; Abedl Tawab, A.H.; Morsy, T.A. The reflection of control programs of parasitic diseases upon gastrointestinal helminthiasis in Dakahlia Governorate, Egypt. *J. Egypt. Soc. Parasitol.* **2006**, *36*, 467–480.
134. Chai, J.Y.; Seo, B.S.; Lee, S.H.; Hong, S.J.; Sohn, W.M. Human infections by *Heterophyes heterophyes* and *H. dispar* imported from Saudi Arabia. *Kisaengchunghak Chapchi* **1986**, *24*, 82–86. [CrossRef]

135. Chai, J.Y.; Jung, B.K. Foodborne intestinal flukes: A brief review of epidemiology and geographical distribution. *Acta Trop.* **2019**, *201*. [CrossRef]
136. El-Gayar, A.K. Studies on some trematode parasites of stray dogs in Egypt with a key to the identification of intestinal trematodes of dogs. *Vet. Parasitol.* **2007**, *144*, 360–365. [CrossRef]
137. El-Azazy, O.M.; Abdou, N.E.; Khalil, A.I.; Al-Batel, M.K.; Majeed, Q.A.; Henedi, A.A.; Tahrani, L.M. Potential Zoonotic Trematodes Recovered in Stray Cats from Kuwait Municipality, Kuwait. *Korean J. Parasitol.* **2015**, *53*, 279–287. [CrossRef]
138. Khalil, M.I.; El-Shahawy, I.S.; Abdelkader, H.S. Studies on some fish parasites of public health importance in the southern area of Saudi Arabia. *Rev. Bras. Parasitol. Vet.* **2014**, *23*, 435–442. [CrossRef] [PubMed]
139. Steinmann, P.; Keiser, J.; Bos, R.; Tanner, M.; Utzinger, J. Schistosomiasis and water resources development: Systematic review, meta-analysis, and estimates of people at risk. *Lancet Infect. Dis.* **2006**, *6*, 411–425. [CrossRef]
140. El-Sayed, H.F.; Rizkalla, N.H.; Mehanna, S.; Abaza, S.M.; Winch, P.J. Prevalence and epidemiology of *Schistosoma mansoni* and *S. haematobium* infection in two areas of Egypt recently reclaimed from the desert. *Am. J. Trop. Med. Hyg.* **1995**, *52*, 194–198. [CrossRef]
141. Odhiambo, G.O. Water scarcity in the Arabian Peninsula and socio-economic implications. *Appl. Water Sci.* **2017**, *7*, 2479–2492. [CrossRef]
142. Bordes, F.; Blasdell, K.; Morand, S. Transmission ecology of rodent-borne diseases: New frontiers. *Integr. Zool.* **2015**, *10*, 424–435. [CrossRef]
143. Eisen, R.J.; Enscore, R.E.; Atiku, L.A.; Zielinski-Gutierrez, E.; Mpanga, J.T.; Kajik, E.; Andama, V.; Mungujakisa, C.; Tibo, E.; MacMillan, K.; et al. Evidence that rodent control strategies ought to be improved to enhance food security and reduce the risk of rodent-borne illnesses within subsistence farming villages in the plague-endemic West Nile region, Uganda. *Int. J. Pest. Manag.* **2013**, *59*, 259–270. [CrossRef]
144. Brown, L.M.; Laco, J. Rodent Control and Public Health: A Description of Local Rodent Control Programs. *J. Environ. Health* **2015**, *78*, 28–29.
145. Kaplan, B.; Kahn, L.H.; Monath, T.P.; Woodall, J. 'ONE HEALTH' and parasitology. *Parasites Vectors* **2009**, *2*, 36. [CrossRef] [PubMed]
146. Centers for Disease Control and Prevention. One Health Basics. Available online: https://www.cdc.gov/onehealth/basics/ (accessed on 2 October 2020).

15

Parasite Occurrence and Parasite Management in Swedish Horses Presenting with Gastrointestinal Disease

Ylva Hedberg-Alm [1,*], Johanna Penell [2], Miia Riihimäki [3], Eva Osterman-Lind [4], Martin K. Nielsen [5] and Eva Tydén [6]

1 Horse Clinic, University Animal Hospital, Swedish University of Agricultural Sciences, 750 07 Uppsala, Sweden
2 Division of Veterinary Nursing, Department of Clinical Sciences, Swedish University of Agricultural Sciences, 750 07 Uppsala, Sweden; Johanna.Penell@slu.se
3 Equine Medicine Unit, Department of Clinical Sciences, Swedish University of Agricultural Sciences, 750 07 Uppsala, Sweden; Miia.Riihimaki@slu.se
4 National Veterinary Institute, Department of Microbiology, Section for Parasitology diagnostics, 751 89 Uppsala, Sweden; eva.osterman-lind@sva.se
5 Maxwell H. Gluck Equine Research Center, Department of Veterinary Science, University of Kentucky, Lexington, KY 40546, USA; martin.nielsen@uky.edu
6 Parasitology Unit, Department of Biomedical Science and Veterinary Public Health, Swedish University of Agricultural Sciences, 750 07 Uppsala, Sweden; eva.tyden@slu.se
* Correspondence: ylva.hedberg.alm@uds.slu.se.

Simple Summary: Abdominal pain, colic, is a common clinical sign in horses, sometimes reflecting life-threatening disease. One cause of colic is parasitic infection of the gut. Various drugs, anthelmintics, can be used to reduce or eliminate such parasites. However, frequent use has led to problems of drug resistance, whereby many countries now allow anthelmintics to be used on a prescription-only basis. In Sweden, this has led to a concern that parasitic-related colic in horses is increasing. This study aimed to investigate whether horses with colic differed in parasitological status compared to horses without colic. A secondary aim was to collect information regarding current parasite control measures used by horse owners. Exposure to *S. vulgaris*, a parasite with the potential to cause life-threatening disease, appeared high as determined by the presence of antibodies in the blood. Horses with inflammation in the abdominal cavity had higher antibody levels than other causes of colic. Despite new legislation, 29% of owners did not use fecal analyses for parasites and the use of extended methods to diagnose specific parasites was low. Also, owners rarely used alternative methods to reduce the pasture parasite burden. The study suggests a need for education in the use of both fecal analyses and pasture management.

Abstract: All grazing horses are exposed to intestinal parasites, which have the potential to cause gastrointestinal disease. In Sweden, there is a concern about an increase in parasite-related equine gastrointestinal disease, in particular *Strongylus vulgaris*, since the implementation of prescription-only anthelmintics approximately 10 years ago. In a prospective case–control study, parasitological status, using fecal analyses for strongyle egg counts, the presence of *Anoplocephala perfoliata* eggs and *S. vulgaris* Polymerase chain reaction (PCR) as well as serology for *S. vulgaris*, were compared between horses presenting with or without gastrointestinal disease at a University hospital during a one-year period. Information regarding anthelmintic routines and pasture management was gathered with an owner-filled questionnaire. Although the prevalence of *S. vulgaris* PCR was 5.5%, 62% of horses were positive in the enzyme-linked immunosorbent assay (ELISA) test and horses with peritonitis showed higher antibody levels for *S. vulgaris*, as compared to other diagnoses or controls. Overall, 36% of the horse owners used only fecal egg counts (FEC), 32% used FEC combined with specific diagnostics for *S. vulgaris* or *A. perfoliata*, and 29% dewormed routinely without prior parasite diagnostics. Effective management methods to reduce the parasitic burden on pastures were rare and considering exposure to *S. vulgaris* appears high; the study indicates a need for education in specific fecal diagnostics and pasture management.

Keywords: horse; colic; gastrointestinal disease; *Strongylus vulgaris*; *Anoplocephala perfoliata*; cyathostominae

---

1. Introduction

Colic in horses is a significant cause of mortality and morbidity and thus, is a major contributing factor to economic loss within the equine industry [1]. A vast number of potential risk factors have been implicated as a cause of gastrointestinal disease in horses, including intestinal parasites [2,3]. As grazing animals, horses are hosts to a large number of internal parasites that, to a varying degree, may result in pathology of the gastrointestinal tract [2].

Of all the equine internal parasites, *Strongylus vulgaris* is regarded as the most pathogenic and was therefore the main target of parasitic control programs in the 1960s, when modern anthelmintic drugs were first introduced [4]. This parasite has a long lifecycle of about six months, of which four months involve migration of larvae in the mesenteric arteries, in particular the cranial mesenteric artery [5]. Due to its larval migration within the mesenteric vasculature, *S. vulgaris* may cause severe arterial inflammation and damage to the otherwise smooth endothelial surface, with subsequent thrombus formation [5]. This potentially leads to the occlusion of arteries and arterioles supplying the intestinal wall, causing intestinal infarction and septic peritonitis. This condition is often fatal and requires surgical resection of the infarcted intestinal segment for a chance of survival [6].

The cestode *Anoplocephala perfoliata* has also been implicated as a cause of colic of varying degrees of severity [7]. This parasite's predilection for the ileocecal junction may cause lesions in this area, such as ileocecal invaginations and ileal impactions, most likely due to parasite-induced intestinal pathology at the site of attachment, but perhaps also secondary to physical obstruction and/or modifications in intestinal motility [8,9]. In addition, studies have demonstrated an association between *A. perfoliata* infection and spasmodic colic [10] as well as colic in general [11].

In contrast to other parasites, small strongyles, cyathostomins, have a direct life cycle and the early third larval stage can be arrested in the gut wall as encysted larvae for prolonged periods of time. The emergence of large numbers of such arrested larval stages can cause a severe inflammatory reaction in the colon and cecum resulting in diarrhea, sometimes with fatal outcomes, predominately in young animals; a condition known as larval cyathostominosis [12,13]. Moreover, large burdens of cyathostomins have been related to ill-thrift and weight-loss [14,15]. However, it is still under debate if cyathostomins are associated with colic in general, and a recent case–control study was unable to demonstrate a connection between cyathostomins and colic [16].

In the 1960s, regular anthelmintic treatment of horses was introduced, and as a result, some previously common parasite-induced gastrointestinal diseases, such as non-strangulating intestinal infarction caused by *S. vulgaris*, appeared to be largely eradicated [2]. However, the increasing reports of anthelmintic resistance in both cyathostomin parasites and *Parascaris* spp. [17,18], have led several countries, including Denmark, Finland, the Netherlands, Italy and Sweden, to implement a prescription-only sale of equine and livestock anthelmintic drugs [19]. In Sweden, the legislation advocates the prescription of anthelmintics to adult horses only after fecal analyses. By treating horses exceeding a chosen cut-off value, often 200 strongyle eggs per gram of feces (EPG), fewer anthelmintic treatments are administered, thus reducing the risk of developing of anthelmintic resistance [19,20]. However, since the implementation of more selective anthelmintic treatment strategies, Denmark and Sweden have recently documented a clear increase in the prevalence of *S. vulgaris* in the equine population in these countries [21,22]. Furthermore, post-mortem studies conducted in Italy indicate that pathological lesions caused by *S. vulgaris* are still widespread and in Denmark, several clinical cases of *S. vulgaris*-associated non-strangulating infarctions with subsequent septic peritonitis with a high mortality rate have been reported [6,23,24].

In Sweden, the legislation restricting anthelmintic products to prescription-only came into effect in October 2007. Just prior to this, only a minority (1%) of Swedish horse owners based anthelmintic treatment on fecal analyses of their horses [25]. As yet, there are few studies investigating how the prescription-only legislation has affected anthelmintic routines in Sweden and its possible effect on parasite-related disease in Swedish horses. Despite similar legislation in several European countries, there appears to be substantial national differences in how the law is implemented in practice [19]. Recently, an *S. vulgaris* prevalence of 61% was demonstrated in Swedish horse farms [22]. Whether this has resulted in an increase in clinical disease in Swedish horses is, however, unknown.

The aim of the present study was to compare the parasitological status between horses presenting for gastrointestinal disease (colic, colitis, peritonitis, weight loss) and horses presenting for non-intestinal disease at a university equine referral hospital during a one-year period, using coprological and serological assays. In addition, a secondary aim was to gather information regarding current anthelmintic treatment routines and pasture management practices using an owner-filled questionnaire at admission.

2. Materials and Methods

The study was approved by the Uppsala animal welfare ethics committee (license number: Dnr 68/16). Owner consent was required for study participation and participating owners were asked to fill in a consent form at admission.

2.1. Project Outline

The study was designed as a prospective case–control study at the Horse Clinic, University Animal Hospital, Swedish University of Agricultural Sciences, over a one-year period (February 2017–February 2018). The Horse Clinic receives both first opinion as well as referred equine cases with an annual case load of approximately 6000 cases. A horse presenting to the clinic and diagnosed with a disease related to the gastrointestinal canal was classified as a case. Each case was matched with a control horse presenting during the same week and, when possible, of same or similar age, and diagnosed with either a disease unrelated to the gastrointestinal canal (e.g., respiratory, skin, eye, cardiac, and orthopedic conditions) or presenting for prophylactic reasons (e.g., general health check, oral examination). Fecal and blood samples were collected by veterinarians from each case and control during the horse´s visit at the clinic. In addition, each owner was asked to respond to a questionnaire for collecting information regarding previous colic history, previous anthelmintic treatment, anthelmintic routines, and pasture management (Table 1). Regarding the question about deworming routines, there were five alternatives for the horse owner with the highest number of treatments being 2–4 times/year (Table 1). The reason for this is that in Sweden the recommendation for adult horses is to perform parasite diagnostics in April/May and only treat individuals exceeding 200 EPG and positive for *S. vulgaris* and/or *A. perfoliata* [26]. It is very rare that adult horses are dewormed more than 4 times/year in Sweden.

Table 1. Questionnaire data collected from participating cases and controls.

Information	Descriptor
Age of horse	Years
Time in ownership	Years
Any previous history of colic [a]	Yes/No
If yes, specify number of colic episodes	Number
Treated for colic by a veterinarian during last 24 months	Yes/No
Signs of diarrhea [b] during last 2 months	Yes/No
Lost weight [c] during last 2 months	Yes/No
Last anthelmintic treatment (months)	0–3; 3–6; 6–12; >12
Drug used during last treatment	FBZ [d]; PYR [e]; IVM [f]; MOX [g]; COMB [h]
Deworming routines applied on the farm	(i) only after FEC [i] (ii) after FEC and *S. vulgaris* diagnostics (iii) diagnostics for *A. perfoliata* at least 1/year (iv) routine deworming once/year (v) routine deworming 2–4 times/year
Presence of parasites in fecal sample during last 24 months	Small strongyles; *S. vulgaris*; *A. perfoliata*; *Parascasris spp*; do not know
Access to separate winter and summer pasture	Yes/No
Grazing with other animals species	Yes/No
Size of pasture or paddock, winter	Hectare
Size of pasture or paddock, summer	Hectare
Number of horses in pasture/paddock, winter	Number
Number of horses in pasture/paddock, summer	Number
Use of fecal removal	Yes/No
If yes, how often are feces removed	Number/week
Hours spent outdoors (paddock), winter	1–24
Hours spent outdoors (pasture), summer	1–24

[a] restlessness and pawing at the ground, irritated kicking to the stomach, rolling or attempting to roll; [b] loose consistency of feces; [c] as subjectively appreciated by owner; [d] fenbendazole; [e] pyrantel; [f] ivermectin; [g] moxidectin; [h] ivermectin/moxidectin and praziquantel; [i] fecal egg count.

2.2. Processing of Samples

Each horse included in the study had a fecal sample collected either at the time of rectal exam (majority of case horses), or from feces passed in the loose box (cases and controls) or transport vehicle in which the horse was brought to the clinic (controls). Fecal samples, approximately 200 g, were stored at 4 °C until parasite analyses the following day. In addition, two serum blood collection tubes (10 mL BD Vacutainer®(BD Technologies, Durham, NC, USA)) were obtained, either by vacutainer technique (20 G × 25 mm) from the jugular vein, or, in some case horses, from a permanent jugular catheter (Extended Use MILACATH® (MILA International Inc, Florence, KY, USA) placed in the jugular vein. In the latter case, at least 10 mL of blood was discarded before obtaining the sample. Blood samples were refrigerated at 4 °C for 12–24 h and then centrifuged at 2000× g for ten minutes. Serum was pipetted off and stored in 1.8 mL cryo tubes at −80 °C until the enzyme-linked immunosorbent assay (ELISA) was performed.

2.3. Parasite Analyses

Strongyle fecal egg counts (FECs) were carried out for each horse using a modified McMaster technique with a minimum detection limit of 50 EPG [27]. Parasite eggs in fecal samples (3 g) were floated using a saturated NaCl solution (SG = 1.18) [27]. Irrespective of FEC, larval cultures for detection of *S. vulgaris* were performed on 50 g feces from each horse according to Bellaw and Nielsen [28]. In brief, feces were mixed with an equal volume of vermiculite (Weibulls, Sweden), tap water was added to obtain a moist condition and samples were cultured at 20 °C for 14 ds. Third stage larvae were harvested after sedimentation for 12–16 h at 20 °C by the inverted Petri dish method [29]. Pellet of harvested L3 was performed by collecting approximately 20 mL of the fluid into a 50 mL Falcon tube, centrifuging at 248× g for three minutes and discarding the supernatant. Larval DNA was extracted with NuceloSpin®Tissue (Macherey-Nagel, Düren, Germany) according to the manufacturer´s instruction. An ITS-2 specific PCR was used for identification of *S. vulgaris* according to Nielsen et al. (2008) and Tydén et al. (2019) [22,30].

Anoplocephala perfoliata were examined on 30 g feces using the modified flotation technique described by Berozoa et al. [31]. Feces were mixed with 60 mL tap water, sieved and collected into four 15 mL test tubes and centrifuged 1000× g for ten minutes. The supernatant was removed and pellet suspended in sugar salt solution (saturated sodium chloride solution with 50% glucose with a density of 1.280) to form a convex meniscus. Cover glasses (18 mm × 18 mm) were put on the top and centrifuged for 5 min at 214× *g* (no brakes) in a swing out centrifuge. Samples were left 5 min after centrifugation and thereafter transferred to microscope slides and microscopically examined at 40–100× magnification.

2.4. *Strongylus vulgaris* Specific ELISA

Serum samples were packed with dry ice and shipped to the Nielsen Parasitology Laboratory at the University of Kentucky. Here, an indirect ELISA using recombinant SvSXP protein as antigen was performed as previously described [32]. Samples were diluted 1:50 and horseradish peroxidase-conjugated goat anti-horse IgG(T) (Bethyl Laboratories, Inc., Montgomery, TX, USA) was used as a secondary antibody at a dilution of 1:40,000. Results were reported as the normalised value, percentage of a positive control to reduce inter-assay variability [32]. The positive control sample was obtained from a horse known to be infected with *S. vulgaris*.

2.5. Statistical Analyses

All statistical analyses were interpreted as statistically significant up to the p-value < 0.05 with the application of Bonferroni correction of the p-value, i.e., the division of the p-value for significance with the number of tests applied, to account for multiple testing, when appropriate. All statistical analyses were performed using Stata SE (version 14.2, StataCorp, College Station, TX, USA).

2.5.1. Data on Horses, Colic Diagnoses and Season

Statistical analyses on data on horses, colic diagnosis and season were performed as follows. Horses were categorised into six age-groups (1–2; 3–5; 6–10; 11–15; 16–20 and >20 years) and gender (mare, stallion, gelding). Gastrointestinal disease was classified into nine categories: impaction (large colon, small colon, and cecal), large intestinal displacement, acute colitis, peritonitis, equine eosinophilic gastroenteritis/enterocolitis, gas distention colic, chronic colitis, undiagnosed, and other. Season was categorised into four seasons (December–February, March–May, June–August, September–November).

Comparisons between diagnostic categories and season was performed using Fisher's exact test. Comparisons between cases and controls regarding demographic profile was done using univariate logistic regression generating crude ORs (for age, as continuous variable) and chi 2 test (for gender), respectively. For cases, comparisons between gastrointestinal diagnoses and age categories were done using univariate logistic regression generating crude ORs.

2.5.2. Questionnaire Data Including Previous Medical History, Anthelmintic Routines and Pasture Management

Comparisons between cases and controls regarding previous medical history (colic, veterinary treated colic, diarrhea, weight loss), anthelmintic routines (last drug used, time since last deworming, farm deworming routine, prevalence of previous parasitic infection) and management factors (use of co-grazing, fecal removal routines in pasture/paddock, time at pasture/in paddock, stocking density) were made using univariate logistic regression generating crude ORs.

2.5.3. Parasitological Status

The parasitological status of each horse was determined for cyathostomins as FECs, and for *S. vulgaris* PCR, *S. vulgaris* ELISA and *A. perfoliata* as positive/not positive. Strongyle egg counts were clustered into the following EPG groups: low egg shedders (EPG $\leq$ 200), medium egg shedders (250–500 EPG) and high egg shedders (>500 EPG) [33]. The difference in distribution of the EPG categories for each determinant, respectively, was investigated using univariate ordered logistic regression generating crude ORs. The *S. vulgaris* ELISA was identified as positive using a cut-off value of 13.47% of positive control according to Andersen et al. [32]. The number of positive samples (i.e., above the positive threshold) were presented as total number and proportion of the total. For *S. vulgaris* PCR, *S. vulgaris* ELISA, and *A. perfoliata*, the association between each parasitological outcome and various determinants (season, case/control, age, previous medical history, anthelmintic routines, gastrointestinal diagnosis and pasture management factors) was evaluated in separate logistic regression models (one per each specific combination of exposure and outcome). Additional analysis using the Wilcoxon matched-pairs signed-rank test for *S. vulgaris* ELISA was performed as distribution plots (using the original continuous data) for cases and controls, respectively, for each gastrointestinal disease category as well as for all cases compared with all controls.

2.5.4. Multivariable Logistic Regression Analysis

Variables with a univariable p value < 0.2 were considered for subsequent inclusion in a multivariable model. To avoid problems associated with collinearity, where variables were considered to be measuring the same exposure or were shown to be highly correlated (Pearson correlation coefficient > 0.8), the most statistically significant or biologically plausible variable was selected for inclusion in the model. Five submodels were initially created for the following dependent variables: cases/controls, strongyle fecal egg counts, *S. vulgaris* PCR, *S. vulgaris* ELISA, *A. perfoliata*. For each model, all variables with $p < 0.20$ from the univariate analysis with the specific dependent variable were added to create the full model. From each model, backward selection of variables was performed: the variable with the highest p-value was removed, one at a time, until all variables remaining in the model had $p < 0.05$.

3. Results

3.1. Data on Horses

A total of 137 cases and 137 controls were included in the study. A total of 66.7% of all presenting gastrointestinal patients at the clinic during the period February 2017 to February 2018 were included in the study. The mean and median ages of the cases and control horses were 10.8 (± SD 5.8) and 11 years and 10.2 (± SD 6.0) and 9 years, respectively, with a range of one to 25 years in both groups. The control population consisted of 74 geldings (54.0%), 58 mares (42.3%) and five stallions (3.6%) and the case population of 62 geldings (45.3%), 65 mares (47.4%) and 10 stallions (7.3%). There were no statistical differences in either age ($p = 0.53$) or gender distribution ($p = 0.83$) between cases and controls. The control horses were represented by 23 different breeds, the majority of which were Warmbloods (54.7%), followed by pony breeds (16.8%), Icelandic Horses (7.3%), Thoroughbreds (5.8%), draft breeds (4.4%), and Standardbreds (1.5%), with 9.5% consisting of various other breeds. Similarly, cases, consisting of 26 different breeds, were predominantly Warmbloods (40.1%), followed by Icelandic Horses (15.3%), pony breeds (13.7%), Standardbreds (7.2%), draft breeds (6.6%) and Thoroughbreds (4.4%), with 10.9% consisting of various other breeds.

3.2. Colic Diagnoses

The diagnoses of cases included impaction colic (large colon, small colon and cecal impactions) (38.0%), acute colitis (10.2%), large intestinal displacement (9.5%), peritonitis (8.0%), gas distention colic (5.8%), eosinophilic enteritis/colitis (3.6%), chronic colitis (2.2%), and other (7.3%). No specific diagnosis was reached in 15.3% of the cases (Table 2). Age had no association with type of diagnosis, with impaction colic common in all ages ($p = 0.32$). Of the horses diagnosed with peritonitis, the underlying etiology was known in three cases; esophageal rupture (n = 1) and non-strangulating intestinal infarction (n = 2). The remainder were classified as idiopathic. Abdominal surgery was performed in 12/137 cases (8.0%). Of the horses that had surgery performed, the final diagnoses were as follows: large colon displacement (4), ileocecal invagination (2), equine eosinophilic gastroenteritis/enterocolitis (2), non-strangulating intestinal infarction (2), gas distention colic (1) and undiagnosed (1). A total of four (2.9%) cases were euthanised, all of which had had abdominal surgery. Of the horses that had abdominal surgery and/or were euthanised, parasitic injuries were found in two cases, both of which were diagnosed with *S. vulgaris*-associated non-strangulating intestinal infarction of the colon. Both cases of ileocecal invagination had abdominal surgery without parasitic findings, e.g., *A. perfoliata*. The final diagnoses and number of cases in each group are presented in Table 2.

Table 2. Distribution of gastrointestinal diagnoses in cases.

Diagnosis	Number of Cases (% of Total Case Load)
Impaction (small colon, large colon, cecal)	52 (38.0%)
Acute colitis	14 (10.2%)
Large colon displacement	13 (9.5%)
Peritonitis	11 (8.0%)
Gas distention colic	8 (5.8%)
Equine eosinophilic gastroenteritis/enterocolitis (EEG)	5 (3.6%)
Chronic colitis	3 (2.2%)
Undiagnosed	21 (15.3%)
Other	10 (7.3%)

3.3. Assocation with Season

A total of 47 horses presented with colic during the winter months (December–February), equivalent to a third (34.3%) of the total number of cases. The most common diagnoses made during this season included different types of impaction colic (31.9%), intestinal displacement (17%), acute colitis (12.8%), peritonitis (10.6%), and equine eosinophilic gastroenteritis/enterocolitis (6.4%). In spring (March–May), 37 cases were included (27% of total caseload), the majority of which were impaction colic (37.8%), peritonitis (10.8%) and intestinal displacement (8.1%). Fewer horses with gastrointestinal disease presented during the summer, with 21 cases (15.3% of total caseload) during the months June–August. Furthermore, during the summer, impaction colic (large intestinal) was most commonly diagnosed (38%). Peritonitis, gas distention colic and acute colitis were each diagnosed in 9.5% of the cases during these three months. Twenty-three percent of the total number of cases presented during the autumn (September–November). Again, impactions were common and were diagnosed in almost half of the colic cases during this time period (46.9%). The second and third most common diagnoses during these months were acute colitis (15.6%) and gas distention colic (12.5%), respectively. No peritonitis cases were diagnosed in the autumn. There was no statistical association with season and the type of colic diagnosed ($p = 0.32$).

3.4. Questionnaire Data

The owner of each horse participating in the study completed a questionnaire on previous colic history, deworming routines and pasture management (Table 1). The overall questionnaire response rate for cases was 92% (126/137) and for control horses, 98% (134/137); however, within the questionnaire, the response rate varied depending on the questions asked (74.5%–98%). The results from the questionnaire are presented in Tables 3–5.

3.5. Previous Medical History

Case horses had been owned by the present owner for a mean of 4.3 years (range of one month to 25 years), and control horses had been in the present ownership for a mean of 4.9 years (range of one month to 25 years). Of the cases, 50.4% (60/119) had previously reported episodes of colic, with an average of 2.2 colic episodes prior to the study (range 1–12). The reported prevalence of previous colic was 23.9% for the controls (32/134), with an average of 1.8 previous colic episodes (range 1–10). Cases were significantly more likely to have had previous episodes of colic, compared to controls ($p < 0.01$) (Table 3). A third of the cases (33.3%) had been attended by a veterinarian due to colic within the previous 24 months, which was significantly more often compared with control horses (8.0%) ($p < 0.01$). In addition, cases were more likely to have had diarrhea within the previous two months compared to controls, although with a conservative Bonferroni correction approach, this difference did not reach statistical significance ($p = 0.03$).

Table 3. Results of questionnaire data: owner-reported previous medical history of cases and controls as outlined in a questionnaire presented after agreement of study participation. The p-value for statistical significance was corrected for the number of analyses (n = 5) according to Bonferroni, i.e., $p < 0.01$ (0.05/5).

Information	Cases	Controls	OR (95% C.I.)	p-Value
Prevalence with previous history of colic [a] (%)	50.4%	23.9%	3.13 (1.83–5.35)	<0.01
Number of previous colic episodes (mean ± SD)	2.2 (± 2.3)	1.8 (± 1.9)	1.09 (0.86–1.39)	0.47
Prevalence treated for colic during last 24 months (%)	33.3%	8%	5.73 (2.78–11.84)	<0.01
Prevalence with diarrhea [b] during last 2 months	15.8%	7.5%	0.42 (0.18–0.94)	0.03
Prevalence with weight loss [c] during last 2 months	9.2%	6.0%	0.45 (0.18–1.10)	0.08

[a] restlessness and pawing at the ground, irritated kicking to the stomach, rolling or attempting to roll; [b] loose consistency of feces; [c] as subjectively appreciated by owner.

3.6. Anthelmintic Routines

Deworming history was known in 88.9% (112/126) of cases and 98.5% (132/134) of controls that responded to the questionnaire, although the overall response rate to individual anthelmintic routine questions again varied (74.5%–98.5%). Anthelmintic treatment was performed at various times prior to presentation: 0–3 months (18.9%), 3–6 months (25.4%), 6–12 months (31.1%) and over 12 months (24.6%). There was no significant difference in time from deworming between cases and controls ($p = 0.46$) (Table 4). Macrocyclic lactones (ML) was the anthelmintic group most commonly used (59%) at the last treatment occasion. In detail, 41.7% had treated with ivermectin (IVM), 3.3% with moxidectin (MOX), 14.2% with a combination of IVM/moxidectin and praziquantel (COMB), 5.4% with pyrantel (PYR) and 3.3% had used fenbendazole (FBZ). Cases and controls showed a tendency to differ in terms of which drug was used at the last treatment, with control horses more often treated with IVM or COMB, and owners of cases, more often unable to recall the drug used ($p = 0.02$) (Table 4). Overall, 32.1% of the owners did not remember which drug they had used on the most recent treatment occasion (cases 43.8%, controls 24.2%).

In this data set, 28.8% of the horses were dewormed routinely without parasitic diagnostics being performed, where 12.3% of the horses were dewormed once per year and 16.5% of the horses 2–4 times per year. Selective treatment based on FECs was used by 35.8% of the owners, and 31.9% of owners used selective treatment based on both FECs and larval culture. Overall, 16% performed routine diagnostics for *A. perfoliata*, but this was more common within the control group (18.7%) compared to cases (13.5%). In addition, routine deworming 2–4 times per year was more often employed by owners of control horses (20.2%) compared to cases (12.7%). However, there were no significant differences between cases and controls in fecal diagnostics and deworming routines ($p = 0.11$–0.99) (Table 4).

One third of all horses were reported to have been infected with cyathostomins within the previous 24 months (cases 29.4%, controls 36.8%). In contrast, only 4.6% of horses were known to have been positive for *S. vulgaris* during the same time period. Case horses showed a higher prevalence of previous *S. vulgaris* infection (6.9% versus 2.6%), although this difference did not reach statistical significance ($p = 0.10$). Infection with *A. perfoliata* and *Parascaris* spp. were rarely reported to have occurred within the previous 24 months, and the data showed same frequency for both parasites (1.4% (1.0% cases, 1.7% controls)), see Table 4. However, previous parasitic infection history was unknown in the majority of horses (59.4% (61.8% cases, 57.3% controls)). Overall, previous parasitic infection was not significantly different between cases and controls ($p = 0.10$–0.79).

Table 4. Result of questionnaire data: anthelmintic routines. The *p*-value for statistical significance was corrected for the number of analyses (n = 4) according to Bonferroni, i.e., $p < 0.01$ (0.05/4).

Information	Cases	Controls	*p*-Value
Time from last helmintic treatment (months) (%)			
0–3	17.9%	19.7%	0.38
3–6	28.6%	22.7%	0.40
6–12	26.8%	34.8%	0.66
>12	26.8%	22.7%	0.51
For the variable (all time groups) cases/controls:			0.46
Drugs used at last treatment (%)			
FBZ [a]	4.5%	2.3%	0.48
PYR [b]	3.6%	6.9%	0.16
MOX [c]	3.6%	3.1%	0.62
IVM [d]	35.5%	46.9%	0.21
COMB [e]	10%	17.7%	0.13
Unknown	42.7%	23.1%	0.94
For the variable (all drug groups) cases/controls:			0.02
Deworming routines applied on the farm (%)			
(i) after FEC [f]	35.7%	35.8%	0.99
(ii) after FEC and *S. vulgaris* diagnostics	30.2%	33.6%	0.55
(iii) diagnostics for *A. perfoliata* at least once/year	13.5%	18.7%	0.26
(iv) routine deworming once/year	13.5%	11.1%	0.57
(v) routine deworming 2–4 times/year	12.7%	20.1%	0.11
Presence of parasites in fecal sample during last 24 months			
Cyathostomins	29.4%	36.8%	0.13
S. vulgaris	6.9%	2.6%	0.10
A. perfoliata	1.0%	1.7%	0.79
Parascaris spp.	1.0%	1.7%	0.79
Do not know	61.8%	57.3%	0.31

[a] fenbendazole; [b] pyrantel; [c] ivermectin; [d] moxidectin; [e] ivermectin/moxidectin and praziquantel; [f] fecal egg count.

3.7. Pasture Management

Regarding pasture management, it was rare for owners to report the use of mixed or alternate grazing with other species (9.8% (cases 10.6%, controls 9.0%)). However, the majority of owners employed the use of separate winter and summer paddocks/grazing areas (64.0% (67.5% cases, 60.9% controls)) (Table 5). Fecal removal was utilised overall by 46.2% of horse owners, with no statistical difference between cases and controls (54.6% and 45.9%, respectively) ($p = 0.17$). However, only a small proportion of owners declared that they removed feces at least twice weekly (7.1%), with almost two thirds of owners (65.3%) reporting that they removed feces less often than once weekly.

All horses had access to pasture during the summer months, with the majority (54.7%) kept at pasture 24 h per day during the summer, with no significant difference in time at pasture during the summer found between cases and controls ($p = 0.96$). Similarly, there were no differences found between the two groups in the number of horses kept solely outdoors in the winter ($p = 0.88$). Cases were more likely to be stabled > 12 h per day in the winter, compared to controls (65% compared to 55.6%), although no statistical difference was found ($p = 0.13$).

Stocking density (hectare/horse) calculated from data regarding paddock size and number of horses/paddocks, was similar between cases and controls in both winter and summer ($p = 0.22$–0.68) (Table 5). The majority of horses, both cases and controls, were kept at stocking densities providing < 0.4 hectare/horse (72.8% winter, 64.7% summer). Overall, season (winter/summer) showed a significant difference in both time at pasture and stocking density, with more horses stabled > 12 h/d and kept at stocking densities providing less than 0.4 hectare/horse during the winter as compared to the summer ($p < 0.01$).

Table 5. Results of questionnaire data: pasture management. The p-value for statistical significance was corrected for the number of analyses (n = 10) according to Bonferroni, i.e., $p < 0.005$ (0.05/10).

Information>	Cases	Controls	p-Value
Access to separate summer/winter paddocks	67.5%	60.9%	0.27
Grazing with other animal species	10.6%	9.0%	0.67
Fecal removal			
Fecal removal from pasture, overall	54.6%	45.9%	0.17
Fecal removal from pasture, ≥2x/week	5.9%	8.1%	0.33
Time stabled/outdoors			
Outdoors 24 h/d, winter	14.2%	14.8%	0.88
Stabled > 12 h/d, winter	65%	55.6%	0.13
Outdoors 24h/d, summer	54.2	54.8%	0.96
Stabled > 12 h/d, summer	26.7%	26.7%	0.93
Stocking density			
Stocking density, summer (hectare/horse)	0.6	0.8	0.68
Stocking density, winter (hectare/horse)	0.4	0.4	0.22

3.8. *Multivariate Model for Cases and Controls*

The multivariate logistic regression model investigating factors associated with being a case resulted in a final model that included three variables: age, treated for colic during last 24 months and stocking density. There was a significantly higher odds of being a case if treated for colic within the last 24 months (OR 7.87 (95% C.I. 3.04–20.34), $p < 0.001$), when adjusting for stocking density and age.

3.9. *Strongyle Fecal Egg Counts*

The overall prevalence of strongyle eggs was 44.9% (123/274) and the prevalence was similar between cases and controls, 47.4% and 42.3%, respectively. The majority, 67.5% (185/274), of the horses were classified as low egg shedders (EPG ≤ 200), with 16.4% denoted as high shedders (>500 EPG). The mean strongyle EPG was 238 ± SD 397 in the case group of which 55.5% (76/137) of the horses were shedding ≤ 50 EPG. The mean strongyle EPG was 320 ± SD 688 in the control group of which 52.6% (72/137) of the horses were shedding ≤ 50. Both the case group and the control group revealed similar number of high egg shedding horses (>500 EPG), 18.2% (25/137) and 14.6% (20/137), respectively. No statistical difference in the number of low, medium and high shedding horses between cases and controls was found ($p = 0.92$). In the study population as a whole, age was associated with egg shedding, with increasing age resulting in an increase in the number of low shedding horses and a decrease in the number of high shedders ($p < 0.01$). No statistically significant association with season and EPG level was found ($p = 0.38$).

Horses with a previous history of weight loss or diarrhea had higher average EPG levels (426 ± SD 778 and 400 ± SD 530, respectively) compared to horses without such complaints (268 ± SD

732 and 262 ± SD 544, respectively); however, these differences were not significant ($p = 0.39–0.49$). EPG levels were not associated with gastrointestinal disease in general ($p = 0.92$) (Table 6), nor with a particular colic diagnosis ($p = 0.61$).

EPG levels were lowest in horses most recently dewormed (0–3 months), with time since deworming overall approaching a significant association with EPG levels ($p = 0.01$). However, previously used anthelmintic drugs were not associated with egg shedding ($p = 0.22$). Although horses whose owners employed the use of FECs, as opposed to regular deworming at least once/year, had higher mean EPG levels, anthelmintic routine had no significant association with EPG level ($p = 0.06$). The result of the previous fecal sample had no statistical relationship with EPG level ($p = 0.50$).

Horses kept in smaller enclosures during the winter, often on their own, were more likely to be low shedders, compared with horses kept in larger paddocks but with more companions, although no statistical significance was shown ($p = 0.01$). No such trend was observed during the summer ($p = 0.22$). Time at pasture, either in the winter or summer, did not influence EPG levels ($p = 0.07–0.49$).

Table 6. Fecal and serology results in cases and controls. The p-value for statistical significance was corrected for the number of analyses (n = 4) according to Bonferroni, i.e., $p < 0.01$ (0.05/4).

Investigated Parameter	Cases n (%)	Controls n (%)	p-Value
EPG [a] level LOW	93 (67.9%)	92 (67.1%)	
EPG [a] level MEDIUM	19 (13.9%)	25 (18.2%)	0.92
EPG [a] level HIGH	25 (18.3%)	20 (14.6%)	
S. vulgaris PCR	7 (5.2%)	8 (5.8%)	0.80
S. vulgaris ELISA	75 (61.5%)	86 (62.8%)	0.83
A. perfoliata	17 (12.4%)	26 (19.0%)	0.14

[a] EPG, eggs per gram of feces.

3.10. *Strongylus Vulgaris PCR*

Seven horses in the case group and eight horses in the control group were PCR positive for *S. vulgaris*. The overall occurrence of *S. vulgaris* in this study was 5.5% (15/274). Seven of these 15 horses (46.7%) were defined as low egg shedders with EPG ≤ 200. Age showed no significant association with the number of positive horses ($p = 0.46$). Fewer positive horses were demonstrated during the winter months, compared to the other seasons, although no statistical association with season was shown ($p = 0.05$).

The majority, 80% (12/15), of the *S. vulgaris*-positive horses were dewormed either between 6–12 months or ≥ 12 months prior to fecal sampling, with almost half (7/15, 46.7%) of the positive horses having been dewormed with an unknown anthelmintic product > 12 months ago. Two horses were dewormed with a macrocyclic lactone (ML) within 3–6 months but were still positive for *S. vulgaris*. In addition, four horses were dewormed either once (3/15) or 2–4 times (1/15) a year but were also positive for *S. vulgaris*. None of the horses that were positive for *S. vulgaris* had reported a positive previous fecal sample for their last sample.

In the *S. vulgaris* PCR positive group, only 20.0% (3/15) of owners (compared to 31.9% overall in the study sample) utilised larval culture at least once yearly, with more horses (46.0%) regularly diagnosed by only performing FECs as compared to the study population as a whole (35.8%). Likewise, horses regularly dewormed once per year were more likely to be positive for *S. vulgaris* compared to horses that received anthelmintic treatment 2–4 times per year and to horses, where specific diagnostics for *S. vulgaris* were used. The majority of owners that performed diagnostics for *A. perfoliata*, also screened for *S. vulgaris* (78.6%). However, the number of horses positive for *S. vulgaris* in each group was low, making true comparisons difficult and no statistically significant association with anthelmintic routine and the number of positive horses was found ($p = 0.32$). There was no association between a positive PCR and gastrointestinal disease ($p = 0.80$) (Table 6) or with a specific diagnosis ($p = 0.76$).

Neither stocking density nor hours at pasture had a significant association with the number of *S. vulgaris*-positive horses ($p = 0.42–0.80$).

3.11. *Strongylus vulgaris* ELISA

The total *S. vulgaris* seroprevalence in this study was 62.2% (161/259). Serum was unavailable in 15 cases. No statistical differences between cases and controls in a number of horses positive in the ELISA test was shown ($p = 0.83$) (Table 6). However, when the separate gastrointestinal diagnoses were compared to controls matched by time of presentation, horses diagnosed with peritonitis showed significantly higher ELISA scores, expressed as a percentage of positive control, than their matched controls ($p < 0.02$) (Figure 1).

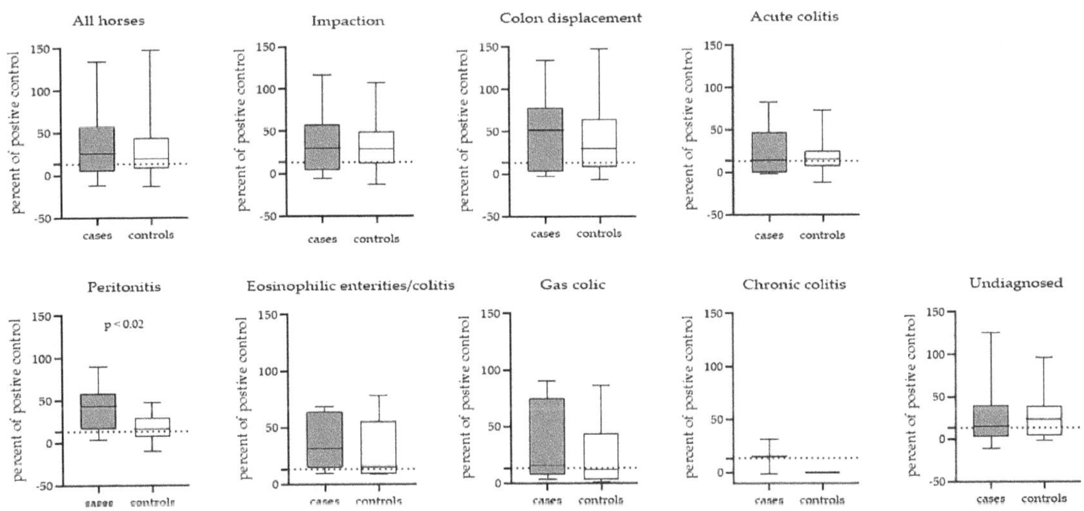

Figure 1. A boxplot illustrating the quantitative enzyme-linked immunosorbent assay (ELISA) values for each colic diagnosis compared with their matched controls. The bold line indicates median, the dotted line indicates the cut-off (13.47) value for positive ELISA.

Overall, there was a trend towards a greater prevalence of positive ELISA tests in older horses (>20) compared to young individuals (≤2 years) (81.3% and 44.4%, respectively), but this difference did not reach significance ($p = 0.04$). Overall, age had no significant association with ELISA score ($p = 0.37$). A lower prevalence was observed during the spring (60%) as compared to the rest of the year (71.4%–81.7%), but overall there was no significant association with season on ELISA score ($p = 0.17$).

Of the ELISA positive horses, 39.8% (64/161) were regularly diagnosed only performing FEC, 29.8% (48/161) of the horses performed FEC combined with *S. vulgaris* diagnostics, 16.1% (26/161) of the horses were dewormed 2–4 times/year and 8.7% (14/161) of the horses were dewormed on a yearly basis. Horses dewormed based on FECs without further diagnostics were more likely to have a positive ELISA score, compared to other anthelmintic routines, although using the conservative Bonferroni correction, statistical significance was not shown ($p = 0.02$). Neither the time from last anthelmintic treatment nor the drug used was associated with a positive ELISA result ($p = 0.37$–0.81).

Stocking density in either season had no significant association with number of positive horses ($p = 0.77$–0.90). Time at pasture during the summer was shown to have a significant association with the outcome of the ELISA test ($p < 0.01$), but no such association was demonstrated during the winter ($p = 0.51$).

3.12. *Anoplocephala perfoliata*

A total of 15.7% (43/274) of the horses were positive for *A. perfoliata*. Seventeen horses (12.4%) were positive for *A. perfoliata* in the case group and 26 horses (19.0%) in the control group, with no significant difference between the two groups ($p = 0.14$). Age had no significant association with *A. perfoliata* prevalence ($p = 0.12$). Although the highest number of positive horses was found in the spring (44.2%), no statistically significant seasonal differences were observed ($p = 0.05$).

No association between gastrointestinal disease and a positive *A. perfoliata* sample was demonstrated ($p = 0.14$) (Table 6). In addition, no specific gastrointestinal diagnosis was associated with a positive *A. perfoliata* sample ($p = 0.96$). Of the only two cases diagnosed with ileocecal invagination, fecal samples were negative for *A. perfoliata* and no tapeworms were found during abdominal surgery.

The time since last deworming was not associated with a positive test for *A. perfoliata* ($p = 0.92$). Three horses were positive for *A. perfoliata* despite treatment with ML combined with praziquantel within the last 3–6 months and for one horse, within 0–3 months. Another horse had been treated with this combination within 6–12 months of fecal sampling. Previous anthelmintic drug use had no overall significant association with the occurrence of *A. perfoliata* ($p = 0.06$). Eight of the 43 positive horses (18.6%) were normally analysed for *A. perfoliata* on a yearly basis. The group with the highest proportion of individuals positive for *A. perfoliata*, were horses whose owners reported the use of specific diagnostics for tapeworm. However, no horse that had a previous sample positive for *A. perfoliata*, had a positive fecal sample in the study. Overall, there was no significant association with anthelmintic routine used and a positive test for *A. perfoliata* ($p = 0.20$).

Although horses with at least 12 h of pasture/paddock access, regardless of time of year, had a higher prevalence of *A. perfoliata*, no statistically significant association with hours at pasture was shown ($p = 0.04$–0.06). The majority of positive horses were kept in paddocks allowing less than 0.4 hectares/horse, but no significant association with stocking density on *A. perfoliata* prevalence was demonstrated ($p = 0.10$–0.67).

3.13. Multivariate Model for Parasite Outcome

The multivariate ordered logistic regression model investigating factors associated with the fecal egg count in categories of low, medium and high egg shedders, resulted in a final model that included four variables: season, stocking density, any previous history of colic and time since deworming ($p < 0.05$ for all). There was an increased odds of a higher fecal egg category when time since deworming increased, with a 7.3 (95% C.I. 2.2 –24.1; $p = 0.001$) times increase in risk found when a horse had received anthelmintic treatment 6–12 months prior to presentation, compared to being treated within 0–3 months, when adjusting for season, stocking density in the winter and known history of previous colic.

When investigated factors associated with a positive PCR result for *S. vulgaris*, the multivariate ordered logistic regression model resulted in one variable: time since deworming. Deworming more than six months prior to sampling, as compared to treatment less than six months before presentation, resulted in an increased likelihood of a positive *S. vulgaris* PCR of 4.4 (95% CI 1.20–15.80; $p = 0.025$).

A multivariate ordered logistic regression for a positive *S. vulgaris* ELISA outcome resulted in a final model that included three variables: time in ownership, stabling > 12 h/d in the summer and deworming only after FECs. Deworming using only FECs was associated with an increased risk of a positive test, when adjusting for time of ownership and stabling > 12 h/d in the summer (OR 2.3 (95% C.I. 1.3–4.1; $p = 0.025$)).

Factors investigated to be associated with presence of *A. perfoliata*, resulted in a final model that included two variables: season and stabled > 12 h/d in the winter. The odds for the presence of *A. perfoliata* in a fecal sample was 2.8 times higher (95% C.I. 1.2–6.4; $p = 0.035$) in March–May when adjusting for time stabled in the winter.

4. Discussion

The present study demonstrated a high percentage of horses (cases and controls) were positive in the *S. vulgaris* ELISA test, amounting to almost two thirds of the horses included, indicating a high frequency of exposure to large strongyles in the population studied. The ELISA test assesses IgG (T) antibodies in *S. vulgaris* excretory proteins with a relatively high specificity (81%), and appears to reflect current infection or recent exposure, within the previous five months [31,34]. The number of positive horses in this study may be a surprisingly high figure, given the low individual *S. vulgaris* prevalence found using fecal PCR analyses (5.5%), but it is equivalent to the recently shown farm prevalence of *S. vulgaris* (61%) in Sweden [22].

Given the known pathogenicity of *S. vulgaris*, horses diagnosed with peritonitis were considered of particular interest to a possible *S. vulgaris* etiology. One case in this group was excluded due to the reason that peritonitis was known (esophageal perforation). However, two cases of peritonitis were confirmed on necropsy to have been caused by non-strangulating infarction secondary to *S. vulgaris* thrombosis. The remaining eight cases of peritonitis were classified as idiopathic and responded successfully to antimicrobial treatment, but none of these cases underwent exploratory laparotomy or necropsy. In addition to causing non-strangulating intestinal lesions, *S. vulgaris* has also been suggested as a possible cause of *Actinobacillus equuli* peritonitis, the most common bacterium isolated from horses presenting with idiopathic peritonitis [35]. The causal relationship, however, cannot be confirmed using fecal analyses, given that peritonitis associated with *S. vulgaris* would be due to the migrating larval stages and not the adult form of the parasite, and therefore before egg excretion is expected. None of the horses presenting with peritonitis in the present study were PCR positive for *S. vulgaris*. However, in the peritonitis group, the percentage of horses positive for the ELISA test was significantly higher (77.8%) than overall, with only two cases being negative (serum was missing in one case). In addition, horses diagnosed with peritonitis had significantly higher ELISA scores as compared to matched controls, which could be suggestive of an *S. vulgaris* etiology ($p < 0.02$). *S. vulgaris*-specific antibodies have been shown to be strongly associated with non-strangulating intestinal infarction, resulting in septic peritonitis; however, not with other types of colic [6,36]. The cause of eosinophilic intestinal lesions is still under debate, and previous studies do not convincingly demonstrate a parasitic etiology [37,38]. Nonetheless, it is interesting to observe that, although few cases were included, all but one case with an eosinophilic intestinal lesion were also positive in the ELISA test (80%, 4/5). In one case of eosinophilic enteritis, although no *S. vulgaris* larvae were found, thrombosed vessels were observed adjacent to the lesion.

In agreement with other case–control studies, no significant differences in parasitological status could be demonstrated using coprological assays between horses presenting with gastrointestinal disease in general and controls [16,36,39]. Overall, the fecal prevalence of *S. vulgaris* as assessed by PCR analyses and the presence of cyathostomins and *A. perfoliata* eggs were either lower or comparable to previously published prevalences of these equine intestinal parasites, as outlined below.

Although a possible role in colic incidence has been suggested [40], cyathostomins appear to be well tolerated without causing disease in most cases, apart from the well-known syndrome of larval cyathostominosis in young animals [12,13]. As in the present study, a recent publication showed no differences in strongyle EPG between non-surgical colic cases and controls [16]. Previous studies have, however, shown an association of cyathostomins with weight loss and diarrhea [12,15,41,42]. In the present study, although horses with a previous history of diarrhea or weight loss within the last two months had higher average EPG levels compared to the rest of the study population, there was considerable variation in EPG levels and this difference was not significant. In the case group, only two cases (2/14) of acute colitis and one case (1/3) of chronic colitis were high shedders (EPG > 500). There are, however, several causes of colitis in horses [43], and even in diarrhea caused by cyathostomins, fecal egg counts are often negative, with the L4 stage present in the feces instead [12,41]. In addition, it has been shown that neither egg nor larval counts correlate well with the horse´s actual worm burden [44].

The prevalence of *A. perfoliata* reported here is in accordance with a previous Swedish case–control study that showed positive samples in 13% (18/134) of horses [11]. Previous studies have shown conflicting results regarding the association of tapeworm infection and general colic [7]. However, *A. perfoliata* has consistently shown to be associated with ileocecal lesions [8,10,45–49]. The present study included few cases with confirmed ileocecal lesions (2/137) and was thus unable to demonstrate such a relationship.

No differences in parasite control strategies between cases and controls were found in the present study. ML was the most commonly used anthelmintic group overall, in accordance with several previous publications from various countries [50–55]. However, within the study population as a whole, differences in anthelmintic routines were present, with 28.8% of the owners deworming their horses on a routine basis without prior parasitic diagnostics. Likewise, in a recently published study 21% of Swedish horse-owners employed routine anthelmintic treatment 1–4 times yearly, without using coproscopic analyses [22]. However, before the prescription-only legislation was implemented, only 1% of owners were reported to use fecal analyses [25]. National differences in anthelmintic routines were recently described, with Denmark showing a much greater use of FECs than Austria, Netherlands, Germany and the United States [19]. Interestingly, the frequencies of use of FECs were very low (1.8% and 3.1%, respectively) in Germany and Austria, although these countries have allowed only the use of prescription anthelmintic drugs since 1975. In Denmark, where the concept was introduced in 1999, the figure was 50% [19]. One reason for this discrepancy was suggested to be differences in administration of the law and perhaps how rigidly the legislation was adhered to [19]. Thus, although almost a third of the owners in the present study did not use fecal analyses, compared to the above countries, the current use of FECs in Sweden appears comparatively high and shows a clear increase since selective treatment was enforced. However, it has to be noted that only approximately one third of owners declared the use of specific diagnostics for *S. vulgaris*, which is concerning, given that, in the present study, the use of FECs alone to determine the need for anthelmintic treatment, without further diagnostics, was associated with an increased odds of horses being positive in the *S. vulgaris* ELISA test.

Regular deworming, once or twice yearly, has been suggested to provide adequate control of *S. vulgaris* [21,56]. However, in the present study, although *S. vulgaris* was more common in horses dewormed six months or more prior to sampling, with time since deworming increasing the odds of a positive *S. vulgaris* sample, a total of six positive horses (40%) had either been dewormed within six months of sampling or were regularly dewormed at least once yearly. A post-mortem study in Sardinian horses demonstrated parasite-induced lesions in the cranial mesenteric arteries in all 46 horses in the study, and *S. vulgaris* larvae in 39%, despite treatment with broad-spectrum anthelmintic drugs at least three times per year [24]. Also, a recent study in Kentucky showed a high level of exposure to *S. vulgaris*, with 95/128 of horses being ELISA positive, despite treatment with anthelmintics on average twice yearly [57]. Considering clinical signs of disease may occur in as early as 2–4 months after infection [58], re-infection resulting in disease is possible despite regular anthelmintic treatment, and indicates that targeting the infected pasture is critical in management, and that eradication of *S. vulgaris* is unlikely using annual or bi-annual anthelmintic treatment, if horses are still allowed to graze in contaminated pastures. In addition, an experimental study in foals indicated that ivermectin may have little or no effect against migrating L5 larvae [59], suggesting that treatment may be less effective than often assumed.

Similar to a previous study on parasite control strategies in Sweden [25], only a minority of owners used alternating grazing species (9.8%), one method to reduce pasture contamination. This is low compared to some countries, such as Ireland, where co-grazing was used by the majority of owners [55]. However, most owners in the present study employed the use of separate winter and summer grazing areas. The regular use of fecal removal from the pasture can be an effective method to reduce parasite burden [60,61] and may be as effective as regular anthelmintic treatment, if performed twice weekly [61]. In the present study, although almost half of the owners reported removing feces from the pasture or paddock, only a minority did so at least twice weekly. The effect of fecal removal done more seldom than once weekly, which was the case in almost two thirds (65.4%) of owners that removed feces, is most likely poor, given that infective larvae will develop from excreted eggs within 2–3 weeks in spring and fall, and in as short as three days under ideal conditions [62]. In addition, most horses, both cases and controls, were kept at high stocking densities, provided with < 0.4 hectare/horse both in summer and winter. A high stocking density, with a large number of horses in paddocks of limited space, increases the risk of parasitic infections [63], and, in general, 1–2 acres/horse (corresponding to 0.4–0.8 hectare) is recommended [64].

Given the prospective nature, the study population in the present study was dependent on whichever gastrointestinal cases presented to the hospital within the set time-frame and, gastrointestinal diagnoses of particular interest with regards to a parasitic etiology, such as non-strangulating intestinal infarctions and ileo-cecal lesions, were, unfortunately, few. In addition, the study included a relatively small number of severe and/or surgical cases, probably because such cases required more urgent attention, resulting in lower consideration for study participation.

5. Conclusions

In conclusion, the present study demonstrated a high level of exposure of Swedish horses to *S. vulgaris*, as shown by the majority of horses, both cases and controls, being positive in the ELISA test. In addition, horses with peritonitis had significantly higher ELISA values as compared to controls and other gastrointestinal diagnoses, suggestive of an *S. vulgaris* etiology in this case group. Future studies addressing the association of *S. vulgaris* and peritonitis in the Swedish horse population is highly desirable, in order to further elucidate the clinical implication of the increasing prevalence of *S. vulgaris* in this country.

Furthermore, the present study revealed important information regarding the current use of anthelmintic treatment regimes in Sweden. For example, although the study showed a clear increase in the use of fecal analyses compared with before the prescription-only law was implemented, such legislation does not, per se, result in all owners using fecal diagnostics prior to treatment. The use of specific diagnostics is still low, indicating a need for education, of both owners and the veterinary profession, on how to best apply the diagnostic tools available. Treating horses annually or bi-annually, did not ensure a negative test result for *S. vulgaris*. Moreover, the study revealed that stocking intensity is often high and practices such as frequent fecal removal or co-grazing with other species were rarely performed. Thus, in addition, educating owners regarding optimal pasture management appears vital. In the advent of the increasing resistance to the anthelmintic drugs available together with the increase in prevalence of *S. vulgaris*, strategies for sustainable control of equine internal parasites are urgently needed, including pasture management.

Author Contributions: This study was performed within a larger project, where E.T. and E.O.-L. are PI. The individual contributions in the present study were as follows: conceptualization Y.H.-A., E.T., J.P., M.R., E.O.-L. and methodology E.T., Y.H.-A., J.P., E.O.-L., M.K.N., M.R.; software Y.H.-A., J.P., E.T.; validation Y.H.-A., J.P., E.T.; formal analysis Y.H.-A., J.P., E.T.; investigation Y.H.-A., E.T., E.O.-L., M.R.; resources E.T. E.O.-L.; data curation Y.H.-A., J.P., E.T.; writing—original draft preparation Y.H.-A., E.T., J.P.; writing—Y.H.-A., E.T., J.P.; M.K.N., E.O.-L. visualization Y.H.-A., E.T., and J.P.; project administration E.T., M.R., Y.H.-A.; funding acquisition E.T., E.O.-L. All authors have read and agreed to the published version of the manuscript.

Acknowledgments: We are greteful for the collaboration with the personel at the Equine Veterinary Clinic at SLU and all horseowners participating in this study.

References

1. Tinker, M.K.; White, N.A.; Lessard, P.; Thatcher, C.D.; Pelzer, K.D.; Davis, B.; Carmel, D.K. Prospective study of equine colic risk factors. *Equine Vet. J.* **1997**, *29*, 454–458. [CrossRef]
2. Reinemeyer, C.R.; Nielsen, M.K. Parasitism and colic. *Vet. Clin. N. Am. Equine Pract.* **2009**, *25*, 233–245. [CrossRef]
3. Curtis, L.; Burford, J.H.; England, G.C.W.; Freeman, S.L. Risk factors for acute abdominal pain (colic) in the adult horse: A scoping review of risk factors, and a systematic review of the effect of management-related changes. *PLoS ONE* **2019**, *14*, e0219307. [CrossRef]

4. Drudge, J.H.; Lyons, E.T. Control of internal parasites of the horse. *J. Am. Vet. Med. Assoc.* **1966**, *148*, 378–383.
5. Duncan, J.L.; Pirie, H.M. The pathogenesis of single experimental infections with *Strongylus vulgaris* in foals. *Res. Vet. Sci.* **1975**, *18*, 82–93. [CrossRef]
6. Pihl, T.H.; Nielsen, M.-K.; Olsen, S.N.; Leifsson, P.S.; Jacobsen, S. Nonstrangulating intestinal infarctions associated with *Strongylus vulgaris*: Clinical presentation and treatment outcome of 30 horses (2008–2016). *Equine Vet. J.* **2018**, *50*, 474–480. [CrossRef]
7. Nielsen, M.K. Equine tapeworm infections—Disease, diagnosis, and control. *Equine Vet. Educ.* **2016**, *28*, 388–395. [CrossRef]
8. Pavone, S.; Veronesi, F.; Piergili Fioretti, D.; Mandara, M.T. Pathological changes caused by *Anoplocephala perfoliata* in the equine ileocecal junction. *Vet. Res. Commun.* **2010**, *34*, 53–56. [CrossRef]
9. Pavone, S.; Veronesi, F.; Genchi, C.; Fioretti, D.P.; Brianti, E.; Mandara, M.T. Pathological changes caused by *Anoplocephala perfoliata* in the mucosa/submucosa and in the enteric nervous system of equine ileocecal junction. *Vet. Parasitol.* **2011**, *176*, 43–52. [CrossRef]
10. Proudman, C.J.; French, N.P.; Trees, A.J. Tapeworm infection is a significant risk factor for spasmodic colic and ileal impaction colic in the horse. *Equine Vet. J.* **1998**, *30*, 194–199. [CrossRef]
11. Back, H.; Nyman, A.; Osterman Lind, E. The association between *Anoplocephala perfoliata* and colic in Swedish horses–a case control study. *Vet. Parasitol.* **2013**, *197*, 580–585. [CrossRef] [PubMed]
12. Lyons, E.T.; Drudge, J.H.; Tolliver, S.C. Larval cyathostomiasis. *Vet. Clin. N. Am. Equine Pract.* **2000**, *16*, 501–513. [CrossRef]
13. Mair, T.S. Outbreak of larval cyathostomiasis among a group of yearling and two-year-old horses. *Vet. Rec.* **1994**, *135*, 598–600.
14. Murphy, D.; Love, S. The pathogenic effects of experimental cyathostome infections in ponies. *Vet. Parasitol.* **1997**, *70*, 99–110. [CrossRef]
15. Love, S.; Murphy, D.; Mellor, D. Pathogenicity of cyathostome infection. *Vet. Parasitol.* **1999**, *85*, 113–122. [CrossRef]
16. Stancampiano, L.; Usai, F.; Marigo, A.; Rinnovati, R. Are small strongyles (Cyathostominae) involved in horse colic occurrence? *Vet. Parasitol.* **2017**, *247*, 33–36. [CrossRef]
17. Kaplan, R.M. Anthelmintic resistance in nematodes of horses. *Vet. Res.* **2002**, *33*, 491–507. [CrossRef]
18. Von Samson-Himmelstjerna, G. Anthelmintic resistance in equine parasites—Detection, potential clinical relevance and implications for control. *Vet. Parasitol.* **2012**, *185*, 2–8. [CrossRef]
19. Becher, A.M.; van Doorn, D.C.; Pfister, K.; Kaplan, R.M.; Reist, M.; Nielsen, M.K. Equine parasite control and the role of national legislation—A multinational questionnaire survey. *Vet. Parasitol.* **2018**, *15*, 259–612. [CrossRef]
20. SJVFS 2010:17 24 § Legislations (In Swedish) Swedish Board of Agriculture. Available online: http://www.jordbruksverket.se/forfattningar/forfattningssamling (accessed on 26 March 2019).
21. Nielsen, M.K.; Vidyashankar, A.N.; Olsen, S.N.; Monrad, J.; Thamsborg, S.M. *Strongylus vulgaris* associated with usage of selective therapy on Danish horse farms-is it reemerging? *Vet. Parasitol.* **2012**, *189*, 260–266. [CrossRef]
22. Tydén, E.; Larsen Enemark, H.; Andersson Franko, M.; Höglund, J.; Osterman-Lind, E. Prevalence of *Strongylus vulgaris* in horses after ten years of prescription usage of anthelmintics in Sweden. *Vet. Parasitol.* **2019**, *2*, 100013. [CrossRef]
23. Stancampiano, L.; Mughini Gras, L.; Poglayen, G. Spatial niche competition among helminth parasites in horse's large intestine. *Vet. Parasitol.* **2010**, *170*, 88–95. [CrossRef] [PubMed]
24. Pilo, C.; Altea, A.; Pirino, S.; Nicolussi, P.; Varcasia, A.; Genchi, M.; Scala, A. *Strongylus vulgaris* (Looss, 1900) in horses in Italy: Is it still a problem? *Vet. Parasitol.* **2012**, *184*, 161–167. [CrossRef] [PubMed]
25. Osterman Lind, E.; Rautalinko, E.; Uggla, A.; Waller, P.J.; Morrison, D.A.; Höglund, J. Parasite control practices on Swedish horse farms. *Acta Vet. Scand.* **2007**, *49*, 25. [CrossRef]
26. Swedish National Veterinary Institute. 2018. Avmaskning av häst. (In Swedish). Available online: http://www.sva.se/djurhalsa/hast/parasiter-hos-hast/avmaskning-av-hast (accessed on 3 March 2020).
27. Coles, G.C.; Bauer, C.; Borgsteede, F.H.; Geerts, S.; Klei, T.R.; Taylor, M.A.; Waller, P.J. World Association for the Advancement of Veterinary Parasitology (W.A.A.V.P.) methods for the detection of anthelmintic resistance in nematodes of veterinary importance. *Vet. Parasitol.* **1992**, *44*, 35–44. [CrossRef]

28. Bellaw, J.L.; Nielsen, M.K. Evaluation of Baermann apparatus sedimentation time on recovery of *Strongylus vulgaris* and *Strongylus edentatus* third stage larvae from equine coprocultures. *Vet. Parasitol.* **2015**, *211*, 99–101. [CrossRef]
29. Van Wyk, J.A.; Mayhew, E. Morphological identification of parasitic nematode infective larvae of small ruminants and cattle: A practical lab guide. *Onderstepoort J. Vet. Res.* **2013**, *80*, 539. [CrossRef]
30. Nielsen, M.K.; Peterson, D.S.; Monrad, J.; Thamsborg, S.M.; Olsen, S.N.; Kaplan, R.M. Detection and semi-quantification of *Strongylus vulgaris* DNA in equine faeces by real-time quantitative PCR. *Int. J. Parasitol.* **2008**, *38*, 443–453. [CrossRef]
31. Beroza, G.A.; Marcus, L.C.; Williams, R.; Bauer, S.M. Laboratory diagnosis of *Anoplocephala perfoliata* infection in horses. *Proc. Am. Assoc. Equine Pract.* **1987**, *32*, 435–439.
32. Andersen, U.V.; Howe, D.K.; Dangoudoubiyam, S.; Toft, N.; Reinemeyer, C.R.; Lyons, E.T.; Olsen, S.N.; Monrad, J.; Nejsum, P.; Nielsen, M.K. SvSXP: A *Strongylus vulgaris* antigen with potential for prepatent diagnosis. *Parasites Vectors* **2013**, *6*, 84. [CrossRef]
33. Nielsen, M.; Mittel, L.; Grice, A.; Erskine, M.; Graves, E.; Vaala, W.; Tully, R.; French, D.; Bowman, R.; Kaplan, R. *AAEP Parasite Control Guidelines*; American Association of Equine Practitioners: Lexington, KY, USA, 2016.
34. Nielsen, M.K.; Vidyashankar, A.N.; Bellaw, J.; Gravatte, H.S.; Cao, X.; Rubinson, E.F.; Reinemeyer, C.R. Serum *Strongylus vulgaris*-specific antibody responses to anthelmintic treatment in naturally infected horses. *Parasitol Res.* **2015**, *114*, 445–451. [CrossRef]
35. Matthews, S.; Dart, A.J.; Dowling, B.A.; Hodgson, J.L.; Hodgson, D.R. Peritonitis associated with *Actinobacillus equuli* in horses: 51 cases. *Aust. Vet. J.* **2001**, *79*, 536–539. [CrossRef]
36. Nielsen, M.K.; Jacobsen, S.; Olsen, S.N.; Bousquet, E.; Pihl, T. Nonstrangulating intestinal infarction associated with *Strongylus vulgaris* in referred Danish equine cases. *Equine Vet. J.* **2016**, *48*, 376–379. [CrossRef]
37. Rötting, A.K.; Freeman, D.E.; Constable, P.D.; Moore, R.M.; Eurell, J.C.; Wallig, M.A.; Hubert, J.D. The effects of *Strongylus vulgaris* parasitism on eosinophil distribution and accumulation in equine large intestinal mucosa. *Equine Vet. J.* **2008**, *40*, 379–384. [CrossRef]
38. Olofsson, K.M. Immunopathological Aspects of Equine Inflammatory Bowel Disease. Ph.D. Thesis, Swedish University of Agricultural Sciences, Uppsala, Sweden, 2016.
39. Trotz-Williams, L.; Physick-Sheard, P.; McFarlane, H.; Pearl, D.L.; Martin, S.W.; Peregrine, A.S. Occurrence of *Anoplocephala perfoliata* infection in horses in Ontario, Canada and associations with colic and management practices. *Vet. Parasitol.* **2008**, *153*, 73–84. [CrossRef]
40. Uhlinger, C. Effects of three anthelmintic schedules on the incidence of colic in horses. *Equine Vet. J.* **1990**, *22*, 251–254. [CrossRef]
41. Smets, K.; Shaw, D.J.; Deprez, P.; Vercruysse, J. Diagnosis of larval cyathostominosis in horses in Belgium. *Vet. Rec.* **1999**, *144*, 665–668. [CrossRef]
42. Steinbach, T.; Bauer, C.; Sasse, H.; Baumgärtner, W.; Rey-Moreno, C.; Hermosilla, C.; Damriyasa, I.M.; Zahner, H. Small strongyle infection: Consequences of larvicidal treatment of horses with fenbendazole and moxidectin. *Vet. Parasitol.* **2006**, *139*, 115–131. [CrossRef]
43. Larsen, J. Acute colitis in adult horses. A review with emphasis on aetiology and pathogenesis. *Vet. Q.* **1997**, *19*, 72–80. [CrossRef] [PubMed]
44. Nielsen, M.K.; Baptiste, K.E.; Tolliver, S.C.; Collins, S.S.; Lyons, E.T. Analysis of multiyear studies in horses in Kentucky to ascertain whether counts of eggs and larvae per gram of feces are reliable indicators of numbers of strongyles and ascarids present. *Vet. Parasitol.* **2010**, *74*, 77–84. [CrossRef]
45. Nilsson, O.; Ljungström, B.L.; Höglund, J.; Lundquist, H.; Uggla, A. *Anoplocephala perfoliata* in horses in Sweden: Prevalence, infection levels and intestinal lesions. *Acta Vet. Scand.* **1995**, *36*, 319–328. [PubMed]
46. Proudman, C.J.; Edwards, G.B. Validation of a centrifugation/flotation technique for the diagnosis of equine cestodiasis. *Vet. Rec.* **1992**, *131*, 71–72. [CrossRef]
47. Proudman, C.J.; Edwards, G.B. Are tapeworms associated with equine colic? A case control study. *Equine Vet. J.* **1993**, *25*, 224–226. [CrossRef] [PubMed]
48. 48 Ryu, S.H.; Bak, U.B.; Kim, J.G.; Yoon, H.J.; Seo, H.S.; Kim, J.T.; Park, J.Y.; Lee, C.W. Cecal rupture by *Anoplocephala perfoliata* infection in a thoroughbred horse in Seoul Race Park, South Korea. *J. Vet. Sci.* **2001**, *3*, 189–193. [CrossRef]

49. Little, D.; Blikslager, A.T. Factors associated with development of ileal impaction in horses with surgical colic: 78 cases (1986–2000). *Equine Vet. J.* **2002**, *34*, 464–468. [CrossRef] [PubMed]
50. Hinney, B.; Wirtherle, N.C.; Kyule, M.; Miethe, N.; Zessin, K.H.; Clausen, P.H. A questionnaire survey on helminth control on horse farms in Brandenburg, Germany and the assessment of risks caused by different kinds of management. *Parasitol. Res.* **2011**, *109*, 1625–1635. [CrossRef]
51. Robert, M.; Hu, W.; Nielsen, M.K.; Stowe, C.J. Attitudes towards implementation of surveillance-based parasite control on Kentucky Thoroughbred farms—Current strategies, awareness and willingness-to-pay. *Equine Vet. J.* **2015**, *476*, 694–700. [CrossRef]
52. Stratford, C.H.; Lester, H.E.; Morgan, E.R.; Pickles, K.J.; Relf, V.; McGorum, B.C.; Matthews, J.B. A questionnaire study of equine gastrointestinal parasite control in Scotland. *Equine Vet. J.* **2014**, *46*, 25–31. [CrossRef]
53. Sallé, G.; Cabaret, J. A survey on parasite management by equine veterinarians highlights the need for a regulation change. *Vet. Rec. Open.* **2015**, *2*, e000104. [CrossRef]
54. Nielsen, M.K.; Branan, M.A.; Wiedenheft, A.M.; Digianantonio, R.; Scare, J.A.; Bellaw, J.L.; Garber, L.P.; Kopral, C.A.; Phillippi-Taylor, A.M.; Traub-Dargatz, J.L. Anthelmintic efficacy against equine strongyles in the United States. *Vet. Parasitol.* **2018**, *259*, 53–60. [CrossRef]
55. Elghryani, N.; Duggan, V.; Relf, V.; de Waal, T. Questionnaire survey on helminth control practices in horse farms in Ireland. *Parasitology* **2019**, *146*, 873–882. [CrossRef] [PubMed]
56. *A Guide to the Treatment and Control of Equine Gastrointestinal Parasite Infections ESCCAP Guidelines*, 1st ed.; ESCCAP: Malvern, UK, 2018; ISBN 978-1-907259-70-8.
57. Scare, J.A.; Steuer, A.E.; Gravatte, H.; Kálmán, C.S.; Ramires, L.; Dias de Castro, L.L.; Norris, J.; Miller, F.; Camargo, F.; Lawyer, A.; et al. Management practices associated with strongylid parasite prevalence on horse farms in rural counties of Kentucky. *Vet. Parasitol.* **2018**, *14*, 25–31. [CrossRef] [PubMed]
58. Borji, H.; Moosavi, Z.; Ahmadi, F. Cranial mesenteric arterial obstruction due to *Strongylus vulgaris* larvae in a Donkey (*Equus asinus*). *Iran. J. Parasitol.* **2014**, *9*, 441–444. [PubMed]
59. Nielsen, M.K.; Scare, J.; Gravatte, H.S.; Bellaw, J.L.; Prado, J.C.; Reinemeyer, C.R. Changes in Serum *Strongylus vulgaris*-Specific Antibody Concentrations in Response to Anthelmintic Treatment of Experimentally Infected Foals. *Front. Vet. Sci.* **2015**, *2*, 17. [CrossRef]
60. Herd, R.P. Epidemiology and control of equine strongylosis at Newmarket. *Equine Vet. J.* **1986**, *18*, 447–452. [CrossRef] [PubMed]
61. Corbett, C.J.; Love, S.; Moore, A.; Burden, F.A.; Matthews, J.B.; Denwood, M.J. The effectiveness of faecal removal methods of pasture management to control the cyathostomin burden of donkeys. *Parasit Vectors* **2014**, *7*, 48. [CrossRef]
62. Ogbourne, C.P. Observations on the free-living stages of strongylid nematodes of the horse. *Parasitology* **1972**, *64*, 461–477. [CrossRef]
63. Proudman, C.; Matthews, J. Control of intestinal parasites in horses. *Pract. BMJ* **2000**, *22*, 90–97. [CrossRef]
64. Singer, J.W.; Bamka, W.J.; Kluchinski, D.; Govindasamy, R. Using the recommended stocking density to predict equine pasture management. *J. Equine Vet. Sci.* **2002**, *22*, 73–76. [CrossRef]

16

Microbiome Shift, Diversity and Overabundance of Opportunistic Pathogens in Bovine Digital Dermatitis Revealed by 16S rRNA Amplicon Sequencing

Hector M. Espiritu [1], Lovelia L. Mamuad [1], Seon-ho Kim [1], Su-jeong Jin [1], Sang-suk Lee [1], Seok-won Kwon [2] and Yong-il Cho [1,*]

1 Department of Animal Science and Technology, Sunchon National University, Suncheon, Jeonnam 57922, Korea; 1193001@s.scnu.ac.kr (H.M.E.); loveliamamuad2306@gmail.com (L.L.M.); mhs0425@daum.net (S.-h.K.); herodias@scnu.ac.kr (S.-j.J.); rumen@scnu.ac.kr (S.-s.L.)

2 Woosarang Animal Hospital, Yongin, Gyeonggi 17026, Korea; gastra00@naver.com

* Correspondence: ycho@scnu.ac.kr.

Simple Summary: Bovine digital dermatitis (BDD) is a foot infection known as the primary cause of lameness in cattle due to painful lesions, posing serious impacts on the productivity and welfare of affected animals. Members of the bacterial group *Treponema* have long been considered as the main causative agents because previous investigations by bacterial isolation, tissue analyses, and high molecular sequencing have persistently identified this group in BDD. However, other studies indicated that the presence of several bacteria on the lesion due to the slurry environment the cattle foot are exposed to, suggests an interdependent polybacterial nature which could also play a role in disease development and progression. Therefore, we analyzed the diversity and relationship of the diverse microbiome in BDD lesions compared to normal skin from cattle foot by using next-generation high throughput sequencing. Based on the results obtained, we concluded that the shift in microbial composition which leads to richer diversity in BDD, and the overabundance of opportunistic bacterial pathogens could be associated with BDD pathogenesis.

Abstract: This study analyzed the diversity and phylogenetic relationship of the microbiome of bovine digital dermatitis (BDD) lesions and normal skin from cattle foot by using 16S rRNA amplicon sequencing. Three BDD samples and a normal skin sample were pre-assessed for analysis. The Illumina Miseq platform was used for sequencing and sequences were assembled and were categorized to operational taxonomic units (OTUs) based on similarity, then the core microbiome was visualized. The phylogeny was inferred using MEGA7 (Molecular evolutionary genetics analysis version 7.0). A total of 129 and 185 OTUs were uniquely observed in normal and in BDD samples, respectively. Of the 47 shared OTUs, 15 species presented increased abundance in BDD. In BDD and normal samples, Spirochetes and Proteobacteria showed the most abundant phyla, respectively, suggesting the close association of observed species in each sample group. The phylogeny revealed the evolutionary relationship of OTUs and the Euclidean distance suggested a high sequence divergence between OTUs. We concluded that a shift in the microbiome leads to richer diversity in BDD lesions, and the overabundance of opportunistic pathogens and its synergistic relationship with commensal bacteria could serve as factors in disease development. The influence of these factors should be thoroughly investigated in future studies to provide deeper insights on the pathogenesis of BDD.

Keywords: bovine digital dermatitis; cattle lameness; microbiome; *Treponema* spp

1. Introduction

Bovine digital dermatitis (BDD) is known as the most important foot infection causing lameness in cattle [1]. This severe lameness, which is the primary clinical manifestation of BDD caused by painful hyperkeratotic lesions [2], poses serious concerns on the welfare of the affected animals [3]. Serious economic impacts have also been implicated with BDD due to significant milk production losses, poor reproductive performance [4,5], and most extremely, premature culling of the affected animals [6].

The first reported case of BDD was in Italy in 1974 by Chelli and Mortellaro [7], and since then, it has been globally reported reaching an endemic state in many countries [8]. Etiological investigations have identified a variety of bacteria in BDD lesions [9], but advancements in sequencing technology have provided essential information on the identity of associated causal agents [8]. In previous investigations, Spirochetes are considered to be the major pathogen in BDD [1,10]. However, studies indicated that the presence of several bacteria on the lesion due to the slurry environment the cattle foot are exposed to [2], suggests a synergistic polybacterial nature [11] which plays a role in disease development and progression [12].

Many reports have attempted to elucidate the association of the microbiome of BDD towards disease development [11,13–15]. Surprisingly, for more than 20 years since it emerged as a major problem in the cattle industry in certain countries, studies on BDD have just recently started in Korea. In a recent report, *Treponema* spp. was established as the dominant pathogen in BDD lesions in Korea [16], but an emphasis on the plethora of bacteria that was observed is still lacking. Although the majority of studies considered that the main pathogen of BDD is *Treponema* spp., its polybacterial nature must also be considered in order to understand its pathogenesis [15]. Therefore, this study analyzed the diversity and phylogenetic relationship of the microbiome of BDD lesions and normal skin from the interdigital space of the cattle using 16S rRNA amplicon sequencing.

2. Materials and Methods

2.1. Sample Collection

This study was performed following general ethical principles and with the consent of farm owners. The collection of samples was done in Holstein–Friesian cattle in housed dairy farm, and was conducted during hoof cleaning, trimming and treatment performed by a professional veterinarian with years of expertise in the field. Inspection was done by anatomic pathological observation of grossly visible active BDD lesions on the proximal border of interdigital space characterized by the presence of ulceration, with hyperkeratosis and proliferative growth with hair-like projections as described by Zinicola et al. (2015) [17]. For normal skin sample, healthy animals with no sign of lameness and no history of BDD were inspected. After thorough cleaning of the foot surface, lidocaine (2%) was subcutaneously injected around the lesion and a 5-mm punch biopsy was taken from the center of the lesion for BDD, while for normal skin, biopsy sample was taken where BDD most often take place. Samples were washed thoroughly with buffered phosphate saline (pH 7.4) and delivered to the laboratory with ice. A total of 66 pre-assessed active BDD samples were subjected to detection of *Treponema* spp. by genus-specific PCR as described in the results of our previous study [16]. Since 100% of the active BDD lesions are positive in PCR, three samples were randomly selected for metagenomics sequencing. A normal sample was provided for BDD negative control. Samples were categorized as Group A for normal skin sample, and Group B for BDD-infected samples.

2.2. Metagenomics Sequencing and Diversity Analysis

The four randomly pre-assessed samples were submitted to Macrogen (Korea) for high-throughput sequencing. DNA samples extracted from lesion and normal sample biopsies were subjected to quality control by Picogreen method before library construction. By targeting the V3-V4 region of the 16S rRNA gene, libraries were constructed and were purified. Sequencing was carried out using Illumina Miseq platform (Illumina, San Diego, CA, USA). The base call binary data produced by Real-Time Analysis (RTA) were converted to FASTQ files by bcl2fastq package (Illumina, San Diego, CA, USA) and were filtered using Scythe (v0.994) (https://github.com/vsbuffalo/scythe) and Sickle (https://github.com/najoshi/sickle) programs to remove adapter sequences. The obtained 16S rRNA sequences were binned into Operational Taxonomic Units (OTUs) based on 97% identity using Quantitative Insights Into Microbial Ecology (QIIME) [18]. The microbiome was visualized using Metagenomics Core Microbiome Exploration Tool (MetaCoMET) [19] using a Biological Observation Matrix format (BIOM) [20] generated using Mothur [21].

2.3. *Divergence and Phylogenetic Analysis*

The phylogeny of the microbiome was inferred by aligning the obtained 16S rRNA sequences of the operational taxonomic units identified using ClustalW [22], and the Newick tree data were obtained from MEGA7 [23] by maximum likelihood method following the general time-reversible model as the fit model for calculating the rate of nucleotide base substitution. The final dendrogram was constructed using Iroki [24]. The divergence distance between OTUs was calculated by Euclidian distance method based on the rate of nucleotide base substitution between OTUs, and presented as a heatmap matrix generated by Heatmapper [25] for the aligned sequences of OTUs using the Euclidean distance method.

3. Results

In total, 66 samples pre-assessed from our previous research [16] were used in this study. From these, one normal skin sample (Group A) and three BDD lesions (Group B) were subjected for analysis.

The Chao1 diversity index shows that Group B has richer species diversity compared to Group A (Figure 1A). The size of the microbiome presented in Figure 1B shows a higher observed OTUs in BDD lesions compared to the normal skin sample. Out of 267 OTUs observed, 138 were uniquely observed in Group B, 82 in Group A, while 47 were overlapping in both groups. Fifteen of these shared OTUs increased their abundance from normal to BDD and includes T. pedis (20.93%), a group of unclassified species (12.4%), Treponema denticola (9.8%), T. medium (6.48%), Porphyromonas levii (1.56%), P. somerae (1.22%), and Acholeplasma vituli (0.89%). OTUs absent in Group A with increased abundance ratio in Group B were as follows in decreasing order: Carboxylicivirga mesophila (5.89%), T. lecithinolyticum (5.35%), A. morum (5.03%), Spirochaeta africana (3.74%), Mycoplasma feliminutum (3.65%), A. modicum (2.77%), Pelobacter propionicus (2.04%), H. sueciensis (1.64%), P. uenonis (1.30%), Falcatimonas natans (1.25%), Devosia confluentis (1.17), Christensenella minuta (1.08%), and M. fermentans (1.30%). Additional information can be accessed in Supplementary Table S1. The shift in abundance ratio of each species from normal to BDD (Figure 1C) shows the drop in abundance of dominant bacteria, Psychrobacter fulvigenes and Pseudomonas caeni from the normal sample, and the increased abundance of Treponema spp., and other bacteria in BDD. In addition, the Euclidian distance heat-map based on OTU abundance between samples and representative phyla (Figure 1D) illustrated the high association of Spirochetes with BDD. Moraxellaceae and Pseudomonadaceae, both under phylum Proteobacteria presented a close relationship with normal tissue. Moreover, Bacteroidetes and Firmicutes are considerably associated in both groups, while Tenericutes is associated with BDD only.

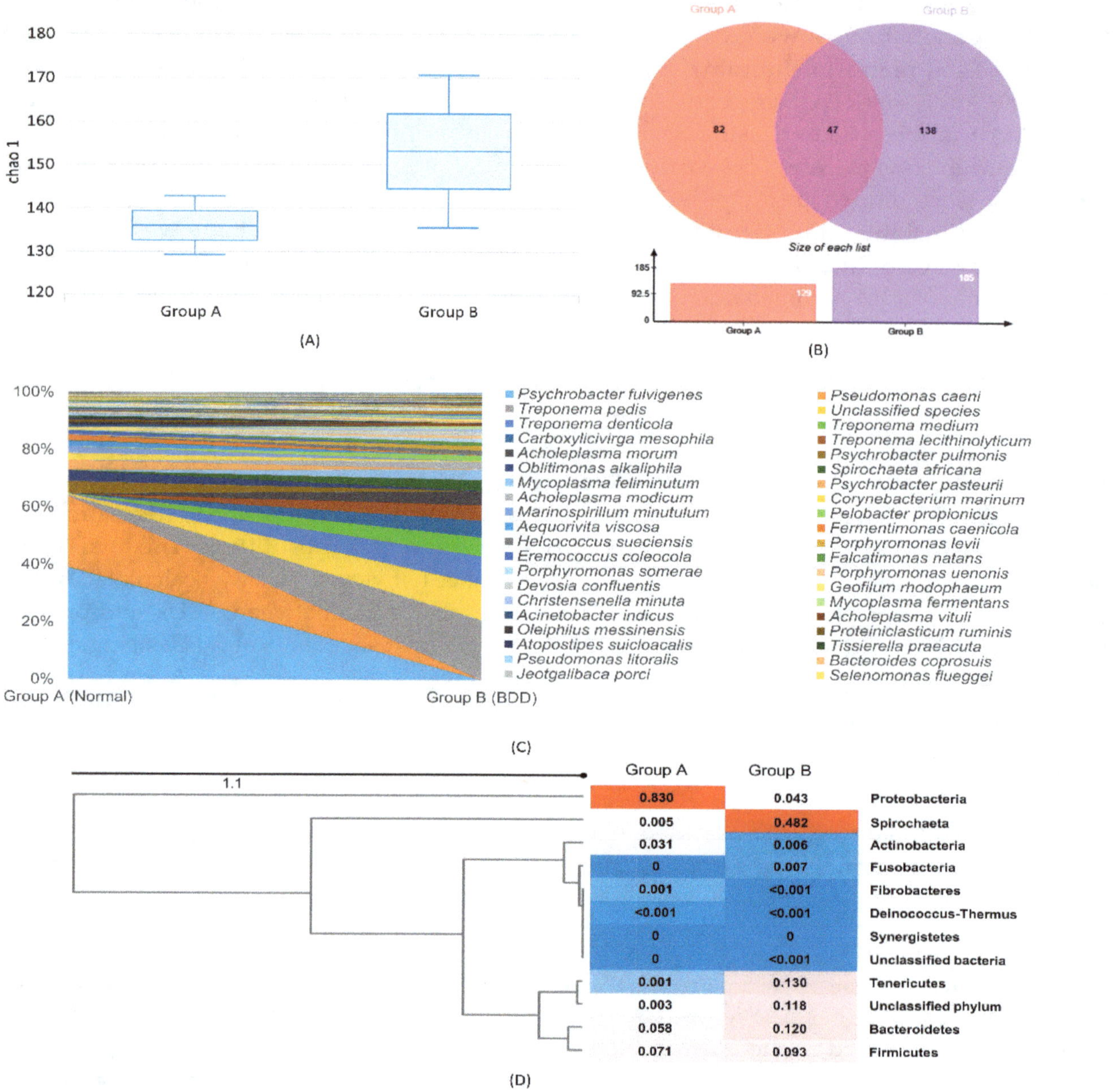

Figure 1. (**A**) Box plot of Chao1 diversity index for bovine digital dermatitis (BDD) (Group A) and normal (Group B), (**B**) the microbiome presenting the number of operational taxonomic units (OTUs) in Group A and Group B showing the unique and shared OTUs between groups, and (**C**) relative abundance of operational taxonomic units from Group A and Group B (legend: 22 most abundant). (**D**) Euclidian distance heatmap presenting the association between phylum and sample groups. Red denotes closer association while blue denotes a lesser association with normal sample and BDD.

The maximum likelihood tree constructed using the general time-reversible model illustrated the phylogenetic relationship of all the OTUs (Figure 2A). The tree showed the phylum classification of the OTUs, and the abundance ratio and OTU count (Figure 2B). Firmicutes was the most diverse phylum representing 41.85% and 37.21% of the observed OTUs in BDD and normal skin, respectively. Spirochetes (which is the most abundant) only represented 3.75% of the over-all observed OTUs. In addition, the Euclidean distance heat map matrix showed the estimates of the evolutionary divergence between OTUs in lesions and normal tissue (Figure 2C), and the frequency distribution of the computed distance of the pairwise comparisons was graphed in Figure 2D. Overall, 63.89% of the pairwise comparisons were above the median distance.

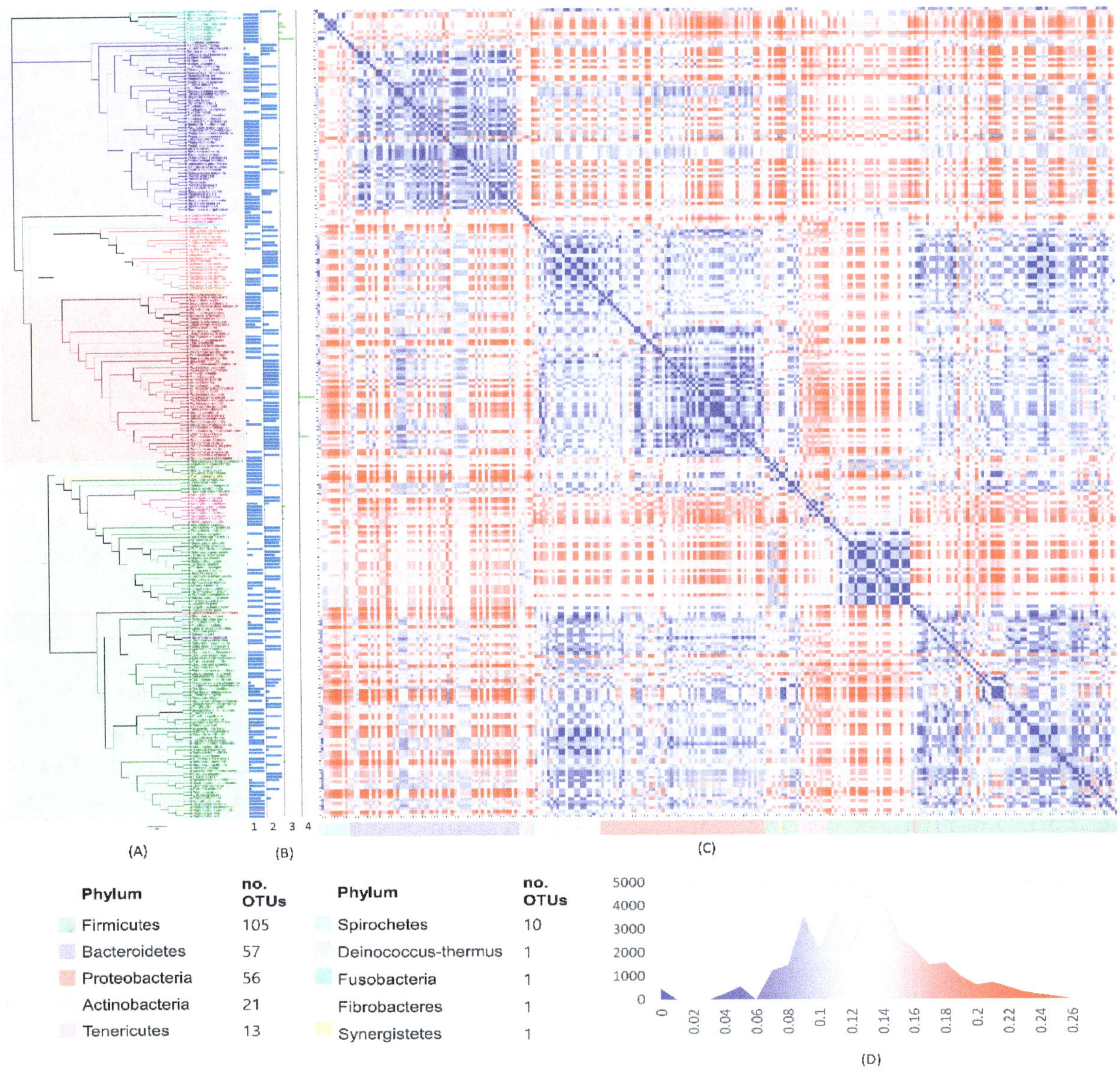

Figure 2. General time-reversible tree representing all observed OTUs in BDD-infected and normal skin samples color-coded based on phylum classification (**A**). The scale value is 2.57. The blue bar graph denotes the abundance ratio of each species on BDD (**B1**) and normal sample (**B2**), while the green bar graph shows the actual count per species (OTU) for BDD (**B3**) and normal (**B4**) sample. Euclidean distance heat map matrix is based on the nucleotide base substitution rate presenting the divergence between all OTUs in BDD and normal sample (**C**). The graph (**D**) shows the frequency distribution of pairwise comparison between OTUs in each calculated distance from low (blue) to high (red).

4. Discussion

This study analyzed the diversity and phylogenetic relationship of the microbiome of BDD lesions compared to normal skin from the interdigital space of the cattle. From our previous study [16], we elucidated the relative abundance of Spirochetes, specifically *Treponema* spp. in BDD lesions and concluded that *Treponema* spp., was the dominant pathogen involved in BDD in Korea. Although the major abundance of *Treponema* spp. in lesions based on several investigations suggest that BDD is polytreponemal, the presence of other bacteria implies that they may also play certain roles in its pathogenesis.

The data analyzed exhibited a change in the microbiome in BDD lesions from the normal skin sample. This altered microbiome has been previously observed by Krull et al., (2014) [13] and Zinicola et al., (2015) [11] by investigating the microbiome of each stage and layer of BDD lesions, respectively. They observed the replacement of species from the normal sample by other species along with the disease progression and the alteration of the microbiome in each layer of lesions. In the current data, the 82 OTUs from the normal sample were replaced in BDD-infected sample by 138 OTUs. This alteration also led to a richer diversity in BDD as opposed to the findings of Krull et al., (2014) where disease progression leads to a drop in diversity [13]. Although samples subjected in our study is categorized only as active BDD, it is recommended to use several normal samples and BDD samples categorized in varying lesion stages to gain more conclusive data. Another interesting finding of this study is the shared OTUs between normal and BDD found in the overlap comprised of three *Treponema* spp. (*T. pedis, T. medium, T. denticola*), along with two *Phorphyromonas* spp. as the five most abundant bacteria in BDD. The increased abundance of these species from normal to BDD, along with others could imply that these bacteria are commensals which later progresses as opportunistic pathological agents which initiates disease development when triggered under favorable conditions.

The abundance data previously presented by Mamuad et al., (2020) [16], to some extent, agree with the reports of Moreira et al., (2018) [14], Zinicola et al., (2015) [11], Beninger et al., (2016) [26], Krull et al., (2014) [13], and Nielsen et al., (2016) [12], that BDD is polybacterial, with *Treponema* spp., as the most abundant genus. However, the dominance and diversity of species under this genus still varies between reports from different geographical locations. Moreira et al., (2018) reported that *Treponema pedis* is the most abundant species in BDD in Brazil, which is in accordance with Mamuad et al., (2020). However, in one study in the USA, *T. denticola* and *T. phagedenis* were the most abundant species in active and inactive lesions, respectively [11]. Additionally, the results of investigation of Beninger et al., (2015) [26] and Krull et al., (2014) [13] were in agreement with each other that the most abundant species in BDD is *T. phagedenis*, which was absent in all samples in our data. This suggests that BDD microbiome has geographical and/or sample-to-sample variation.

Given that certain members of genus *Treponema* are recognized as the abundant bacteria, and considered as major contributors in the development and progression of the disease, other bacterial genera have also been reported in BDD from other countries as also in this study such as *Porphyromonas* [14], *Campylobacter*, *Acholeplasma* [11], *Peptoniphilus* and *Romboutsia* [27]. In this study, a major abundance of *Carboxylicivirga mesophila* and *Treponema lecithinolyticum* was observed as the fourth and fifth most abundant identified bacteria in BDD, respectively, which were not observed from previous studies. Further investigation is required to verify if these bacteria have actual involvement with the disease, since *C. mesophila* was first isolated from tidal flat sediment in Korea [28], while *T. lecithinolyticum* was commonly found in human oral microbiome [29].

The distance heat map between phyla and samples based on OTU count and taxonomy showed the close relationship of the observed species under phylum Spirochetes and Proteobacteria in BDD and normal skin, respectively. Phylum Bacteroidetes and Firmicutes can be associated in both groups, while Tenericutes is associated only with BDD which agrees with Nielsen et al., (2016) [12]. In a study by Bay et al., (2018) Firmicutes was the most abundant phylum in other polybacterial foot infections in bovine models such as interdigital hyperplasia, interdigital phlegmon, sole ulcer, toe necrosis, and white line disease, with Spirochetes being the fifth most abundant phylum overall, after Bacteroidetes, Actinobacteria, and Proteobacteria [27]. This suggests that there are variations on the major pathogens between these diseases.

The GTR tree shows the phylogenetic relationship of all OTUs present in both BDD-infected and normal skin samples, classified under 10 phyla, with Firmicutes representing the highest diversity. This large number of Firmicutes was supported by the findings of Yano et al., (2010) [30] and Santos et al., (2012) [31] in both normal and BDD-infected samples, regardless of its relative abundance. In this study, Spirochetes with the highest abundance in BDD have lower diversity both before and during infection. Compared with Firmicutes with highest diversity in normal and BDD, there was no increase in its abundance before and during infection. This suggests that diversity richness of a certain phylum may be irrelative with the abundance or its pathogenic involvement in BDD. The microbiome of BDD in this study was verified to be highly diverse, thus, we hypothesize that synergism between overabundant opportunistic pathogens and the diversity of commensals makes the disease more complicated. The pairwise distances of OTUs based on the computed rate of nucleotide substitution show higher frequencies for above-median distances between species found in all samples. This supports the idea that bacterial diversity is evolutionarily diverged.

5. Conclusions

We concluded that a shift in the microbiome leads to richer diversity in BDD lesions, and the overabundance of opportunistic pathogens and its possible synergistic relationship between less abundant commensal bacteria could serve as factors in disease development and progression. Spirochetes is the most abundant phylum associated with BDD in other previous studies, and in this study, we deliberated that the abundance of species on each of the observed phylum varied between reports, suggesting either geographical or sample-to-sample variation. The influence of the overabundance of opportunistic species and the synergistic interaction of the plethora of commensal bacteria should be thoroughly investigated in future studies by including additional samples categorized to varying degree of the severity of infection, not just in BDD, but also in other lameness-related foot diseases, to provide deeper insights on the pathogenesis and microbiome relationship of these debilitating diseases.

Author Contributions: Conceptualization, Y.-i.C.; methodology, H.M.E., L.L.M., S.-j.J., S.-h.K., and S.-w.K. software, H.M.E. and L.L.M.; validation, Y.-i.C.; formal analysis, H.M.E. and L.L.M.; investigation, H.M.E. and L.L.M.; resources, Y.-i.C. and S.-w.K.; data curation, H.M.E. and L.L.M.; writing—original draft preparation, H.M.E. and L.L.M.; writing—review and editing, Y.-i.C., and S.-s.L.; visualization, H.M.E. and L.L.M.; supervision, Y.-i.C., and S.-s.L.; project administration, S.-j.J.; funding acquisition, Y.-i.C. All authors have read and agreed to the published version of the manuscript.

References

1. Evans, N.J.; Murray, R.D.; Carter, S.D. Bovine digital dermatitis: Current concepts from laboratory to farm. *Vet. J.* **2016**, *211*, 3–13. [CrossRef]
2. Demirkan, I.; Evans, N.J.; Singh, P.; Brown, J.M.; Getty, B.; Carter, S.D.; Timofte, D.; Hart, C.A.; Vink, W.D.; Birtles, R.J.; et al. Association of unique, isolated treponemes with bovine digital dermatitis lesions. *J. Clin. Microbiol.* **2009**, *47*, 689–696. [CrossRef]
3. Klitgaard, K.; Nielsen, M.W.; Ingerslev, H.C.; Boye, M.; Jensen, T.K. Discovery of bovine digital dermatitis-associated *Treponema* spp. in the dairy herd environment by a targeted deep-sequencing approach. *Appl. Environ. Microbiol.* **2014**, *80*, 4427–4432. [CrossRef] [PubMed]
4. De Jesús Argáez-Rodríguez, F.; Hird, D.W.; Hernández De Anda, J.; Read, D.H.; Rodríguez-Lainz, A. Papillomatous digital dermatitis on a commercial dairy farm in Mexicali, Mexico: Incidence and effect on reproduction and milk production. *Prev. Vet. Med.* **1997**, *32*, 275–286. [CrossRef]
5. Read, D.H.; Walker, R.L. Papillomatous digital dermatitis (footwarts) in California dairy cattle: Clinical and gross pathologic findings. *J. Vet. Diagn. Investig.* **1998**, *10*, 67–76. [CrossRef]
6. Elliott, M.K.; Alt, D.P.; Zuerner, R.L. Lesion formation and antibody response induced by papillomatous digital dermatitis-associated spirochetes in a murine abscess model. *Infect. Immun.* **2007**, *75*, 4400–4408. [CrossRef] [PubMed]
7. Cheli, R.; Mortellaro, C. Digital dermatitis in cattle. In Proceedings of the 8th International Conference Diseases of Cattle, Milan, Italy, 9–13 September 1974; pp. 208–213.

8. Palmer, M.A.; O'Connell, N.E. Digital dermatitis in dairy cows: A review of risk factors and potential sources of between-animal variation in susceptibility. *Animals* **2015**, *5*, 512–535. [CrossRef]
9. Nally, J.E.; Hornsby, R.L.; Alt, D.P.; Whitelegge, J.P. Phenotypic and proteomic characterization of treponemes associated with bovine digital dermatitis. *Vet. Microbiol.* **2019**, *235*, 35–42. [CrossRef]
10. Wilson-Welder, J.H.; Alt, D.P.; Nally, J.E. Digital dermatitis in cattle: Current bacterial and immunological findings. *Animals* **2015**, *5*, 1114–1135. [CrossRef]
11. Zinicola, M.; Lima, F.; Lima, S.; Machado, V.; Gomez, M. Altered microbiomes in bovine digital dermatitis lesions, and the gut as a pathogen reservoir. *PLoS ONE* **2015**, 1–23. [CrossRef]
12. Nielsen, M.W.; Strube, M.L.; Isbrand, A.; Al-Medrasi, W.D.H.M.; Boye, M.; Jensen, T.K.; Klitgaard, K. Potential bacterial core species associated with digital dermatitis in cattle herds identified by molecular profiling of interdigital skin samples. *Vet. Microbiol.* **2016**, *186*, 139–149. [CrossRef] [PubMed]
13. Krull, A.C.; Shearer, J.K.; Gorden, P.J.; Cooper, V.L.; Phillips, G.J.; Plummera, P.J. Deep sequencing analysis reveals temporal microbiota changes associated with development of bovine digital dermatitis. *Infect. Immun.* **2014**, *82*, 3359–3373. [CrossRef] [PubMed]
14. Moreira, T.F.; Facury Filho, E.J.; Carvalho, A.U.; Strube, M.L.; Nielsen, M.W.; Klitgaard, K.; Jensen, T.K. Pathology and bacteria related to digital dermatitis in dairy cattle in all year round grazing system in Brazil. *PLoS ONE* **2018**, *13*, 1–15. [CrossRef] [PubMed]
15. Hesseling, J.; Legione, A.R.; Stevenson, M.A.; McCowan, C.I.; Pyman, M.F.; Finochio, C.; Nguyen, D.; Roic, C.L.; Thiris, O.L.; Zhang, A.J.; et al. Bovine digital dermatitis in Victoria, Australia. *Aust. Vet. J.* **2019**, *97*, 404–413. [CrossRef]
16. Mamuad, L.L.; Joo, B.; Al, S.; Espiritu, H.M.; Jeong, S.; Kim, W.; Lee, S.; Cho, Y. *Treponema* spp., the dominant pathogen in the lesion of bovine digital dermatitis and its characterization in dairy cattle. *Vet. Microbiol.* **2020**, *245*, 108696. [CrossRef]
17. Zinicola, M.; Higgins, H.; Lima, S.; Machado, V.; Guard, C.; Bicalho, R. Shotgun metagenomic sequencing reveals functional genes and microbiome associated with bovine digital dermatitis. *PLoS ONE* **2015**, *10*, 1–17. [CrossRef]
18. Caporaso, J.G.; Kuczynski, J.; Stombaugh, J.; Bittinger, K.; Bushman, F.D.; Costello, E.K.; Fierer, N.; Peña, A.G.; Goodrich, J.K.; Gordon, J.I.; et al. QIIME allows analysis of high- throughput community sequencing data intensity normalization improves color calling in SOLiD sequencing. *Nat. Methods* **2010**, *7*, 335–336. [CrossRef]
19. Wang, Y.; Xu, L.; Gu, Y.Q.; Coleman-Derr, D. MetaCoMET: A web platform for discovery and visualization of the core microbiome. *Bioinformatics* **2016**, *32*, 3469–3470. [CrossRef]
20. McDonald, D.; Clemente, J.C.; Kuczynski, J.; Rideout, J.R.; Stombaugh, J.; Wendel, D.; Wilke, A.; Huse, S.; Hufnagle, J.; Meyer, F.; et al. The Biological Observation Matrix (BIOM) format or: How I learned to stop worrying and love the ome-ome. *Gigascience* **2012**, *464*, 1–6. [CrossRef]
21. Schloss, P.D.; Westcott, S.L.; Ryabin, T.; Hall, J.R.; Hartmann, M.; Hollister, E.B.; Lesniewski, R.A.; Oakley, B.B.; Parks, D.H.; Robinson, C.J.; et al. Introducing mothur: Open-source, platform-independent, community-supported software for describing and comparing microbial communities. *Appl. Environ. Microbiol.* **2009**, *75*, 7537–7541. [CrossRef]
22. Thompson, J.D.; Higgins, D.G.; Gibson, T.J. CLUSTAL W: Improving the sensitivity of progressive multiple sequence alignment through sequence weighting, position-specific gap penalties and weight matrix choice. *Nucl. Acids Res.* **1994**, *22*, 4673–4680. [CrossRef] [PubMed]
23. Kumar, S.; Stecher, G.; Tamura, K. MEGA7: Molecular evolutionary genetics analysis version 7.0 for bigger datasets. *Mol. Biol. Evol.* **2016**, *33*, 1870–1874. [CrossRef] [PubMed]
24. Moore, R.M.; Harrison, A.O.; McAllister, S.M.; Polson, S.W.; Wommack, K.E. Iroki: Automatic customization and visualization of phylogenetic trees. *PeerJ* **2020**, *8*, e8584. [CrossRef]
25. Babicki, S.; Arndt, D.; Marcu, A.; Liang, Y.; Grant, J.R.; Maciejewski, A.; Wishart, D.S. Heatmapper: Web-enabled heat mapping for all. *Nucl. Acids Res.* **2016**, *44*, W147–W153. [CrossRef] [PubMed]
26. Beninger, C.; Naqvi, S.A.; Naushad, S.; Orsel, K.; Luby, C.; Derakhshani, H.; Khafipour, E.; De Buck, J. Associations between digital dermatitis lesion grades in dairy cattle and the quantities of four *Treponema* species. *Vet. Res.* **2018**, *49*, 10–12. [CrossRef] [PubMed]

27. Bay, V.; Griffiths, B.; Carter, S.; Evans, N.J.; Lenzi, L.; Bicalho, R.C.; Oikonomou, G. 16S rRNA amplicon sequencing reveals a polymicrobial nature of complicated claw horn disruption lesions and interdigital phlegmon in dairy cattle. *Sci. Rep.* **2018**, *8*, 1–12. [CrossRef]
28. Yang, S.H.; Seo, H.S.; Woo, J.H.; Oh, H.M.; Jang, H.; Lee, J.H.; Kim, S.J.; Kwon, K.K. *Carboxylicivirga* gen. nov. in the family Marinilabiliaceae with two novel species, *Carboxylicivirga mesophila* sp. nov. and *Carboxylicivirga taeanensis* sp. nov., and reclassification of *Cytophaga fermentans* as *Saccharicrinis fermentans* gen. nov., comb. nov. *Int. J. Syst. Evol. Microbiol.* **2014**, *64*, 1351–1358. [CrossRef]
29. Belkacemi, S.; Khalil, J.B.; Ominami, Y.; Hisada, A.; Fontanini, A.; Caputo, A.; Levasseur, A.; Lagier, J.C.; Khelaifia, S.; Raoult, D. Passive filtration, rapid scanning electron microscopy, and matrix-assisted laser desorption ionization–time of flight mass spectrometry for *Treponema* culture and identification from the oral cavity. *J. Clin. Microbiol.* **2019**, *57*. [CrossRef]
30. Yano, T.; Moe, K.K.; Yamazaki, K.; Ooka, T.; Hayashi, T.; Misawa, N. Identification of candidate pathogens of papillomatous digital dermatitis in dairy cattle from quantitative 16S rRNA clonal analysis. *Vet. Microbiol.* **2010**, *143*, 352–362. [CrossRef]
31. Santos, T.M.A.; Pereira, R.V.; Caixeta, L.S.; Guard, C.L.; Bicalho, R.C. Microbial diversity in bovine Papillomatous digital dermatitis in Holstein dairy cows from upstate New York. *FEMS Microbiol. Ecol.* **2012**, *79*, 518–529. [CrossRef]

17

Identification of *Sarcocystis* spp. in One-humped Camels (*Camelus dromedarius*) from Riyadh and Dammam, Saudi Arabia, via Histological and Phylogenetic Approaches

Dina M. Metwally [1,2,*], Tahani T. Al-Otaibi [3], Isra M. Al-Turaiki [4], Manal F. El-Khadragy [5,6] and Reem A. Alajmi [1]

1 Department of Zoology, College of Science, King Saud University, Riyadh 11451, KSA; ralajmi@ksu.edu.sa
2 Department of Parasitology, Faculty of Veterinary Medicine, Zagazig University, Zagazig 44519, Egypt
3 Department of Biology, Al-Nairiyah University College, University of Hafr Al-Batin, Hafr Al-Batin 31991, Saudi Arabia; ttaalotaibi@gmail.com
4 Department of Information Technology, College of Computer and Information Sciences, King Saud University, Riyadh 11451, Saudi Arabia; ialturaiki@ksu.edu.sa
5 Department of Biology, Faculty of Science, Princess Nourah Bint Abdelrahman University, Riyadh 84428, Saudi Arabia; manalelkhadragy@yahoo.com
6 Department of Zoology and Entomology, Faculty of Science, Helwan University, Cairo 11795, Egypt
* Correspondence: dhasanin@ksu.edu.sa

Simple Summary: In the present work, we explored the existence of *Sarcocystis* spp. in samples of camels obtained from abattoirs in Riyadh, Saudi Arabia. We examined tissues of the tongue, heart, esophagus, diaphragm, and skeletal muscle by macroscopic assessments, optical microscopy of tissues, optical microscopy of digested sediment, Transmission Electron Microscopy (TEM), and Polymerase chain reaction (PCR) followed by gene sequencing. The results identified *Sarcocystis cameli* (*S. cameli*) and *S. camelicanis*. *Sarcocystis* spp. were detected in Saudi Arabian camels by molecular analysis. *S. levinei* and *S. miescheriana* were most closely related.

Abstract: *Sarcocystis (S.)* spp. are intracellular protozoan parasites that infect birds and animals, resulting in substantial commercial losses. *Sarcocystis* spp. have an indirect life cycle; canines and felines are known to act as final hosts, and numerous domestic and wild animals act as intermediate hosts. The presence of sarcocysts in camel meat may diminish its commercial quality. There is limited knowledge regarding the taxonomy and diagnosis of *Sarcocystis* spp. that infect camels in Saudi Arabia. In this study, transmission electron microscopy (TEM) revealed *S. cameli* and *S. camelicanis* (*camelicanis*) in *Camelus (C.) dromedarius*. This is the first report of *S. camelicanis* in Saudi Arabia and is considered a significant finding. Based on cytochrome c oxidase subunit I gene (COX1) sequences, two samples of *Sarcocystis* spp. isolated from *C. dromedarius* in Riyadh and Dammam were grouped with *S. levinei* hosted by *Bubalus bubalis* in India, *S. rangi* hosted by *Rangifer tarandus* in Norway, *S. miescheriana* hosted by *Sus scrofa* in Italy and *S. fayeri* hosted by *Equus caballus* in Canada. The sequences obtained in this study have been deposited in GenBank.

Keywords: *Sarcocystis* spp.; COX1; Camelus dromedarius

1. Introduction

Sarcocystis (S.) is a genus of intracellular coccidian parasites that was first identified in 1843 [1]. More than 200 species have been identified and were demonstrated to infect a wide range of domestic and wild animals, resulting in significant losses in farm animals worldwide [2,3]. *Sarcocystis* spp. accomplish their life cycles in two hosts, a final and an intermediate host, and are known to have a high level of host specificity with regard to their intermediate hosts as opposed to their final hosts [4]. The asexual stages of *Sarcocystis* development occur in intermediate hosts (herbivorous animals, such as sheep, cattle and camels, and primates, such as humans, poikilothermic animals and birds), where sarcocysts generally become visible in skeletal muscles and in the striated muscles of the heart, diaphragm and esophagus [5,6] but are rarely found in the smooth muscle of the intestine and the central nervous system [4–7]. The final hosts (e.g., canids, felids, marsupials and primates) become infected by eating intermediate host tissue infected with mature sarcocysts. Next, a stage of sexual reproduction occurs in the final host, after which oocysts/sporocysts are expelled into the environment through feces to be eaten by appropriate intermediate hosts.

The one-humped camel *Camelus dromedarius* is broadly distributed in the hot, arid regions of the Middle East, South Asia, Africa, the Canary Islands, and Central Australia. Compared to beef, lamb, and ostrich meat, camel meat is favored in several countries due to its reduced fat and cholesterol contents [8,9]. However, the presence of sarcocysts in camel meat may decrease its value for human utilization because camels act as intermediate hosts for at least two *Sarcocystis* spp.; furthermore, such infection is a general phenomenon in the one-humped camel due to its worldwide distribution [10–12]. The presence of sarcocysts in the musculature decreases the economic value of the musculature, especially if macroscopic cysts are detected, as their presence leads to condemning the product for consumption [13,14]. Microscopic cysts, on the other hand, may cause serious pathological conditions in infected animals, especially in the case of acute forms, and result in heavy production losses [15–17].

Infected camels generally exhibit subclinical infections, although *Sarcocystis* spp. can produce extensive pathology or death in these animals [12,18].

The diagnosis of acute sarcocystosis in camels is an onerous task because of the absence of an industrial standard indicator test, asymptomatic features of the infection, and the presence of microscopic sarcocysts. Muscle squash, pepsin digestion, trypsin digestion and histopathological examination have been used for the analysis of microscopic sarcocysts in camels [11,12,18,19]. Ultrastructural analysis of the cyst wall is quite useful in the identification of sarcocysts in camels. Transmission electron microscopy (TEM) has demonstrated that *S. cameli* has a primary cyst wall that appears as a thin wall with finger-like villar protrusions and rows of knob-like projections. *S. ippeni* was defined in Egypt [20], wherein the authors of that study observed cyst walls harboring cone-like villar protrusions. *S. camelicanis* was also defined in Egypt [19], wherein the authors found that the primary cyst wall appeared as a thick layer and had finger-like protrusions with a blunt apex. Furthermore, another study defined *S. miescheri* in Egypt [10], in which the primary cyst wall appeared as a thick electron-dense layer with spine-like protrusions.

Although molecular analysis might be an alternative technique for the identification of *Sarcocystis* spp., there is a limitation of such data for camels. The first molecular identification of *S. cameli* sarcocysts was performed in camels in Iran, wherein the 18S rRNA gene fragment was amplified from bradyzoite DNA using conventional polymerase chain reaction (PCR), followed by sequencing (GenBank: GU074011.1) and restriction fragment length polymorphism (RFLP) analysis [21,22]. However, the RFLP technique was found to be more expensive than DNA sequencing or electron microscopy techniques. In another study, the 18S rRNA gene was amplified from microscopic sarcocysts in camels, although no phylogenetic analysis was reported [12]. Therefore, in the present study, a molecular marker, cytochrome oxidase subunit I (COX1), was used to identify different *Sarcocystis* spp. infecting camels from Riyadh and Dammam, Saudi Arabia.

2. Materials and Methods

2.1. Sample Collection

Between February and October 2018, veterinarians collected samples of tissues (diaphragm, skeletal muscle, cardiac muscle, tongue, and esophagus) during postmortem investigations of slaughtered animals in the West Abattoir and Dammam Slaughterhouses in Riyadh and Dammam, Saudi Arabia, respectively. Tissue samples were collected from 37 (27 in Riyadh and 10 in Dammam) male camels aged >5 years and transported to the laboratory in boxes containing ice packs. This study (IRB number: KSU-SE-18-33) secured the approval of the Institutional Committee of Postgraduate Studies and Research at King Saud University (Saudi Arabia).

2.2. Macroscopic Examination

On the same day as the tissues were collected, a macroscopic analysis was performed. In this process, a scalpel was used to make as many as five transverse incisions on organs, such as the heart and the tongue, for the purpose of revealing the cysts (macroscopic). A macroscopic analysis of the entire esophagus was also performed to examine the external and internal walls; the lumen was exposed after longitudinal sectioning [23].

2.3. Microscopic Examination

Microscopic evaluation of cysts was performed using the squashing method [24]. Distinct fragments of each tissue with a thickness of approximately 5 mm were squashed robustly from both slides, after which an optical microscope was used to analyze the specimen. For all tissues, the procedure was performed in triplicate. *Sarcocystis* spp. were also examined by light microscopy and DNA analyses.

2.4. Digestion Method

For all tissues, approximately 20 g were minced before digestion for a period of 30 min in 100 mL at a temperature of 40 °C; the digestion solution comprised pepsin (1.3 g), HCl (3.5 mL) and NaCl (2.5 g) in distilled water (500 mL) [25]. After digestion, the mixture was centrifuged at 3500× *g* for 3 min, followed by Giemsa staining and optical microscopy evaluation [26].

2.5. Histopathological Examination

Small specimens of muscles and organs were collected, fixed in 10% neutral buffered formalin, serially dehydrated in increasing concentrations of ethanol (30%, 70% and 95% absolute) and embedded in paraffin. Three 5-μm-thick sections of each of the abovementioned organs and muscles were prepared, stained with hematoxylin and eosin and examined under an ECLIPSE NI-4 (Nikon, Tokyo, Japan) [27].

2.6. Transmission Electron Microscopy (TEM)

Six *Sarcocystis* spp. cysts embedded in the tissues were collected from organs, fixed in 0.1 M sodium cacodylate buffer (pH 7.4) supplemented with 3% glutaraldehyde solution for 4 h at 4 °C and stored at 4 °C until processing. After fixation, the samples were washed in 0.1 M sodium cacodylate buffer, fixed with 2% osmium tetroxide for 24 h and rewashed four to five times in the buffer (10–15 min each) [19]. The samples were serially dehydrated in increasing concentrations of acetone (30%, 40%, 50%, 70%, 90% and 100%) and blocked with buffer supplemented with 1% phosphotungstic acid and 1% uranyl acetate. Next, the 100% acetone solution was replaced with Polybed resin, followed by paraffin embedding and polymerization in an oven at 60 °C [28]. Moderately thin sections were prepared to observe *Sarcocystis* spp. cysts under a microscope (CX31, Olympus Corporation, Tokyo, Japan). Ultrathin sections were stained with uranyl acetate and lead citrate and examined using a JEM-1400 transmission electron microscope (JEOL, Tokyo, Japan) at 80 kV.

2.7. Molecular Analysis

2.7.1. DNA Extraction and PCR Amplification

From all the microscopic *Sarcocystis* isolates, six isolates were selected and washed five times in distilled water (sterile). gDNA from tissue was extracted using a DNA Mini Kit (QIAGEN GmbH, Hilden, Germany) (Cat. No. 51304) according to the manufacturer's instructions. Amplification of the

COX1 gene was performed using the primer pairs mentioned in Table 1 [28,29] and a thermocycler (Veriti® 96-well Thermal Cycler, Model 9902, Biosystem). This procedure was conducted in a mixture (20 μL) containing 4 μL of master mix (5×), 12 μL of RNase-free water and DNA template (2 μL). The PCR program consisted of denaturation at 95 °C for 5 min, followed by 40 cycles of denaturation for 45 s at 95 °C, annealing for 45 s at 54 °C and extension for 10 min at 72 °C. The PCR products were analyzed by 1.5% agarose gel electrophoresis.

Table 1. List of primers used for the amplification of cytochrome c oxidase subunit I (COX1) gene in *Sarcocystis* spp.

Gene	Primers	Sequences	References
COX1	SF1	5′-ATG GCG TAC AAC AAT CAT AAA GAA-3′	[28–30]
	SR9	5′-ATA TCC ATA CCR CCA TTG CCC AT-3′	

2.7.2. DNA Sequencing

The aforementioned PCR products were first purified and then sequenced in the reverse and forward directions (only) using a Genetic Analyzer at the Central Laboratory of King Saud University.

The sequences were analyzed using Geneious Prime Build [31]. All sequences were truncated slightly using the error probability method with a limit of 0.05 at both ends. A Basic Local Alignment Search Tool (BLAST) search was performed to identify related sequences. Multiple sequence alignments were generated using CLUSTAL Omega [32]. The maximum likelihood trees were constructed using PhyML 3.3 with 100 bootstraps [33].

2.8. *Statistical Analysis*

Statistical analysis was performed using the Statistical Package for Social Sciences (SPSS) software (version 17, SPSS, Inc., Chicago, IL, USA). The lengths and widths of at least five cysts from each organ (diaphragm, skeletal muscle, cardiac muscle, tongue, and esophagus) were determined by light microscopy and expressed as the mean sizes and amplitudes of variation.

3. Results

3.1. *Macroscopic Examination*

No macroscopic cysts were detected by the naked eye during the inspection of carcasses or collected samples.

3.2. *Microscopic Examination*

A compression technique with a light microscope was used for microscopic examination, in which 15 of 37 slaughtered camels (40.54%) were found to be positive for microscopic cysts. In particular, the numbers of positive cases for diaphragm, skeletal muscle, cardiac muscle, tongue, and esophagus samples were 14/37 (37.83%), 10/37 (27.01%), 9/37 (24.32%), 8/37 (21.62%), and 3/37 (8.10%), respectively. Thin-walled sarcocysts and thick-walled sarcocysts were observed. In contrast to the tissue squash method, the pepsin–hydrochloric acid digestion technique revealed a greater number of animals that were positive.

3.2.1. Thin-Walled Microscopic Sarcocysts

Unstained sarcocysts were found to have thin walls, to be elongated and spindle-like in shape, and to be present within the muscle fibers. The sarcocysts measured 197.9–405.6 μm in length (mean 301.75 μm) and 57.3–125.6 μm in breadth (mean 91.45 μm) (Figure 1A). Stained sarcocysts are shown in Figure 1B. Histopathological sections revealed that the cysts measured 83.50–135.50 μm in length (mean 109.5 μm). The cyst wall consisted of two layers, an outer striated layer and an inner homogenous layer. The cystic cavity was divided into several compartments by fine trabeculae originating from the cyst wall (Figure 1C). Ultrastructural analysis of the cyst wall showed that *S. cameli* sarcocysts (shown in Figure 1D) have an outer cyst wall (Ocw) that is in close contact with the cyst wall, ground substance, metrocytes, and bradyzoites or merozoites. The primary cyst wall (Pcw) displayed irregular folded nonbranched finger-like villar protrusions with fibrillar elements originating from the ground substance at a distance of 0.54 μm below the primary cyst wall and protruding into it. The villar protrusions measured 0.93 μm in length and 0.77 μm in width at the base and 0.35 μm at the apex. The distance between each villar protrusion measured 1.7 μm. The finger-like process (Flp) was generally surrounded by numerous scattered host cell mitochondria. The ground substance was located directly under the primary cyst wall with a diameter of 1.27–1.7 μm (mean: 1.48 μm). The space between the primary cyst wall (Pcw) and the contents of the cyst was primarily fine, showing dense homogenous granules and fibrillar elements folding into the primary cyst wall. The ground substance extended into the interior of the cyst, forming a thin septum separating the entire cyst into compartments enclosing the metrocytes and bradyzoites or merozoites.

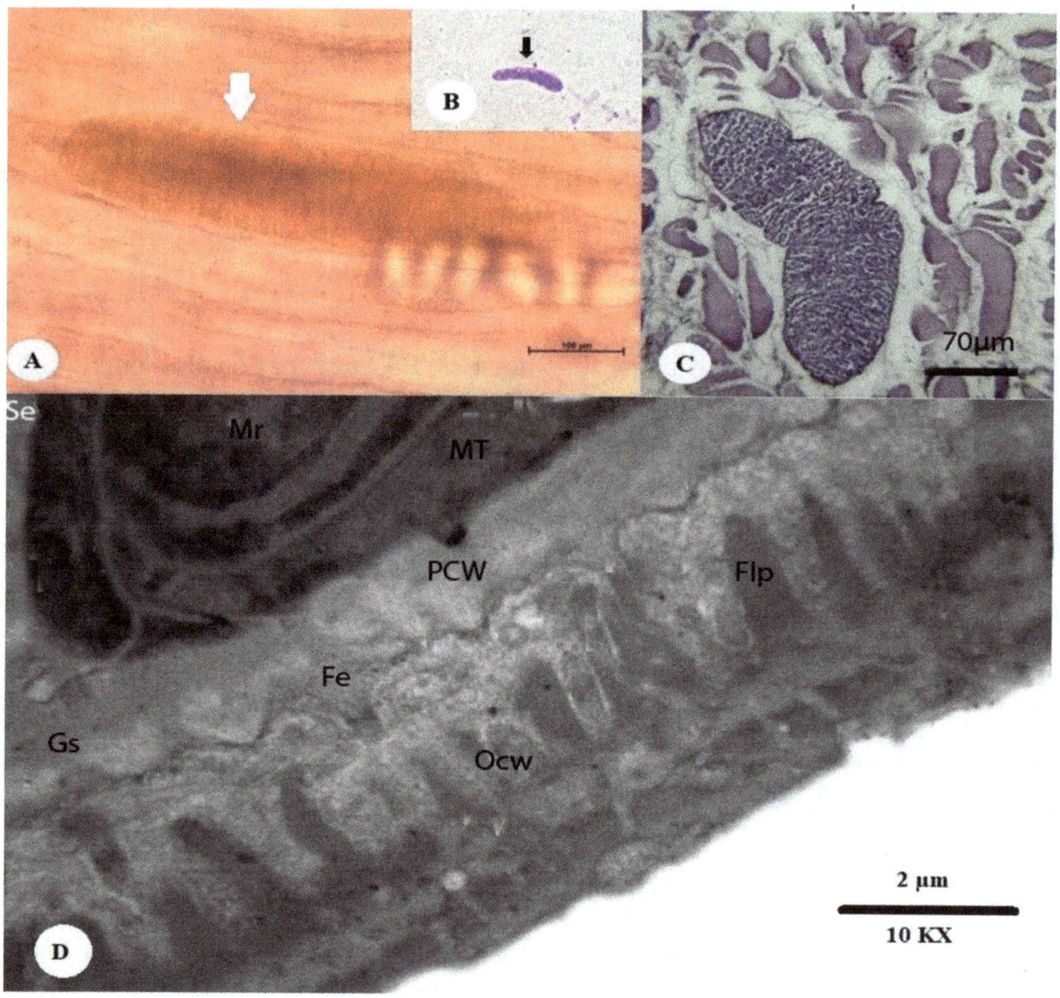

Figure 1. Morphology of a sarcocyst of *S. cameli* from the esophageal muscles of a camel (*Camelus dromedarius*). (**A**) Microscopic thin-walled *S. cameli* (white arrow) (bar = 100 μm). (**B**) Cysts stained with Giemsa after pepsin–hydrochloric acid digestion (black arrow). (**C**) Histopathological section of camel esophageal muscles showing the thin cyst wall (CW) of *S. cameli* (H&E) (bar = 70 μm). The thin and smooth cyst wall and the clearly visible septum are shown. (**D**) The cyst wall in detail, containing an outer cyst wall (Ocw), a primary cyst wall (Pcw), ground substance (Gs), septae (Se), merozoites (Mr), fibrillar elements (Fe), metrocytes (Mt), and finger-like process (Flp) (10,000×).

3.2.2. Thick-walled Microscopic Sarcocysts

The sarcocysts appeared fusiform or spindle-shaped, measuring 151–449 μm in length (mean 300 μm) and 65–140 μm in breadth (mean 102.5 μm) (Figure 2A). Cysts after pepsin–hydrochloric acid digestion are depicted in Figure 2B. Histopathological sections demonstrated that the cysts had a thick wall composed of two layers: an outer striated layer and an inner smooth layer. The cyst cavity was divided into compartments by a narrow septum originating from the wall in the periphery of the cyst (Figure 2C). Ultrastructural analysis (Figure 1D) of the cyst wall revealed an outer cyst wall connected to the primary cyst wall (Pcw), ground substance (Gs), metrocytes, and bradyzoites for *S. camelicanis*.

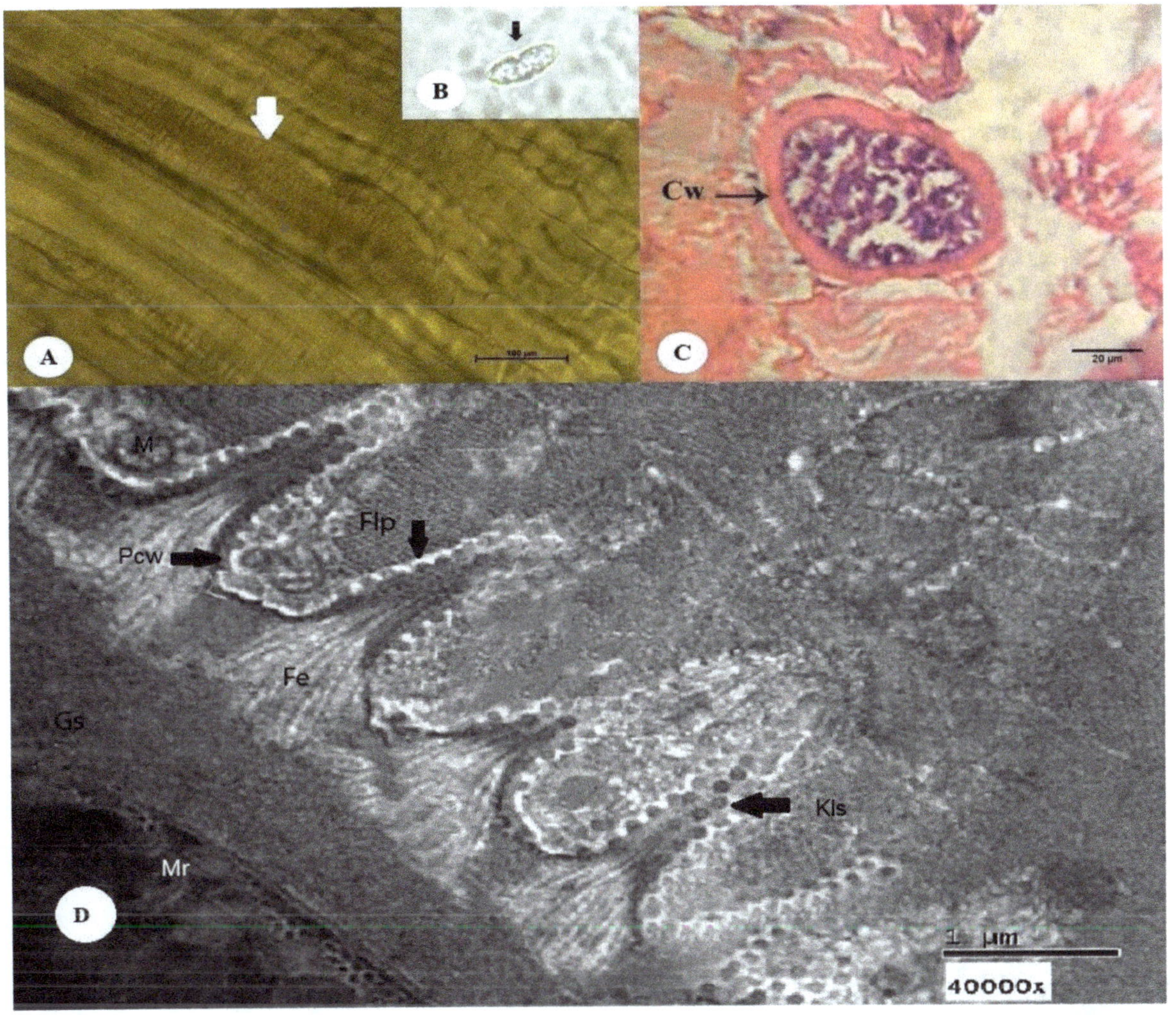

Figure 2. Morphology of a sarcocyst of *S. camelicanis* from the skeletal muscles of a camel (*Camelus dromedarius*). (**A**) Microscopic thick-walled *S. camelicanis* (white arrow) (bar = 100 μm). (**B**) Cysts after pepsin–hydrochloric acid digestion (small black arrow). (**C**) A histopathological section of the skeletal muscles of a camel shows the thick cyst wall (Cw) (black arrow) of *S. camelicanis* and a clearly visible septum (H&E; bar = 20 μm). (**D**) A *Sarcocystis camelicanis* thick-walled cyst showing the primary cyst wall (Pcw) (black arrow), ground substance (Gs), fibrillar elements (Fe), finger-like process (Flp), knoblike structures (Kls) (black arrow), Mitochondria (M), and merozoites (Mr) (40,000×).

The primary cyst wall (Pcw) is a thick, dense layer adjacent to the Gs. Fibrillar elements (Fe) originating from the Gs at 0.60 μm below the Pcw aggregated towards the Pcw and embedded into it, forming finger-like protrusions (Flp). The cyst measured 2.15–2.91 μm (mean 2.53 μm) in length and 0.52–0.60 μm (mean 0.56 μm) in breadth. Each Flp carried characteristic multiple numerous knob-like structures (Kls), which were spherical in shape with a diameter of 0.10–0.14 μm (mean 0.12 μm); their number varied from 19 to 25 on each protrusion. The distance between each Flp was 0.71–0.89 μm (mean 0.80 μm), and they were generally surrounded by numerous dispersed host cell mitochondria (M). The Gs was found to be 1.25–1.60 μm (mean 1.42 μm) below the Pcw and in between the Pcw and metrocytes. It appeared as a homogeneous substance and extended to the interior of the cyst by a septum separating the entire cyst into a number of compartments enclosing the metrocytes, merozoites and other structures.

3.3. Genetic Characteristics

Genomic DNA extracted from four *Sarcocystis* spp. isolates, D7S (thin-walled cyst), D10S (thick-walled cyst), R10C (thick-walled cyst) and R16C (thin-walled cyst), were used for the amplification of 1000-bp COX1 sequences.

The first two were isolated from the skeletal muscle of a Dammam camel, and the last two were isolated from the cardiac muscle of a Riyadh camel. These sequences were 692, 513, 194, and 205 nucleotides in length, respectively, and shared a pairwise identity of 63.1%. All sequences obtained in this study have been deposited in GenBank under accession numbers MK948444 (D7S), MK948443 (D10S), MK948442 (R10C), and MK948441 (R16C).

BLAST results showed that the D7S sequence had similarity to *S. levinei* hosted by *Bubalus bubalis* (heart tissue) in India, accession numbers MH255774–MH255777, with 86.5% pairwise identity and 89.6% coverage. The D7S sequence also displayed similarity to *S. rangi* hosted by *Rangifer tarandus* in Norway, accession numbers KC209662–KC209666, with 85.2% pairwise identity and 87.57% coverage.

Furthermore, the D10S sequence exhibited similarity to *S. miescheriana*, accession number MH404202, hosted by *Sus scrofa* in Italy, with 80.7% pairwise identity and 43% coverage. The D10S sequence was also similar to *S. fayeri*, accession number LC171854, hosted by *Equus caballus* in Canada, with 79.1% pairwise identity and 43% coverage. The phylogenetic tree with bootstrap proportions is illustrated in Figure 3. *Toxoplasma gondii* (JX473253) was used as an outgroup. For R10C and R16C, '194 and 205' are very short sequences inappropriate for analysis. The tree shows that MK948444 (D7S) and MK948442 (R10C) are placed in a clade with *S. levinei*. MK948443 (D10S) is grouped with *Sarcocystis miescheriana*. MK948441 (R16C) is grouped with *Sarcocystis fayeri*.

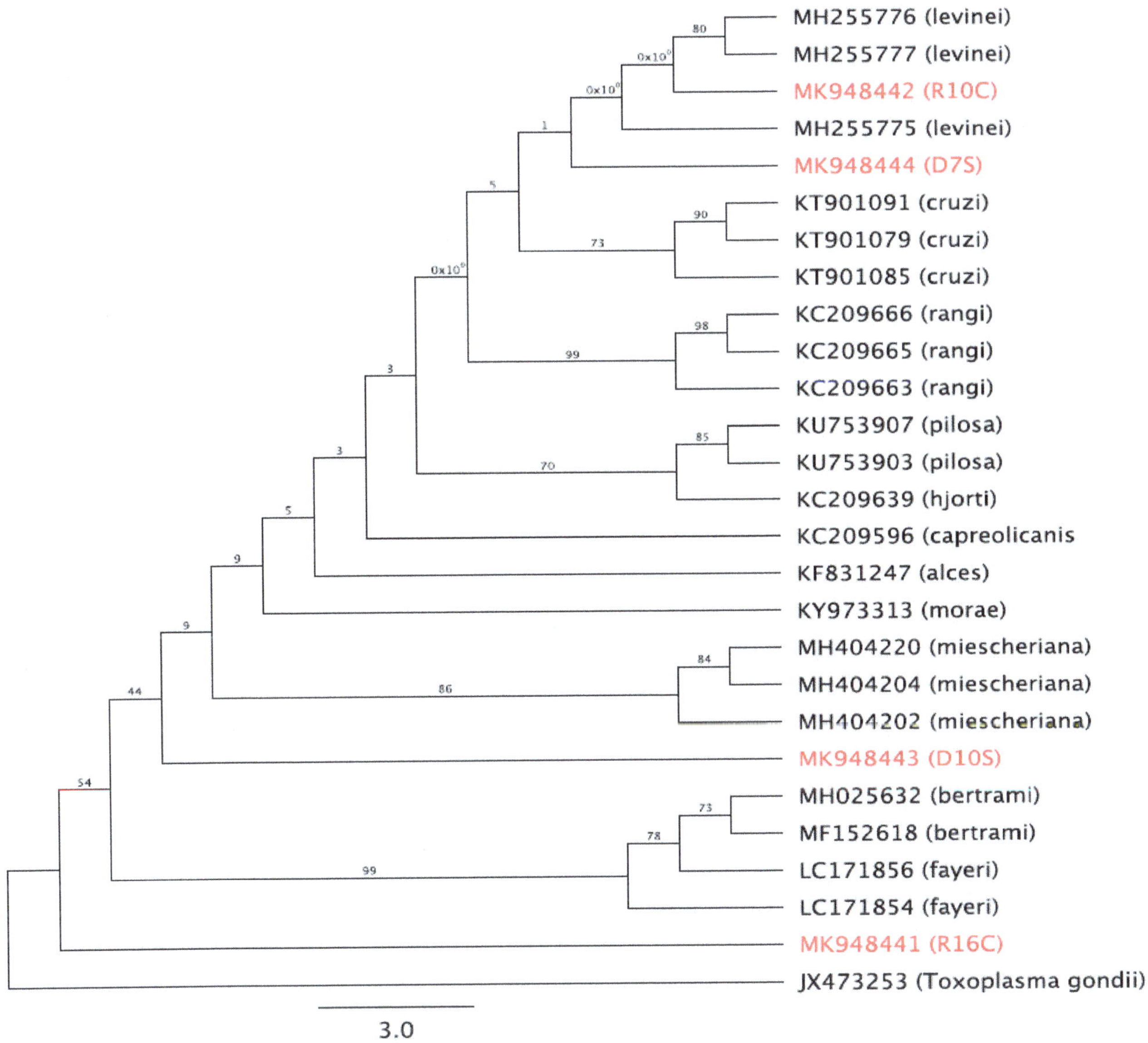

Figure 3. Genetic relationships of our samples isolated from camels in Saudi Arabia (highlighted in pink) with other *Sarcocystis* spp. retrieved from GenBank based on the COX1 region.

4. Discussion

To establish the occurrence of *Sarcocystis* spp., this study examined the esophagus, tongue, diaphragm, skeletal muscle, and heart tissue from 37 camel specimens (27 from Riyadh and 10 from Dammam). The results showed that the overall prevalence rates of *Sarcocystis* spp. were 40.74% (11/27) in Riyadh specimens and 40% (4/10) in Dammam specimens.

In the present study, macroscopic cysts were not detected. However, macroscopic cysts have been reported to be less common in some esophageal samples [34,35]. In this study, the squashing and pepsin-hydrochloric acid digestion methods accompanied by light microscopy were used, wherein the technique of pepsin-hydrochloric acid digestion revealed a greater number of positive animals. Cysts from esophageal and skeletal muscle samples appeared in a cylindrical and spindle-like shape.

Cysts were found to have thin and smooth or thick walls divided internally into several compartments by trabeculae. Thin-walled cysts have been identified in the esophagus and diaphragm of camels slaughtered at Al-Ahsa Abattoir, Saudi Arabia [36]; in the esophagus, diaphragm, heart, shoulder, and masseter muscles of one-humped camels slaughtered in southern Ethiopia [37]; in the esophagus, diaphragm, heart, skeletal muscles, and tongue of one-humped camels slaughtered in Iran [18], and in the esophagus of one-humped camels slaughtered in Egypt [38].

Thick-walled cysts were found in the esophagus of one-humped camels slaughtered in Egypt [10]; in the esophagus, diaphragm, heart, skeletal muscles, and tongue of one-humped camels slaughtered in Egypt [19]; in the esophagus of one-humped camels slaughtered in Egypt [39], and in the esophagus, skeletal muscles, and tongue of one-humped camels slaughtered in Egypt [40]. Similarly, both thin- and thick-walled *Sarcocystis* cysts have been suggested to be at different stages in the same parasite and have been termed *S. cameli* [41]. In addition, thick-walled cysts were found repeatedly and termed *S. cameli*, whereas thin-walled cysts were unnamed [18,25,36].

Sarcocystis spp. isolated from *C. dromedarius* from Dammam and Riyadh grouped alongside *S. levinei* hosted by *B. bubalis* (heart tissue) in India (accession numbers MH255774–MH255777) [42], *S. rangi* hosted by *R. tarandus* in Norway (accession numbers KC209662–KC209666) [43], *S. miescheriana* hosted by *S. scrofa* in Italy (accession number MH404202) [44], and *S. fayeri* hosted by *E. caballus* in Canada (accession number LC171854) [45].

In the present study, four partial sequences of the COX1 gene were analyzed. Two samples, R10C (thick-walled cyst) and D7S (thin-walled cyst), isolated from *C. dromedarius* in Riyadh and Dammam, Saudi Arabia, respectively, were identified by histological and TEM approaches as *Sarcocystis* spp. The phylogenetic tree shows that these two samples are related to *S. mansoni* hosted by South American camelids, *S. levinei* hosted by water buffaloes, and *S. miescheriana* hosted by pigs, suggesting that camels are receptors of *Sarcocystis* spp. from other intermediate hosts.

The main limitation of this study lies in the other two samples, D10S and R16C. These two samples were identified by histological and TEM approaches as *Sarcocystis* spp. (D10S, thick-walled cyst; and R16C, thin-walled cyst). However, in the phylogenetic tree, they were not grouped in a clade with R10C and D7S. Through a deeper analysis of the raw data, it was found that the samples were of lower quality than R10C and D7S. This low quality affected the process of phylogenetic tree construction.

5. Conclusions

In this study, our results highlight the necessity to reinforce a more in-depth phylogenetic analysis and identification of *Sarcocystis* spp. with more taxa and different molecular markers. For instance, amplification of the 18S rRNA gene should be performed to further distinguish among the closely related *Sarcocystis* spp.

Author Contributions: Conceptualization: D.M.M. Data curation: I.M.A.-T. Formal analysis: T.T.A.-O. Funding acquisition: D.M.M. Investigation: D.M.M. and T.T.A.-O. Methodology: T.T.A.-O. Project administration: D.M.M. and R.A.A. Resources: T.T.A.-O. and M.F.E.-K. Software: I.M.A.-T. Supervision: D.M.M. and R.A.A. Validation: D.M.M. Visualization: M.F.E.-K. Writing: original draft: D.M.M. Writing, reviewing and editing: D.M.M., R.A.A., M.F.E.-K., T.T.A.-O. and I.M.A.-T. All authors have read and agreed to the published version of the manuscript.

References

1. Miescher, F. Über eigenthümliche Schläuche in den Muskeln einer Hausmaus. *Ber. Verhandl Nat. Gesell Basel* **1843**, *5*, 198–202.
2. Tenter, A.M. Current research on Sarcocystis species of domestic animals. *Int. J. Parasitol.* **1995**, *25*, 1311–1330. [CrossRef]
3. Dubey, J. Foodborne and waterborne zoonotic sarcocystosis. *Food Waterborne Parasitol.* **2015**, *1*, 2–11. [CrossRef]
4. Fayer, R. Sarcocystis spp. Human Infections. *Clin. Microbiol. Rev.* **2004**, *17*, 894–902. [CrossRef]

5. Hidron, A.; Vogenthaler, N.; Santos-Preciado, J.I.; Rodriguez-Morales, A.J.; Franco-Paredes, C.; Rassi, A. Cardiac Involvement with Parasitic Infections. *Clin. Microbiol. Rev.* **2010**, *23*, 324–349. [CrossRef]
6. Dubey, J.P.; Calero-Bernal, R.; Rosenthal, B.M.; Speer, C.A.; Fayer, R. *Sarcocystosis of Animals and Humans*; CRC Press: Boca Raton, FL, USA, 2015.
7. Miller, M.; Barr, B.; Nordhausen, R.; James, E.; Magargal, S.; Murray, M.; Conrad, P.; Toy-Choutka, S.; Jessup, D.; Grigg, M. Ultrastructural and molecular confirmation of the development of Sarcocystis neurona tissue cysts in the central nervous system of southern sea otters (Enhydra lutris nereis). *Int. J. Parasitol.* **2009**, *39*, 1363–1372. [CrossRef]
8. Kadim, I.; Mahgoub, O.; Purchas, R. A review of the growth, and of the carcass and meat quality characteristics of the one-humped camel (Camelus dromedaries). *Meat Sci.* **2008**, *80*, 555–569. [CrossRef] [PubMed]
9. Kadim, I.T.; Mahgoub, O.; Mbaga, M. Potential of camel meat as a non-traditional high quality source of protein for human consumption. *Anim. Front.* **2014**, *4*, 13–17. [CrossRef]
10. Mandour, A.M.; Rabie, S.A.; Mohammed, N.; Hussein, N.M. On the presence of Sarcocystis miescheri sp. nov. in camels of Qena Governorate. *Egypt. Acad. J. Boil. Sci. E. Med Èntomol. Parasitol.* **2011**, *3*, 1–7. [CrossRef]
11. Hamidinejat, H.; Hekmatimoghaddam, S.; Jafari, H.; Sazmand, A.; Molayan, P.H.; Derakhshan, L.; Mirabdollahi, S. Prevalence and distribution patterns of Sarcocystis in camels (Camelus dromedarius) in Yazd province, Iran. *J. Parasit. Dis.* **2012**, *37*, 163–165. [CrossRef]
12. Omer, S.A.; Alzuraiq, A.A.; Mohammed, O.B. Prevalence and molecular detection of Sarcocystis spp. infection in the dromedary camel (Camelus dromedarius) in Riyadh city, Saudi Arabia. *Biomed. Res.* **2017**, *28*, 4962–4965.
13. Oryan, A.; Moghaddar, N.; Gaur, S.N. The distribution pattern of Sarcocystis species, their transmission and pathogenesis in sheep in Fars Province of Iran. *Veter. Res. Commun.* **1996**, *20*, 243–253. [CrossRef]
14. Dubey, J.P.; Lindsay, D.S.; Speer, C.A.; Fayer, R.; Livingston, C.W. Sarcocystis arieticanis and Other Sarcocystis Species in Sheep in the United States. *J. Parasitol.* **1988**, *74*, 1033. [CrossRef]
15. Fayer, R. Economic losses to Sarcocystis. *Natl. Wool. Grow.* **1976**, *66*, 22–28.
16. Munday, B. The effect of Sarcocystis ovicanis on growth rate and haematocrit in lambs. *Veter. Parasitol.* **1979**, *5*, 129–135. [CrossRef]
17. Munday, B. Effects of different doses of dog-derived Sarcocystis sporocysts on growth rate and haematocrit in lambs. *Veter. Parasitol.* **1986**, *21*, 21–24. [CrossRef]
18. Valinezhad, A.; Oryan, A.; Ahmadi, N. Sarcocystis and Its Complications in Camels (Camelus dromedarius) of Eastern Provinces of Iran. *Korean J. Parasitol.* **2008**, *46*, 229–234. [CrossRef]
19. Abdel-Ghaffar, F.; Mehlhorn, H.; Bashtar, A.-R.; Al-Rasheid, K.; Sakran, T.; El-Fayoumi, H. Life cycle of Sarcocystis camelicanis infecting the camel (Camelus dromedarius) and the dog (Canis familiaris), light and electron microscopic study. *Parasitol. Res.* **2009**, *106*, 189–195. [CrossRef]
20. Entzeroth, R.; A Ghaffar, F.; Chobotar, B.; Scholtyseck, E. Fine structural study of Sarcocystis sp. from Egyptian camels (Camelus dromed arius). *Acta Veter. Acad. Sci. Hung.* **1981**, *29*, 335–339.
21. Motamedi, G.R.; Dalimi, A.; Nouri, A.; Aghaeipour, K. Ultrastructural and molecular characterization of Sarcocystis isolated from camel (Camelus dromedarius) in Iran. *Parasitol. Res.* **2010**, *108*, 949–954. [CrossRef] [PubMed]
22. Eslampanah, M.; Motamedi, G.R.; Dalimi, A.; Noori, A.; Habibi, G.R.; Aghaeepour, K.; Niroumand, M. Study of camel and goat Sarcocystis by electron microscopic and PCR-RFLP. *Vet. Res. Biol. Prod.* **2016**, *29*, 77–84.
23. Bittencourt, M.V.; Meneses, I.D.S.; Ribeiro-Andrade, M.; De Jesus, R.F.; De Araújo, F.R.; Gondim, L.F. Sarcocystis spp. in sheep and goats: Frequency of infection and species identification by morphological, ultrastructural, and molecular tests in Bahia, Brazil. *Parasitol. Res.* **2016**, *115*, 1683–1689. [CrossRef] [PubMed]
24. Odening, K.; Stolte, M.; Bockhardt, I. On the diagnostics of Sarcocystis in cattle: Sarcocysts of a species unusual for Bos taurus in a dwarf zebu. *Veter. Parasitol.* **1996**, *66*, 19–24. [CrossRef]
25. Dubey, J.; Speer, C.; Charleston, W. Ultrastructural differentiation between sarcocysts of Sarcocystis hirsuta and Sarcocystis hominis. *Veter. Parasitol.* **1989**, *34*, 153–157. [CrossRef]
26. Hamidinejat, H.; Moetamedi, H.; Alborzi, A.; Hatami, A. Molecular detection of Sarcocystis species in slaughtered sheep by PCR–RFLP from south-western of Iran. *J. Parasit. Dis.* **2013**, *38*, 233–237. [CrossRef]
27. Carleton, H.M. *Histological Technique for Normal and Pathological Tissues and the Identification of Parasites*, 3rd ed.; Oxford University Press: London, UK, 1957.

28. Gjerde, B. Phylogenetic relationships among Sarcocystis species in cervids, cattle and sheep inferred from the mitochondrial cytochrome c oxidase subunit I gene. *Int. J. Parasitol.* **2013**, *43*, 579–591. [CrossRef]
29. Gjerde, B. Sarcocystis species in red deer revisited: With a re-description of two known species as Sarcocystis elongata n. sp. and Sarcocystis truncata n. sp. based on mitochondrial cox1 sequences. *Parasitology* **2013**, *141*, 441–452. [CrossRef]
30. Metwally, D.M.; Al-Damigh, M.A.; Al-Turaiki, I.; El-Khadragy, M.F. Molecular Characterization of Sarcocystis Species Isolated from Sheep and Goats in Riyadh, Saudi Arabia. *Animals* **2019**, *9*, 256. [CrossRef] [PubMed]
31. Geneious Prime. Available online: http://www.geneious.com/ (accessed on 7 April 2020).
32. Sievers, F.; Wilm, A.; Dineen, D.; Gibson, T.J.; Karplus, K.; Li, W.; López, R.; McWilliam, H.; Remmert, M.; Soeding, J.; et al. Fast, scalable generation of high-quality protein multiple sequence alignments using Clustal Omega. *Mol. Syst. Boil.* **2011**, *7*, 539. [CrossRef] [PubMed]
33. Guindon, S.; Lefort, V.; Anisimova, M.; Hordijk, W.; Gascuel, O.; Dufayard, J.-F. New Algorithms and Methods to Estimate Maximum-Likelihood Phylogenies: Assessing the Performance of PhyML 3.0. *Syst. Boil.* **2010**, *59*, 307–321. [CrossRef] [PubMed]
34. Wahba, A.A. Morphobiological Studies on Cryptosporidia and Sarcocystis in Animals and Their Impact on Their Health. Ph.D. Thesis, Faculty of Veterinary Medicine, Zagazig University, Zagazig, Egypt, 1994.
35. Fatani, A.; Hilali, M.A.; Al-Atiya, S.; Al-Shami, S. Prevalence of Sarcocystis in camels (Camelus dromedarius) from Al-Ahsa, Saudi Arabia. *Veter. Parasitol.* **1996**, *62*, 241–245. [CrossRef]
36. Al-Quraishy, S.A.; Bashtar, A.R.; Al-Rasheid, K.; Abdel-Ghaffar, F. Prevalence and ultrastructure of Sarcocystis species infecting camels (Camelus dromedarius) slaughtered in Riyadh city Saudi Arabia. *Saudi J. Biol. Sci.* **2004**, *11*, 135–141.
37. Woldemeskel, M.; Gumi, B. Prevalence of sarcocysts in one-humped camel (Camelus dromedarius) from Southern Ethiopia. *J. Vet. Med. Ser. B* **2001**, *48*, 223–226. [CrossRef] [PubMed]
38. Hilali, M.; Mohamed, A. The dog (Canis familiaris) as the final host of Sarcocystis cameli (Mason, 1910). *Trop. Parasitol.* **1980**, *31*, 213–214.
39. Abd-Elmalek, B.S.; Abed, G.H.; Mandour, A.M. Study on Sarcosystis sp. By Light and Electron Microscopy in Camel Muscles at Assiut Governorate. *J. Veter. Sci. Technol.* **2015**, *6*. [CrossRef]
40. Mason, F.E. Sarcocysts in the camel in Egypt. *J. Comp. Pathol. Ther.* **1910**, *23*, 168–176. [CrossRef]
41. Moré, G.; Regensburger, C.; Gos, M.L.; Pardini, L.; Verma, S.K.; Ctibor, J.; Serrano-Martínez, E.; Dubey, J.P.; Venturini, M.C. Sarcocystis masoni, n sp. (Apicomplexa: Sarcocystidae), and redescription of Sarcocystis aucheniae from llama (Lama glama), guanaco (Lama guanicoe) and alpaca (Vicugna pacos). *Parasitology* **2016**, *143*, 617–626.
42. Singh, D.; Kumar, B. UP Pandit Deen Dayal Upadhyaya Pashu-Chikitsa Vigyan Vishwavidyalaya Evam Go Anusandhan Sansthan. Ph.D. Thesis, Mathura, Mathura, India, 2018.
43. Gjerde, B.; Luzón, M.; Alunda, J.M.; De La Fuente, C. Morphological and molecular characteristics of six Sarcocystis spp. from red deer (Cervus elaphus) in Spain, including Sarcocystis cervicanis and three new species. *Parasitol. Res.* **2017**, *116*, 2795–2811. [CrossRef]
44. Gazzonis, A.L.; Gjerde, B.; Villa, L.; Minazzi, S.; Zanzani, S.A.; Riccaboni, P.; Sironi, G.; Manfredi, M.T. Prevalence and molecular characterisation of Sarcocystis miescheriana and Sarcocystis suihominis in wild boars (Sus scrofa) in Italy. *Parasitol. Res.* **2019**, *118*, 1271–1287. [CrossRef]
45. Murata, R.; Suzuki, J.; Hyuga, A.; Shinkai, T.; Sadamasu, K. Molecular identification and characterization of Sarcocystis spp. in horsemeat and beef marketed in Japan. *Parasite* **2018**, *25*, 27. [CrossRef]

18

Pathological, Bacteriological and Virological Findings in Sudden and Unexpected Deaths in Young Dogs

Giuseppe Piegari [1,*], Lorena Cardillo [2], Flora Alfano [2], Lucia Vangone [2], Valentina Iovane [3] and Giovanna Fusco [2]

1 Department of Veterinary Medicine and Animal Production, Unit of Pathology, University of Naples Federico II, 80137 Naples, Italy

2 Istituto Zooprofilattico Sperimentale del Mezzogiorno, Portici, 81100 Naples, Italy; lorena.cardillo85@gmail.com (L.C.); flora.alfano@cert.izsmportici.it (F.A.); lucia.vangone@izsmportici.it (L.V.); giovanna.fusco@izsmportici.it (G.F.)

3 Department of Pharmacy, University of Salerno, 84084 Fisciano, Italy; viovane@unisa.it

* Correspondence: giuseppe.piegari@unina.it

Simple Summary: "Sudden death" has been defined by the World Health Organization as a non-violent, unexpected death occurring less than 24 h from the onset of symptoms. The causes of sudden death have been widely investigated in human forensic medicine. In contrast, few studies have been reported in the veterinary literature. This study aimed to investigate the frequency of sudden deaths in young dogs in different age ranges. A secondary aim was to collect information regarding clinical symptoms, and pathological and microbiological findings related to sudden death in young dogs. The results of the present study demonstrate that the highest frequency of sudden death occurs in animals in an age range from 10 days to 1 month and from 6 to 12 months. The most frequently observed clinical symptoms in cases of sudden death were acute respiratory symptoms. Furthermore, *Canine parvovirus type 2, E. coli, Canine Distemper Virus, Clostridium perfringens type A, and Pasteurella* spp. were the main causes of death observed in the present study. The results reported in the present study could provide a reference basis to better investigate sudden death in veterinary clinical practice.

Abstract: In human medicine, "sudden death" has been defined by the World Health Organization (WHO) as a non-violent, unexpected death occurring less than 24 h from the onset of symptoms. The aims of this study were: (1) to estimate the proportional mortality ratio for "sudden and unexpected death" (SUD) in young dogs; (2) to investigate the pathological and microbiological findings in SUD cases in young dogs. For these purposes, a retrospective study of a total of 145 cases of young dead dogs was performed. For each case, we collected information about the age, medical history and the gross and microbiological findings of the animals. The results of this study found 21 cases of SUD. The most frequently observed clinical symptoms in the cases of sudden death were acute respiratory symptoms, followed by acute gastroenteric symptoms, non-specific symptoms and neurological symptoms. The evaluation of necropsy reports allowed us to observe enteritis in 18 out of 21 cases and pneumonia in seven out of 21 cases. Viral infection with *Canine parvovirus type 2* was the most common cause of SUD observed. These results could provide a valuable tool for the investigation of sudden death in young dogs.

Keywords: post-mortem microbiology; veterinary forensic pathology; sudden death; young dogs

1. Introduction

In human medicine, "sudden death" has been defined by the World Health Organization (WHO) as a non-violent, unexpected death occurring less than 24 h from the onset of symptoms [1]; in particular, the term "sudden and unexpected infant death" (SUID) is used to describe deaths that occur relatively suddenly and unexpectedly in children less than 1 years old [2,3]. Infections are reported in the literature as an important cause of SUID, followed by metabolic or molecular disorders [2–5]. The main pathogens reported in SUID cases are as follows: *Staphylococcus aureus, Escherichia coli, Streptococcus pyogenes, Streptococcus agalactiae, Streptococcus pneumoniae, Group B Streptococci (GBS), Respiratory Syncytial Virus (RSV), Cytomegalovirus (CMV) and Adenovirus* [2,6,7]. However, a broad range of pathogens has been reported in the literature as being causes or a co-factors in SUID, such as *Parvovirus B19, Epstein-Barr virus, Influenza A virus* and *Mycobacterium tuberculosis* [2,6,8,9]. Furthermore, recent studies reported the relatively benign Coxsackie virus A16 as a possible contributing factor in SUID in humans [10]. For these reasons, the current SUID autopsy protocol in the UK and the international guidelines advocate for a multidisciplinary approach to the investigation of all cases of SUID, which should be based not only on the findings of the macroscopic examination, but also on a broad range of ancillary investigations, such as bacteriological and virological analyses [11,12]. Sudden infant death syndrome (SIDS) is considered to be a sub-class of SUID, in which the cause of death remains unexplained even after the forensic necropsy, ancillary tests and evaluation of the anamnestic data and crime scene analysis [1,2]. Indeed, among the cases of SUID, only 20% have a clear cause, while most cases remain unexplained and are categorized as SIDS [1,5,13]. Although the cause is unknown, specific genetic mutations or mild infections could be involved in the genesis of the syndrome [5]. Mild infections have been suggested to play a key role, as demonstrated by altered levels of immunoglobulin or cytokine and the high frequency of mild tracheal infections commonly observed during post-mortem examinations of the subjects with a final diagnosis of SIDS [5]. Although, in human medicine, the concept of sudden death, SUID and SIDS has been well defined by the WHO, in veterinary medicine, a universal definition is lacking. Some authors have defined sudden death in animals as death that occurs in a few minutes or several hours, due to pre-existing disease or a functional disorder [14]. However, in the opinion of the authors, this definition should be avoided, because it lacks a well-defined temporal reference range. In contrast, even if not yet validated in veterinary medicine, the WHO definition provides an important temporal reference range useful for the identification of cases of sudden death in veterinary clinical practice.

Over the last few years, many studies have investigated the cause of death in animals. In particular, infectious diseases that affect the gastrointestinal system are reported to be the main cause of death in puppies and young dogs [15,16]. In contrast, neoplastic diseases appear to be the prevalent cause of death in adult dogs [15]. Among the infections, *canine parvovirus type 2* (CPV-2) is reported to be one of the most common and important causes of morbidity and mortality in young dogs [17,18]. Moreover, this virus is considered to be an important pathogen responsible for acute gastroenteritis and myocarditis in dogs [17,18]. However, with regards to sudden and unexpected deaths, despite the underlying causes having been sporadically investigated in dogs [19], to the best of our knowledge, no study has evaluated the microbiological findings in cases of sudden death in young dogs. In light of these observations, the aims of this study were as follows: (1) to estimate the proportional mortality ratio (PMR) for "sudden and unexpected death" in puppies and young dogs; (2) to investigate the pathological, bacteriological, and virological findings in sudden and unexpected death in young dogs; and (3) to introduce a standardized microbiological protocol for the diagnostic investigation of cases of sudden death in veterinary medicine

2. Materials and Methods

2.1. Study Design

An observational retrospective study of a total of 145 cases of young dead dogs, consecutively presented by veterinary practitioners, owners, or law enforcement to the "Istituto Zooprofilattico del Mezzogiorno" (IZSM) of Portici city, Southern Italy, was performed over a 3-year period (2015–2017). The submission forms were collected to obtain information about the medical history and age of the animals. On the basis of the medical history, the animals were divided into groups as follows:

- (Sudden and unexpected death group—SUD group): dogs with a clinical diagnosis of sudden and unexpected death. According to the WHO, sudden and unexpected death (SUD) cases were considered to be a non-violent and unexpected death that occurs less than 24 h after the onset of symptoms;
- (Expected death group—ED group): dogs without a clinical history of sudden and unexpected death

On the basis of age, the available data were categorized as follows: (Group 1) 10 days–4 weeks; (Group 2) 4 weeks–6 weeks; (Group 3) 6 weeks–2 months; (Group 4) 2–3 months; (Group 5) 3–6 months; (Group 6) 6–12 months. Each examined case was subjected to a complete necropsy and bacteriological and virological investigations; however, for the purposes of this study, only the necropsy and microbiological reports from animals in the SUD group were included. Furthermore, the microbiological investigations were restricted to molecular tests for the virological analysis, and microbiological cultures for the bacteriological examinations. In all assessed cases, molecular tests were performed using a real-time polymerase chain reaction assay (RT-PCR) for *canine parvovirus (CPV), canine coronavirus, canine adenovirus, herpesvirus, and canine distemper virus*. Furthermore, in all cases positive for *canine parvovirus type 2*, multiplexed PCR panels were used to distinguish between wild-type and vaccine CPV-2 and to identify the pathogen subtype (CPV-2a; CPV2b; CPV 2c) [20]. The analyzed samples included the liver, lung, kidney, spleen, heart, brain and intestine. Microbiological results and necropsy reports were both extracted from the IZSM information system (SIGLA). Animals that tested positive in the toxicological investigations, or that had died from trauma, were excluded from the study.

2.2. Necropsy Protocol

All necropsies were performed in the necropsy room of the "Istituto Zooprofilattico Sperimentale del Mezzogiorno" (IZSM), Portici, Italy, with a standard necropsy protocol [21]. All SUD cases were stored at 4 °C before necropsy. The period between death and necropsy was between 12 and 36 h. During the necropsy, according to internal institute protocol, all samples were taken in rigorous asepsis conditions using sterile instruments and transported to the laboratory of microbiology. Furthermore, to obtain uncontaminated specimens, a sterilization of the body and organs surfaces was performed before sampling. Finally, the mean time between sample collection and transport to the reference laboratory was under 3 h.

2.3. Analytical Validation of the Results

For each case of sudden and unexpected death, the clinical history, necropsy report and microbiological findings were reviewed, and the final cause of death was categorized as "explained" or "unexplained". However, since determining the pathological significance of the microorganisms isolated during necropsy is often difficult, as has been frequently reported in the literature [22,23]. For the purposes of this study, viruses detected by PCR were considered to be the cause of death, only when associated with the typical macroscopic changes observed during the anatomopathological examination. In addition, the bacteriological and virological findings were interpreted considering a broad range of variables, such as the location of pathogen detection, the capacity of pathogens for virulence, the correlation with injuries observed during the necropsy, the multisite location of the pathogens, the age of the dog and the composition of the normal flora.

2.4. Statistical Analysis

The frequencies of sudden and unexpected death (SUD), expected death (ED), and total deaths (SUD + ED) were evaluated and stratified by age classes. Furthermore, we estimated the proportional mortality ratio (PMR) for "SUD" in each assessed age group. The Chi-square test was used to assess differences in the distributions of ED and SUD among age groups.

3. Results

Out of the 145 examined reports, we found 21 cases of SUD and 124 cases of ED during the 3-year study period. The PMR of SUD was therefore 14.48%, while the ED was 85.52%. Furthermore, the Chi-square test showed a significant difference in the frequencies of ED and SUD among the assessed age groups ($p < 0.05$). All SUD cases were submitted by Italian veterinary practitioners. The highest frequencies of expected death were observed in animals in Group 2 (100% of the cases), Group 3 (87.7% vs. 12.5%), Group 4 (97.2% vs. 12.8%) and Group 5 (93.3% vs. 6.7%). In contrast, the highest frequencies of SUD were found in animals in Group 1 (58.8% vs. 41.2%) and Group 6 (37.5% vs. 62.5%). Table 1 summarizes the frequencies and percentages of SUD and ED and the frequency of total deaths (SUD + ED) stratified by age classes. Overall, of the 21 SUD cases, 10 out of 21 (47.61%) dogs were less than 4 weeks old (Group 1), 0 out of 21 were between 4 weeks and 6 weeks old (Group 2), five out of 21 (23.8%) were between 6 weeks and 2 months old (Group 3), one out of 21 (4.76%) was between 2 and 3 months old (Group 4), two out of 21 (9.51%) were between 3 and 6 months old (Group 5), and three out of 21 (14.28%) were between 6 months and 1 year old (Group 6).

Table 1. Frequency and percentage of sudden and unexpected deaths, expected deaths and the frequency of total deaths stratified by age groups.

Age Group	Sudden Death	Expected Death	Total Deaths
Group 1	10 (58.8%)	7 (41.2%)	17
Group 2	0	14 (100%)	14
Group 3	5 (12.5%)	35 (87.5%)	40
Group 4	1 (2.8%)	35 (97.2%)	36
Group 5	2 (6.7%)	28 (93.3%)	30
Group 6	3 (37.5%)	5 (62.5%)	8
Total	21	124	145

3.1. Clinical Background and Gross Findings

The most frequently observed clinical symptoms in cases of sudden death were as follows: acute respiratory symptoms in 12 out of 21 cases, followed by acute gastroenteric symptoms (a single or few episodes of vomiting or diarrhea) in six out of 21 cases, neurological symptoms in one case, and finally, non-specific symptoms in two out of 21 cases. The evaluation of necropsy reports allowed us to observe haemorrhagic gastroenteritis in 12 out of 21 cases, pneumonia in seven out of 21 cases, and catarrhal enteritis in five out of 21 cases (Figure 1). Pulmonary oedema or multiorgan congestion were also observed in 19 out of 21 cases.

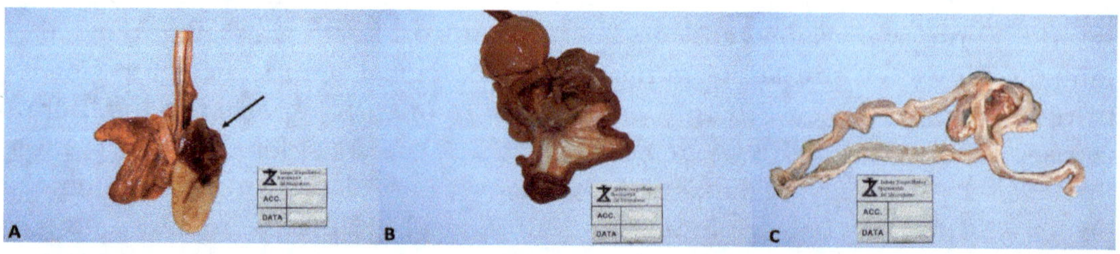

Figure 1. Pathological lesions in cases of sudden death. (**A**): pneumonia (arrows) (**B**): haemorrhagic gastroenteritis (**C**): catarrhal enteritis.

3.2. Microbiological Examination

In all animals dead for sudden and unexpected death, virological investigations were performed with a panel of viruses tested by PCR (*Canine parvovirus, Canine coronavirus, Canine adenovirus, Canine herpesvirus* and *Canine distemper virus*), and a bacteriological examination was performed with microbiological cultures. The retrospective analysis showed positive microbiological results in 18 out of 21 cases (Table 2).

Table 2. Viruses or bacteria detected in cases of sudden and unexpected death.

Pathogen	NO. of Cases
Canine Parvovirus	10
E. Coli	7
Clostridium perfringens type A	6
Adenovirus	3
Canine Distemper Virus	2
Streptococcus sanguinis	2
Pasteurella spp.	2
Streptococcus dysgalactiae	1
Rotavirus	1

However, for the purposes of this study, the microbiological findings were interpreted considering a broad range of variables. In particular, the location of pathogen detection, the capacity of pathogens for virulence and the correlation of that microorganisms with the observed macroscopic injuries were the most important parameters assessed in this study. Therefore, after the review of the necropsies and microbiological reports, the detected pathogens were considered the main cause of death in only 14 out of 21 cases. In particular, among the evaluated cases, the main cause of death was viral infection with *Canine parvovirus type 2* (8/21), followed by viral infection with *Canine parvovirus type 2*, and co-infection with *E. coli* (2/21), bacterial co-infection with *Clostridium perfringens* type A and *E. coli* (2/21) and viral and bacterial co-infection with the *Canine distemper virus* and *Pasteurella* spp. (2/21). Finally, in seven out of 21 cases, the microbiological results did not explain the injuries observed during the necropsy. Therefore, the causative agent of infection was considered undetermined after the microbiological examination. Table 3 summarizes the clinical backgrounds, pathological findings, microbiological results and causes of death of the cases of sudden death.

Table 3. Microbiological and anatomopathological findings of the studied dogs.

Group	Sex	Clinical Background	Pathological Findings	Virological Examination	Bacteriological Examination	Cause of Death
1	M	Acute respiratory insufficiency	Visceral congestion, pulmonary edema, hemorrhagic gastroenteritis	*Canine parvovirus type 2a* (wild type)—detected in the lung, liver, heart, brain, and intestine	*Streptococcus dysgalactiae*—isolated in the lung	Viral infection
	M	Acute respiratory insufficiency	Visceral congestion, pulmonary edema, severe broncho-pneumonia, catarrhal enteritis	No viruses detected	*Streptococcus sanguinis*—isolated in the intestine	Undetermined: severe pneumonia due to unexplained causes
	M	Acute respiratory insufficiency	Visceral congestion, pulmonary edema, severe broncho-pneumonia, catarrhal enteritis	No viruses detected	*Streptococcus sanguinis*—isolated in the intestine	Undetermined: severe pneumonia due to unexplained causes
	F	Acute respiratory insufficiency	Visceral congestion, multifocal pulmonary hemorrhages, hemorrhagic enteritis	*Canine parvovirus type 2b and 2c* (wild type)—detected in the lung, liver, spleen, heart, and intestine	*Clostridium perfringens*, Detection of *Clostridium perfringens* alpha toxin—isolated in the intestine	Viral infection
	M	Acute respiratory insufficiency	Lobar pneumonia, pulmonary edema, catarrhal enteritis	*Canine distemper virus*—detected in the lung, liver, and brain	Pasteurella spp.—detected in the lung	Viral and bacterial infection
	F	Acute respiratory insufficiency	Visceral congestion, multifocal pulmonary hemorrhages, hemorrhagic enteritis	*Canine parvovirus type 2b and 2c* (wild type)—detected in the lung, liver, brain, heart, and intestine	*E. coli*, *Clostridium perfringens*, Detection of *Clostridium perfringens* alpha toxin—isolated in the intestine	Viral infection
	M	Acute respiratory insufficiency	Visceral congestion, pulmonary edema, focal broncho-pneumonia, hemorrhagic gastroenteritis	*Canine distemper virus*—detected in the lung, liver, and brain	*Pasteurella* spp.—detected in the lung	Viral and bacterial co-infection
	M	Acute respiratory insufficiency	Visceral congestion, pulmonary edema, hemorrhagic gastroenteritis	No viruses detected	No bacteria detected	Undetermined
	M	Acute respiratory insufficiency	Visceral congestion, pulmonary edema, severe broncho-pneumonia	No viruses detected	No bacteria detected	Undetermined
	M	Acute respiratory insufficiency	Visceral congestion, hemorrhagic enteritis	*Canine parvovirus type 2a* (wild type)—detected in the heart, spleen, and intestine	No bacteria detected	Viral infection

Table 3. *Cont.*

Group	Sex	Clinical Background	Pathological Findings	Virological Examination	Bacteriological Examination	Cause of Death
3	M	Sialorrhea, unilateral eye swelling, muscle stiffness, a single episode of vomiting	Visceral congestion, pulmonary edema, hemorrhagic enteritis	No virus detected	*E. coli; Clostridium perfringens* Detection of *Clostridium perfringens* alpha toxin—detected in the intestine and lung	Bacterial infection
	M	Neurological symptoms	Visceral congestion, bi-lateral pneumonia, pulmonary edema segmental catarrhal enteritis	Rotavirus (detected in the intestine)	*E. coli*—isolated in the intestine	Undetermined: severe pneumonia due to unexplained causes
	F	Acute gastrointestinal symptoms	Visceral congestion, hemorrhagic enteritis, focal pneumonia	*Canine parvovirus type 2a*, (wild type)—detected in the lung, liver, and intestine; *Adenovirus*—detected in intestine	*Clostridium perfringens* Detection of *Clostridium perfringens* alpha toxin—isolated in the intestine	Viral infection
	F	Vomiting	Visceral congestion, hemorrhagic enteritis, focal pneumonia	*Canine parvovirus type 2a* (wild type)—detected in the lung, liver, heart, and intestine	*E. coli*—isolated in intestine and lung	Viral and bacterial co-infection
	M	Vomiting	Visceral congestion, pulmonary congestion, enteritis, abdominal, thoracic and pericardial effusion, multifocal pulmonary hemorrhage	No virus detected	*E. coli*—isolated in intestine	Undetermined: insufficient findings to explain death
4	F	Acute respiratory insufficiency	Multifocal hemorrhage, abdominal, thoracic and pericardial effusion, hemorrhagic enteritis	No virus detected	*E. coli*—detected in the liver, lung, and intestine *Clostridium perfringens* Detection of *Clostridium perfringens* alpha toxin—detected in the intestine and lung	Bacterial infection
5	M	Acute respiratory insufficiency	Pulmonary congestion, segmental catarrhal enteritis	*Canine parvovirus type 2a* (wild type)—detected in lung, liver, and intestine	*E. coli*—isolated in the intestine	Viral infection
	F	A single episode of diarrhea	Pulmonary congestion, pulmonary edema, segmental hemorrhagic enteritis	*Canine parvovirus type 2a* (wild type)—detected in lung, liver, intestine, and spleen *Adenovirus*—detected in the lung	No bacteria detected	Viral infection

Table 3. *Cont.*

Group	Sex	Clinical Background	Pathological Findings	Virological Examination	Bacteriological Examination	Cause of Death
6	F	Lack of appetite	Thoracic effusion, visceral congestion, multifocal hemorrhage, severe hemorrhagic enteritis	*Canine parvovirus type 2a* (vaccinal) and *2c* (wild type)—detected in lung, liver, intestine, and spleen *Canine distemper virus-detected in lung* *Adenovirus—detected in lung*	No bacteria detected	Viral infection
	F	Lack of appetite and fever for 12 h	Multifocal hepatic necrosis, hemorrhagic enteritis	*Canine parvovirus type 2b* (wild type)—detected in the lung, liver, brain, and intestine	*E. coli. Clostridium perfringens*, Detection of *Clostridium perfringens* alpha toxin (isolated in lung, liver, and intestine)	Viral and bacterial infection
	F	Single episode of diarrhea	Congestion of the spleen, abdominal effusion	No viruses detected	No bacteria detected	Undetermined: insufficient findings to explain death

4. Discussion

In human forensic pathology, the autopsy for cases of SUID are primarily performed according to the "Kennedy Report" [11]. This protocol and the published international guidelines advocate a multidisciplinary approach to investigations of all cases of SUID, which should be based not only on the findings of the post-mortem macroscopic examination, but also on a broad range of ancillary investigations, such as bacteriological and virological analyses. Although a broad range of tests have been proposed in cases of SUID in human forensic medicine, in the present study, we focused on the pathological and post-mortem microbiology findings in cases of sudden death in young dogs. The results of this study show a low frequency of sudden deaths in young dogs, accounting for 14.48% of the total observed deaths. Furthermore, the Chi-squared test showed a significant difference in the frequencies of ED and SUD among the assessed age groups ($p < 0.05$). In particular, the highest frequency of sudden death was observed in dogs younger than 4 weeks old. In contrast, the highest frequency of ED was observed in animals in Groups 2–5. This difference could be due to the immaturity of the immune system of puppies younger than 6–12 weeks of age [24]. Indeed, the endotheliochorial placentation of this species is relatively impenetrable to the transfer of maternal immunoglobulin [24]. Thus, the immune protection of the puppies during the first weeks of life depends on the ingestion of maternal colostrum antibodies (MCA) [24]. In the absence of the passive transfer of MCA, newborn puppies are only able to develop an immune response to antigens at 2–3 weeks of age. Therefore, any delay in colostrum intake or reduction of colostrum ingestion leads to a reduction in the immune protection of the animals [24–26]. Under these conditions, viruses or bacteria can replicate and spread quickly, leading to the death of the puppies, without the development of characteristic symptoms. Furthermore, congenital malformation or maternal malnutrition could be considered additional causes of sudden death in this age range. In contrast, after 2–3 weeks of age, the immune system of puppies, although immature, is able to develop a mild immune response against pathogens, avoiding the rapid spread of the pathogens and allowing the development of characteristic symptoms of the pathology. In addition, in our study, the most frequently observed gross injuries in cases of sudden death were haemorrhagic gastroenteritis in 12 out of 21 cases, pneumonia in seven out of 21 cases, and catarrhal enteritis in five out of 21 cases. Pulmonary oedema or multiorgan congestion were also observed in 19 out of 21 cases. Intra-abdominal and respiratory lesions have been previously reported in the literature as two important causes of sudden and unexpected infant death in human forensic pathology [27]. Indeed, respiratory tract lesions, although mild, can easily lead to serious complications and sudden death of the subjects [27]. Similarly, acute gastroenteric lesions can cause severe dehydration and serum electrolyte disturbance, which have the potential to cause sudden and unexpected death in children [27]. Overall, in our study, positive microbiological results were observed in 18 out of 21 cases. However, as frequently highlighted in the human literature, the isolation of pathogens in cases of sudden death does not necessarily imply a correlation between those pathogens and the death. In particular, this correlation must be confirmed by the observation of severe and specific injuries during the anatomopathological examination [6]. Therefore, after the review of the necropsy findings, detected pathogens were considered the main cause of death in only 14 out of 21 cases, while in the remaining seven cases, the microbiological results did not explain the injuries observed during the necropsy. The negative findings observed in our study could suggest: (1) a non-infectious cause of death of the assessed animals; or (2) a death due to viruses or other pathogens not detected by the virological panel in use in this study. Indeed, there are a wide range of viruses that are potentially pathogenic in young dogs, including both DNA and RNA viruses. However, our virological panel was limited to the detection of the following five specific viruses: *canine parvovirus, canine coronavirus, canine adenovirus, canine herpesvirus* and *canine distemper virus.* With regard to the positive results, viral infection due to *canine parvovirus type 2* (wild type) was the most common cause of death observed in our study. Overall, *CPV-2* is a causative agent of acute gastroenteritis and myocarditis [17,18]. Furthermore, it is reported in the literature to be one of the most common and important causes of morbidity and mortality in young dogs [17,18]. Usually, the clinical symptoms of the infection are as follows: anorexia, depression, lethargy and fever, followed by vomiting and diarrhea [17,18,28]. However, it is also reported to be a cause of sudden cardiac death in puppies between 4 and 8 weeks of age [17,29,30]. Interestingly, we also observed two cases of sudden death due to *Canine distemper virus* and *Pasteurella* spp. co-infection. *Canine distemper virus* is a member of the genus *Morbillivirus*, which can cause a large variety of disorders in dogs including rhinitis, pneumonia, demyelinating leukoencephalitis, necrotizing bronchiolitis and enteritis [31]. *Canine distemper virus* is not reported in the veterinary literature as a cause of sudden death in animals. However, *Canine distemper virus* causes immunosuppression by targeting cells that express the CD150 protein (signaling lymphocyte activation molecule (SLAM)) [31]. Previous studies showed that this immunosuppression favors secondary infections caused by pathogens, such as *Bordetella bronchiseptica* or *C. piliforme* [32]. Therefore, it is possible to suppose that opportunistic pathogens could complicate a sub-clinical *Canine distemper virus* infection, replicating and spreading quickly, and leading to the death of the puppies without the development of characteristic symptoms. With regards to the bacteriological examination, the most common isolated bacteria were *C. perfringens* type A (6/19) and *E. coli* (6/19). However, they were considered the cause of death in only two cases. Indeed, *C. perfrigens* and *E. coli* are considered normal components of canine intestinal flora [33,34]. Similarly, the alpha toxin gene of *C. perfringens* may be found in asymptomatic dogs as part of the normal intestinal microflora [33]. However, in some cases, *E. coli* can cause pleuro-pneumonitis [35], gastroenteritis [36], urogenital infections, cholangitis, cholangiohepatitis and septicaemia [37] in both humans and other animals. Similarly, *C. perfringens* type A has been associated with gastro-enteric disease, such as haemorrhagic enteritis in dogs and abomasitis in ruminants [38–40]. Furthermore, this bacterium has been reported in the literature as a cause of sudden and unexpected death in dogs [39]. Unfortunately, no specific test for the diagnosis of enteritis due to *C. perfringens* is described in the literature [40]. Thus, generally, the clinical signs, the pathological findings, the microbiological analysis, and the absence of other pathogens must be examined before confirming the diagnosis [40]. In our case, the multisite locations of the pathogens, the absence of other viruses or bacteria and the specific anatomopathological findings of haemorrhagic enteritis supported the diagnosis of enteritis due to *C. perfringens* and *E. coli* as the final cause of death.

Finally, this study allowed the detection of a wide range of pathogens that, after the review of the necropsy and microbiological reports, were not considered the main cause of death of the animals, such as *Canine Adenovirus, Rotavirus, Streptococcus sanguinis, Streptococcus dysgalactiae* and, in some cases, *E. coli* and *C. perfringens*. Therefore, further studies will be needed to evaluate the possible contributions of these pathogens to cases of sudden and unexpected death in young dogs.

5. Conclusions

Sudden death is an uncommon cause of death in young dogs. However, the high frequencies of viruses and bacteria detected in our study highlights the importance of performing complete bacteriological and virological analyses in all cases of sudden death in young dogs. The results of this study suggest that our PCR panel combined with a bacteriological analysis could facilitate the rapid detection and type-specific identification of the pathogenic causes or co-factors of death in most cases of sudden death in young dogs. Finally, these results could provide a valuable epidemiological tool for the investigation of sudden death in young dogs.

Author Contributions: The individual contributions in the present study were as follows: conceptualization and methodology G.P., G.F., L.C.; validation F.A., L.V., V.I.; investigation G.P., L.C.; data curation G.P.; writing—original draft preparation G.P.; project administration G.F.; funding acquisition G.F. All authors have read and agreed to the final version of the manuscript.

References

1. Byard, R.W. Sudden death—An overview. In *Sudden Death in Infancy, Childhood, and Adolescence*, 1st ed.; Byard, R.W., Cohle, S.D., Eds.; Cambridge University Press: Cambridge, UK, 1994; pp. 1–4.
2. Kruger, M.M.; Martin, L.J.; Maistry, S.; Heathfield, L.J. A systematic review exploring the relationship between infection and sudden unexpected death between 2000 and 2016: A forensic perspective. *Forensic Sci. Int.* **2018**, *289*, 108–119. [CrossRef]
3. Prtak, L.; Al-Adnani, M.; Fenton, P.; Kudesia, G.; Cohen, M.C. Contribution of bacteriology and virology in sudden unexpected death in infancy. *Arch. Dis. Child.* **2010**, *95*, 371–376.
4. Tajiri, T.; Tate, G.; Miura, K.; Masuda, S.; Ohike, N.; Kunimura, T.; Mitsuya, T.; Morohoshi, T. Sudden death caused by fulminant bacterial infection: Background and pathogenesis of Japanese adult cases. *Intern. Med.* **2008**, *47*, 1499–1504. [CrossRef] [PubMed]
5. Kinney, H.C.; Thach, B.T. The Sudden Infant Death Syndrome. *N. Engl. J. Med.* **2012**, *8*, 795–805.
6. Fernández-Rodríguez, A.; Ballesteros, S.; De Ory, F.; Echevarría, J.E.; Alvarez-Lafuente, R.; Vallejo, G.; Gómez, J. Virological analysis in the diagnosis of sudden children death: A medico-legal approach. *Forensic Sci. Int.* **2006**, *161*, 8–14. [CrossRef]
7. Yagmur, G.; Ziyade, N.; Elgormus, N.; Das, T.; Sahin, M.F.; Yildirim, M.; Ozgun, A.; Akcay, A.; Karayel, F.; Koc, S. Postmortem diagnosis of cytomegalovirus and accompanying other infection agents by real-time PCR in cases of sudden unexpected death in infancy (SUDI). *J. Forensic Leg. Med.* **2016**, *38*, 18–23. [CrossRef]
8. Dettmeyer, R.; Baasner, A.; Schlamann, M.; Padosch, S.A.; Haag, C.; Kandolf, R.; Madea, B. Role of virus-induced myocardial affections in sudden infant death syndrome: A prospective postmortem study. *Pediatr. Res.* **2004**, *55*, 947–952. [CrossRef]
9. Dempers, J.; Ann, S.M.; Wadee, S.A.; Kinney, H.C.; Odendaal, H.J.; Wright, C.A. Progressive Primary Pulmonary Tuberculosis Presenting as the Sudden Unexpected Death in Infancy: A Case Report. *Forensic Sci. Int.* **2011**, *206*, 27–30. [CrossRef]
10. Astrup, B.S.; Johnsen, I.B.G.; Engsbro, A.L. The role of Coxsackievirus A16 in a case of sudden unexplained death in an infant—A SUDI case. *Forensic Sci. Int.* **2016**, *259*, 9–13. [CrossRef]
11. Kennedy, H. *Sudden Unexpected Death in Infancy. A Multi-Agency Protocol for Care and Investigation*, 1st ed.; The Report of a Working Group Convened by the Royal College of Pathologists and the Royal College of Paediatrics and Child Health; The Royal College of Pathologists/The Royal College of Paediatrics and Child Health: London, UK, 2014.
12. Bajanowski, T.; Vege, A.; Byard, R.W.; Krous, H.F.; Arnestad, M.; Bachs, L.; Banner, J.; Blair, P.S.; Borthne, A.; Dettmeyer, R.; et al. Sudden infant death syndrome (SIDS)—Standardized investigations and classification: Recommendations. *Forensic Sci. Int.* **2007**, *165*, 129–143. [CrossRef]
13. Vennemann, M.; Bajanowski, T.; Butterfass-Bahloul, T.; Jorch, G.; Brinkmann, B.; Mitchell, E.A. Do risk factors differ between explained sudden unexpected death in infancy and sudden infant death syndrome? *Arch. Dis. Child.* **2007**, *92*, 133–136. [CrossRef] [PubMed]
14. Parry, N.M. Medicine: Sudden and unexpected death in small animal patients: Part 1. *Companion Anim.* **2008**, *13*, 23–30. [CrossRef]
15. Fleming, J.M.; Creevy, K.E.; Promislow, D.E.L. Mortality in North American Dogs from 1984 to 2004: An Investigation into Age-, Size-, and Breed-Related Causes of Death. *J. Vet. Intern. Med.* **2011**, *25*, 187–198. [CrossRef]
16. Eleni, C.; Panetta, V.; Scholl, F.; Scaramozzino, P. Causes of death in dogs in the province of Rome (Italy). *Vet. Ital.* **2014**, *50*, 137–143. [PubMed]
17. Nandi, S.; Kumar, M. *Canine Parvovirus*: Current Perspective. *Indian J. Virol.* **2010**, *21*, 31–44. [CrossRef]
18. Mylonakis, M.E.; Kalli, I.; Rallis, T.S. Canine parvoviral enteritis: An update on the clinical diagnosis, treatment, and prevention. *Vet. Med.* **2016**, *11*, 91–100. [CrossRef]
19. Olsen, T.F.; Allen, A.L. Causes of sudden and unexpected death in dogs: A 10-year retrospective study. *Can. Vet. J.* **2000**, *41*, 873–875.
20. Kaur, G.; Chandra, M.; Dwivedi, P.N.; Narang, D. Multiplex real-time PCR for identification of canine parvovirus antigenic types. *J. Virol. Methods* **2016**, *233*, 1–5. [CrossRef]
21. Brownlie, H.W.; Munro, R. The Veterinary Forensic Necropsy: A Review of Procedures and Protocols. *Vet. Pathol.* **2016**, *53*, 919–928. [CrossRef]

22. Wilson, S.J.; Wilson, M.L.; Reller, L.B. Diagnostic utility of postmortem blood cultures. *Arch. Pathol. Lab.* **1993**, *117*, 986–988.
23. Morris, J.A.; Harrison, L.M.; Partridge, S.M. Postmortem bacteriology: A re-evaluation. *J. Clin. Pathol.* **2006**, *59*, 1–9. [CrossRef] [PubMed]
24. Day, M.J. Immune System Development in the Dog and Cat. *J. Comp. Path.* **2007**, *137*, 10–15. [CrossRef] [PubMed]
25. Decaro, N.; Buonavoglia, C. *Canine parvovirus*—A review of epidemiological and diagnostic aspects, with emphasis on type 2c. *Vet. Microbiol.* **2012**, *155*, 1–12. [CrossRef] [PubMed]
26. Mila, H.; Grellet, A.; Desario, C.; Feugier, A.; Decaro, N.; Buonavoglia, C.; Chastant-Maillard, S. Protection against *canine parvovirus type 2* infection in puppies by colostrum-derived antibodies. *J. Nutr. Sci.* **2014**, *3*, 54.
27. Byarnt, V.A. Natural Diseases Causing Sudden Death in Infancy and Early Childhood. In *SIDS Sudden Infant and Early Childhood Death: The Past, the Present and the Future*, 1st ed.; Duncan, J.R., Byard, W.R., Eds.; The University of Adelaide: Adelaide, Australia, 2018; pp. 300–312.
28. Stann, S.E.; DiGiacomo, R.F.; Giddens, W.E.; Evermann, J.F. Clinical and pathological features of parvoviral diarrhoea in dogs. *J. Am. Vet. Med. Assoc.* **1984**, *185*, 651–654. [PubMed]
29. Hayes, M.A.; Russell, R.G.; Babiuk, L.A. Sudden death in young dogs with myocarditis caused by *parvovirus*. *J. Am. Vet. Med. Assoc.* **1979**, *174*, 1197–1203. [PubMed]
30. Ridgway, E.J.; Harvey, D. The hospital autopsy: A manual of fundamental autopsy practice. In *The Hospital Autopsy*, 3rd ed.; Burton, J., Rutty, G., Eds.; Hodder Education: London, UK, 2009.
31. Beineke, A.; Puff, C.; Seehusen, F.; Baumgärtner, W. Pathogenesis and immunopathology of systemic and nervous *canine distemper*. *Vet. Immunol. Immunopathol.* **2009**, *127*, 1–18. [CrossRef]
32. Headley, S.A.; Oliveira, T.E.S.; Pereira, A.H.T.; Moreira, J.R.; Michelazzo, M.M.Z.; Pires, B.G.; Marutani, V.H.B.; Xavier, A.A.C.; Di Santis, W.G.; Garcia, J.L.; et al. *Canine morbillivirus (canine distemper virus)* with concomitant *canine adenovirus, canine parvovirus-2*, and *Neospora caninum* in puppies: A retrospective immunohistochemical study. *Sci. Rep.* **2018**, *8*, 13477. [CrossRef]
33. Goldstein, M.R.; Kruth, S.A.; Bersenas, A.M.E.; Holowaychuk, M.K.; Weese, J.S. Detection and characterization of *Clostridium perfringens* in the feces of healthy and diarrheic dogs. *Can. J. Vet. Res.* **2012**, *76*, 161–165.
34. Bettelheim, K.A.; Goldwater, P.N. *Escherichia coli* and Sudden Infant Death Syndrome. *Front. Immunol.* **2015**, *6*, 343. [CrossRef]
35. Handt, L.K.; Stoffregen, D.A.; Prescott, J.S.; Pouch, W.J.; Ngai, D.T.; Anderson, C.A.; Gatto, N.T.; DebRoy, C.; Fairbrother, J.M.; Motzel, S.L.; et al. Clinical and microbiologic characterization of hemorrhagic pneumonia due to extraintestinal pathogenic *Escherichia coli* in four young dogs. *Comp. Med.* **2003**, *53*, 663–670. [PubMed]
36. Astrid, B.K.; Anthony, P.C.; Casey, M. Gaunt Enteropathogenic *Escherichia coli* (EPEC) infection in association with acute gastroenteritis in 7 dogs from Saskatchewan. *Can. Vet. J.* **2016**, *57*, 964–968.
37. Beutin, L. *Escherichia coli* as a pathogen in dogs and cats. *Vet. Res.* **1999**, *30*, 285–298. [PubMed]
38. Sasaki, J.; Goryo, M.; Asahina, M.; Makara, M.; Shishido, S.; Okada, K. Hemorrhagic enteritis associated with *Clostridium perfringens type A* in a dog. *J. Vet. Med. Sci.* **1999**, *61*, 175–177. [CrossRef]
39. Schlegel, J.B.; Dreumel, T.D.; Slavić, D.; Prescott, J.F. *Clostridium perfringens type A* fatal acute hemorrhagic gastroenteritis in a dog. *Can. Vet. J.* **2012**, *53*, 555–557.
40. Marks, S.L.; Kather, E.J. *Clostridium perfringens*- and *Clostridium difficile*-associated diarrhea. In *Infectious Diseases of the Dog and Cat*, 3rd ed.; Greene, C.E., Ed.; Saunders Elsevier: St Louis, MO, USA, 2016; pp. 363–366.

19

Host-Parasite Interaction in *Sarcoptes scabiei* Infestation in Porcine Model with a Preliminary Note on its Genetic Lineage

Arun Kumar De [1,*,†], Sneha Sawhney [1,†], Samiran Mondal [2], Perumal Ponraj [1], Sanjay Kumar Ravi [1], Gopal Sarkar [2], Santanu Banik [3], Dhruba Malakar [4], Kangayan Muniswamy [1], Ashish Kumar [5], Arvind Kumar Tripathi [1], Asit Kumar Bera [6] and Debasis Bhattacharya [1]

1 Animal Science Division, ICAR-Central Island Agricultural Research Institute, Port Blair 744101, India; snehasawhney88@gmail.com (S.S.); perumalponraj@gmail.com (P.P.); skravivet@gmail.com (S.K.R.); swamy02_vet@yahoo.co.in (K.M.); akt9@rediffmail.com (A.K.T.); debasis63@rediffmail.com (D.B.)

2 Department of Veterinary Pathology, West Bengal University of Animal and Fishery Sciences, Kolkata 700037, India; vetsamiran@gmail.com (S.M.); gsarkar999@gmail.com (G.S.)

3 Department of Animal Genetics and Breeding, ICAR-National Research Centre on Pig, Guwahati 781131, India; sbanik2000@gmail.com

4 Animal Biotechnology Centre, National Dairy Research Institute, Karnal 132001, India; dhrubamalakar@gmail.com

5 CTARA, IIT Bombay, Mumbai 400076, India; ashish7@iitb.ac.in

6 Reservoir and Wetland Fisheries Division, ICAR-Central Inland Fishery Research Institute, Barrackpore, Kolkata 700120, India; asitmed2000@yahoo.com

* Correspondence: biotech.cari@gmail.com.

† These authors contributed equally to this paper.

Simple Summary: Scabies or mange caused by *Sarcoptess cabiei* is the latest addition of WHO's list oftropical neglected diseases. It causes severe itching to the host. It has a wide host range including humans, farm animals, companion animals, and wild animals. It is anemerging/re-emerging disease with high prevalence in underdeveloped and developing countries. The disease has zoonotic importance and is of significant public health concern as cross-transmission or species jumping is very common. To date, fifteen *Sarcoptes* varieties have been reported as per host origin. Differential diagnosis at variety level is very crucial for epidemiological study and scratching future eradication program of the disease. As morphotaxonomy fails to differentiate varieties, use of molecular markers is crucial. Moreover, it is very important to understand the host-parasite interaction at the systemic level for a better understanding on the pathogenicity of the disease. Here, we report the genetic characterization of *S. scabiei* from India and host-parasite interaction in a porcine model.

Abstract: The burrowing mite *Sarcoptes scabiei* causes scabies in humans or mange in animals. It infests a wide range of mammalian species including livestock, companion animals, wild animals, and humans. Differential diagnosis of *Sarcoptes* varieties is key for epidemiological studies and for formulation of an eradication program. Host-parasite interaction at the systemic level is very important to understand the pathogenicity of the mite. This communication deals with the preliminary report on the genetic characterization of *S. scabiei* from India. Moreover, the effect of *S. scabiei* infestation on host physiology with special emphasis on serum biochemical parameters, lipid profile, oxidant/antioxidant balance, stress parameters, and immune responses were evaluated in a porcine model. Cytochrome C oxidase 1 and voltage-sensitive sodium channel based phylogenetic study could distinguish human and animals isolates but could not distinguish host or geographical specific isolates belonging to animal origin. An absence of host-specific cluster among animal isolates argues against the hypothesis of delineating *S. scabiei* as per host origin. Elevated levels of markers of liver function such as albumin, AST, ALT, ALP, and LDH in infested animals indicated impaired liver function in infested animals. *S. scabiei* infestation induced atherogenic dyslipidemia indicated by elevated levels of total cholesterol, low-density lipoprotein cholesterol and triglycerides, and a decreased level of high-density lipoprotein cholesterol. Oxidative stress in infested animals was indicated by a high level of nitric oxide and serum MDA as oxidative stress markers and low antioxidant capacity. *S. scabiei* triggered stress response and elevated levels of serum cortisol and heat shock proteins were recorded in infested animals. *S. scabiei* infestation increased the serum concentration of immunoglobulins and was associated with up-regulation of IL-2, IFN-γ, IL-1β, and IL-4 indicating both Th1 and Th2 response. The results of the study will be helpful for a better understanding of host-parasite interaction at the systemic level in crusted scabies in pigs.

Keywords: *Sarcoptes scabiei*; host-parasite interaction; molecular characterization; lipid profile; antioxidant

---

1. Introduction

Scabies in human, or mange in animals, caused by the burrowing mite *Sarcoptes scabiei*, is a neglected tropical infectious disease and is prevalent worldwide especially in developing and under-developed countries [1,2]. It infests more than 100 mammalian species including livestock, companion animals, wild animals, and humans [3–5]. Mange is considered as an emerging/re-emerging infectious disease and imparts huge economic loss to the livestock industry due to devastating morbidity and reduced production [3,5]. It is regarded as a significant public health concern in underdeveloped and developing countries as it is frequently associated with bacterial super-infection, which may sometimes be fatal especially in children if not treated in time [6]. Worldwide, around 300 million people are estimated to be infested with scabies every year [7] and its prevalence among children in Africa and indigenous communities of Northern Australia is astoundingly high ranging from 25 to 80% [8–10]. Scabies is broadly categorized into two forms, ordinary scabies with low mite burden (<20) or crusted scabies with high mite load and hyper-keratosis of the skin [11]. The mite *S. scabiei* causes inflammation of the skin which is associated with an exudate which forms crusts on the surface [12].

Controversy and conflicting opinion exist regarding speciation of *S. scabiei*; some believe that *S. scabiei* infesting different hosts are monospecific whereas others claim that they belong to different species or subspecies [13,14]. Currently, there is a broad consensus that the species *Sarcoptes* is divided into different varieties as per its host origin [13,15] and to date, more than 15 diverse varieties have been reported [2,16]. Of recent, this hypothesis has been challenged as cross-transmission or species jumping is very common in some varieties [17]. Therefore, differential diagnosis of *Sarcoptes* varieties is crucial for epidemiological studies [18] and formulating eradication strategies [15]. Morphotaxonomy has failed to differentiate between varieties as they share similar morphology [19]. Molecular diagnosis based on ribosomal DNA spacer region has been unsuccessful in identifying *S. scabiei* to the host level [20] and immunological diagnosis is also very challenging as different varieties produce immunologically identical proteins [21]. Recently, mitochondrial cytochrome oxidase 1 (COX1) based marker has shown promising results in varieties level confirmation of *S. scabiei* infestation. No information on genetic characterization or molecular confirmation in *S. scabiei* is available from India. The present study seems to be the first report on the genetic characterization of *S. scabiei* from India.

Sarcoptic mange is a very common ectoparasite disease in pigs [22,23]. It affects growth rate and reproductive performance in pigs and increases piglet mortality [24–26] leading to significant economic loss to the swine industry. A rare probability of zoonotic potential of *S. scabiei* var suis cannot be ignored [27]; it may be transmitted to affect a variety of different animal host species as well as pig handlers [28,29] causing severe itching. As pigs in semi-intensive systems in developing and under-developed countries are generally reared by tribes who keep a close association with the animals, there is a chance of transmission to humans, especially children and immunocompromised adults [4]. Moreover, in developed countries, pigs have been kept as pets which can transmit the disease to humans. Sarcoptic mange is a very common problem in the pig rearing regions of India, especially Northeast and Eastern parts of India [30]. In the Andaman and Nicobar Islands, Nicobari pigs are reared by Nicobarese tribal people and close association between tribal people and pigs is observed.

S. scabiei modulates host immunity, inflammatory, and complement reactions in order to be established to the host skin [31–33]. *S. scabiei* infestation triggers multiple reactions including allergic reactions, inflammation, innate immune reactions, and activation of immune components in the skin [34]. The salivary solutions of burrowing mites contain different bioactive compounds with potential to influence host physiological functions [35]. Mites are reported to influence the cytokine and chemokine secretion from keratinocytes and dermal fibroblasts [31,33] and disturb the balance between Th1 and Th2 immune responses [36]. In addition, *S. scabiei* has been reported to disturb the antioxidant defense system in mammalian hosts [37,38]. However, the studies were mostly in vitro using skin equivalents [31]. Little is known about the host parasite interaction in *S. scabiei* infestation at the systemic level. Therefore, the study aims at genetic characterization of *S. scabiei* isolated from Nicobari pigs and a better understanding on host parasite interactions with special emphasis on serum biochemical parameters, lipid profile, oxidant/antioxidant balance, stress parameters, and immune responses.

2. Materials and Methods

2.1. Ethics Approval

This research has been approved by the Institute Animal Ethics Committee (IAEC) of ICAR-Central Island Agricultural Research Institute (ICAR-CIARI), Port Blair, Andaman and Nicobar Islands, India on 12 January 2020 and the ethical approved project identification code is 'ICAR-CIARI/AS/AICRP-Pig/IAEC/4960 dated 12 January 2020'. All the methods were performed in accordance with the relevant national guidelines and regulations.

2.2. Study Area and the Animals

The study was conducted on Nicobari pigs maintained at the institute pig farm of ICAR-CIARI (11.6060° N, 92.7058° E). Sarcoptic mange infestation in pigs was identified during a routine visit to the farm. Fifteen *S. scabiei*-infested animals (5–6 months old, 8 male and 7 female) participated in the present study. Ten healthy animals (5–6 months old, 5 male and 5 female) were treated as control. Absence of *S. scabiei* infestation in control animals was confirmed by dermatological and microscopic examination. All the animals were examined for presence of fleas, lice, ticks, or any other ectoparasite, and animals negative for these were only considered in the study. Coproscopic examination for light and heavy eggs [12] confirmed that the animals were free from gastrointestinal parasites and the animals were serologically negative for classical swine fever which is endemic to the Andaman and Nicobar Islands. Both control and infested animals were maintained in 12-h light-dark cycle on concrete floor in separate pens to avoid chance of transmission of sarcoptic mange and fed with a commercial diet containing 18% crude protein, 2% crude fat, 6% crude fiber, 4% acid insoluble ash and 10% moisture. The animals were offered water ad libitum.

2.3. Collection and Processing of Clinical Samples for Microscopic Analysis

Skin scrapings were collected from the infested Nicobari pigs using surgical blades. Mineral oil was applied on the surgical blades and scrapings were taken from the crusted area of skin till little blood appeared. Collected material was boiled in 10% sodium hydroxide (NaOH) (*w*/*v*) solution to dissolve the keratinized tissue and was centrifuged at 500× *g* for five minutes and the sediment was examined under 100× magnification in a light microscope (Trinocular Compound Microscope, Quasmo,

Ambala, Haryana, India 180129/53268). Photographs of different stages of mite and eggs present were taken at 400× magnification.

2.4. DNA Extraction

DNA from skin scrapings was isolated by a commercial kit (DNeasy Blood and Tissue kit, Cat. No. 69504, Qiagen, Hilden, Germany). Briefly, 25 mg of skin scrapping was ground in lysis buffer using a sterile pestle and motor. For cell lysis, proteinase K was added to the ground scrapings and it was incubated at 56 °C in a water bath overnight. The completely lysed samples were used for genomic DNA extraction as per protocol recommended by the manufacturer. The DNA samples were kept at −80 °C until further use.

2.5. Amplification and Sequencing of Cytochrome C Oxidase Subunit 1 (COX1) and Voltage Sensitive Sodium Channel (VSSC) Gene Segments

For molecular identification and characterization of the mite, two gene segments namely COX1 and VSCC were chosen [34]. COX1 and VSCC gene fragments were amplified using primers described earlier by Erster et al. [34]. The PCR was performed in Thermocycler (Eppendorf, Hamburg, Germany) with the cycling conditions mentioned previously [34]. The amplicons were purified using a commercial kit (MinElute PCR Purification Kit, Cat. No. 28004, Qiagen, Hilden, Germany) as per manufacturer's protocol and sequence information was generated by dideoxy fingerprinting.

2.6. Sequence Analysis

Representative COX1 and VSSC sequences of *S. scabiei* from different hosts distributed in different geographical regions were retrieved from GenBank (www.ncbi.nlm.nih.gov) and a summary of the information has been depicted in Table S1. Alignment of the sequences was done by ClustalW [39] in MEGAX [40]. Phylogenetic tree was constructed in MEGAX using Maximum Likelihood method and Tamura–Nei model [41]. The reliability of the tree was judged by 1000 bootstrap replications. For phylogenetic tree construction, we trimmed extra nucleotides from our sequences and GenBank retrieved sequences to make a homogeneous length of 193 bp for COX1 and 436 bp for VSSC. Evolutionary relationship among different sequences was deduced by median-joining networks constructed in Network v 10 with default settings [42].

2.7. Estimation of Biochemical Parameters

Commercially available kits (TBL, Solan, India) were used for estimation of serum biochemical parameters such as total protein, albumin, globulin, glucose, aspartate aminotransferase (AST), alanine aminotransferase (ALT), alkaline phosphatase (ALP), lactate dehydrogenase (LDH) and creatine kinase (CK). The parameters were assessed in an automated clinical chemistry analyzer (Transasia Biomedical Limited, Mumbai, India). The reference values of the parameters are presented in Table S2.

2.8. Estimation of Oxidative Stress Parameters

To investigate the oxidant/antioxidant balance in serum following *S. scabiei* infestation, the markers of oxidative stress such as serum level of total nitric oxide (NO), total serum antioxidant activity, malonyldialdehyde (MDA) concentration, as well as the levels of antioxidant enzymes; superoxide dismutase (SOD), glutathione-S-transferase (GSH), catalase were determined and compared to control animals.

NO level was evaluated by a commercial kit (EZAssay^{TM} Nitric Oxide Estimation kit, HiMedia Laboratories Pvt. Ltd., Nashik, India) according to the manufacturer's instructions. The principle of the assay is the reduction of NO_3 which was then converted to a blue-colored azo compound. The absorbance was recorded at 630 nm.

Antioxidant activity in serum was estimated by a colorimetric kit (EZAssay^{TM} Antioxidant Activity Estimation kit, HiMedia Laboratories Pvt. Ltd., Nashik, India) following the protocol recommended by the manufacturer.

Level of lipid peroxidation was measured by measurement of malonyldialdehyde (MDA). Levels of MDA in serum were measured by a commercial colorimetric based assay kit (EZAssay^{TM} TBARS estimation kit for lipid peroxidation, HiMedia Laboratories Pvt. Ltd., Nashik, India).

Serum levels of catalase, superoxide dismutase, glutathione-S-transferase were measured by ELISA based methodology using catalase assay kit, superoxide dismutase assay kit, and glutathione assay kit (Cayman chemicals, Ann Arbor, MI, USA) as per manufacturer's protocol.

2.9. Estimation of HSPs in Serum

Serum levels of four heat shock proteins (HSP20, HSP40, HSP70, and HSP90) in infested and control animals were measured by ELISA-based methodology on biotin double antibody sandwich technology using commercial kits (Porcine HSP20, HSP40, SHP70 and HSP90 ELISA kit, Arsh Biotech Pvt. Ltd., Life Technologies, Delhi, India). Briefly, serum samples were added to the wells pre-coated with the respective HSP monoclonal antibodies. This was followed by the addition of respective anti-HSP antibodies labeled with biotin-streptavidin-HRP complex. Washing was done to remove the unbound proteins. This was followed by the addition of substrates and measurement of absorbance at 450 nm using a microplate reader (SpectraMax Plus, Molecular Devices, San Jose, CA, USA).

2.10. Measurement of Cortisol in Serum

Cortisol level in serum was measured by ELISA, based on biotin double antibody sandwich technology using a commercial kit (Porcine Cortisol ELISA kit, Arsh Biotech Pvt. Ltd., Life Technologies, Delhi, India) as per the protocol of the manufacturer. Briefly, serum samples were added to cortisol monoclonal antibodies pre-coated wells. This was followed by the addition of anti-cortisol antibodies labeled with biotin-streptavidin-HRP complex. Washing was done to remove the unbound proteins. This was followed by the addition of substrates and measurement of absorbance at 450 nm using a microplate reader (SpectraMax Plus, Molecular Devices, San Jose, CA, USA). The reference value of cortisol is presented in Table S2.

2.11. Lipid Profile Analysis

Serum levels of total cholesterol (TC), high-density lipoprotein cholesterol (HDLc), low-density lipoprotein cholesterol (LDLc), and triglycerides (TG) were evaluated. Levels of TC, HDLc, and TG were determined by enzymatic methods using commercially available kits (Jeev Diagnostics Pvt. Ltd., Chennai, India; Pathozyme Diagnostics, Kholapur, India; and Spinreact, S.A., Spain respectively). The concentration of LDL was deduced by the following formula: LDL = TC − HDL − (TG ÷ 5) [43]. Moreover, we calculated cardiac risk factor (CRF) and atherogenic index (AI) using the following formulas: CRF =TC/HDL [44] and AI = (TC − HDL)/HDL [45]. The reference values of the parameters are presented in Table S2.

2.12. Estimation of Serum Immune Parameters

The concentrations of total IgG, IgA, and IgM in serum were determined using quantitative ELISA kits (Arsh Biotech Pvt. Ltd., Delhi, India) according to the manufacturer's instructions.

Serum levels of cytokines (IL-2, IL-4, IL6, IL-8, IL-12, IL-1β, IFN-γ) in the serum of *S. scabiei*-infested and control animals were measured by sandwich ELISA methodology using commercial kits from Life Technologies, New Delhi, India.

2.13. *Estimation of Apoptotic Markers*

Serum concentrations of three apoptotic markers (Caspase-3, Caspase-7, and Casepase-8) were estimated by Nori® porcine ELISA kits (Life Technologies Pvt. Ltd., Delhi, India) according to the manufacturer's manual.

2.14. *Histopathology*

Skin scrapings from infested animals were collected and fixed in formalin solution (10%) at room temperature and a routine process was adopted for histopathology. In brief, samples were passed through ascending grades of alcohol (70–100%) for dehydration. The dehydrated samples were then cleared in benzene, transferred to melted paraffin (60 °C) for impregnation, and paraffin blocks were finally prepared in metal molds. Sections were prepared by using microtome (Leica, Wetzlar, Germany; Catalogue No. RM2235) at 5μM Slides were prepared as per standard protocol and were stained with hematoxylin and eosin.

2.15. *Statistical Analysis*

Data were presented as mean ± standard deviation and were normally distributed. Differences among control and infested groups were calculated by *t*-test using GraphPad Prism software (San Diego, CA, USA) (http://www.graphpad.com). The mean values with a significance of $p < 0.05$ were considered to be statistically significant.

3. Results

3.1. *Clinical Signs of the Infested Animals*

Clinical examination showed intense pruritus associated with hyperkeratosis and crusts in the skin. Skin of the animals was thickened and wrinkled in appearance which was a characteristic feature of crusted scabies/Norwegian scabies. Alopecia in the affected area was observed (Figure 1a).

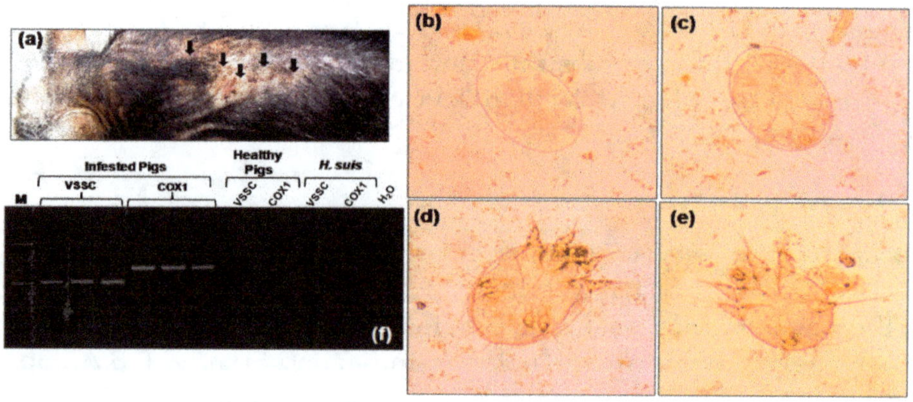

Figure 1. *Sarcoptes scabiei* infestation in Nicobari pig. (**a**) An infested animal with thickened and wrinkled skin and hair loss (black arrows), (**b**) mite egg (400× magnification), (**c**) mite egg containing larvae (400× magnification), (**d**) mite nymph (400× magnification), (**e**) larval stage of mite (400× magnification), (**f**) amplification of cytochrome C oxidase subunit 1 (COX1) and voltage sensitive sodium channel (VSSC) gene segments. Infested animals were positive for both of the gene fragments whereas control animals were negative. Primer specificity was verified using the lice (*Haematopinus suis*) DNA as negative control.

3.2. *Microscopic Examination*

On the basis of clinical symptoms, skin scrapings from infested animals were examined under microscope for the presence of mites. Microscopic examination confirmed the presence of eggs, eggs with six-legged larvae, and nymphal stage of *S. scabiei* (Figure 1b–e). The nymphal stages had short legs. The third and fourth pair of legs never projected beyond the body. Morphologically the mites were indistinguishable from *Sarcoptes* [12].

3.3. Molecular Identification and Characterization of *S. scabiei*

For molecular confirmation, one mitochondrial gene (COX1) and one nuclear gene (VSSC) were amplified using *Sarcoptes* specific primers and amplicons of both the genes were detected in infested pigs whereas in control pig, no amplicons were observed (Figure 1f). Specificity of the PCR was verified by using pig lice (*Haematopinus suis*) DNA as a negative control for both the genes (Figure 1f).

For differential diagnosis and molecular characterization, we generated partial sequence information of COX1 (2 samples) and VSSC (one sample) and the sequences were deposited in GenBank and obtained accession number MN986997-MN986998 for COX1 and MN986999 for VSSC. The sequences of COX1 and VSSC were 686 bp and 498 bp in length respectively. For phylogenetic analysis, we retrieved representative *S. scabiei* COX1 and VSSC sequences from different hosts distributed in different geographical regions. COX1 based phylogenetic tree (Figure 2a) indicated three distinct clades; two for human isolates (Clade A and B) and one for animal isolates (Clade C). In Clade A, two clearly defined clusters were detected; one includes human isolates from Hong Kong, South Korea, China and the other includes human isolates from France and Australia. Clade B contains human isolates from Panama. On the contrary, no host or region-specific clusters were observed in animal clade (Clade C). From the phylogenetic tree, it was evident that the Andaman isolates were phylogenetically close to pig isolate of Israel. A median-joining network was constructed to understand the evolutionary relationship of *S. scabiei* isolates. Two human-specific clades and one animal-specific clade were detected (Figure 2b).

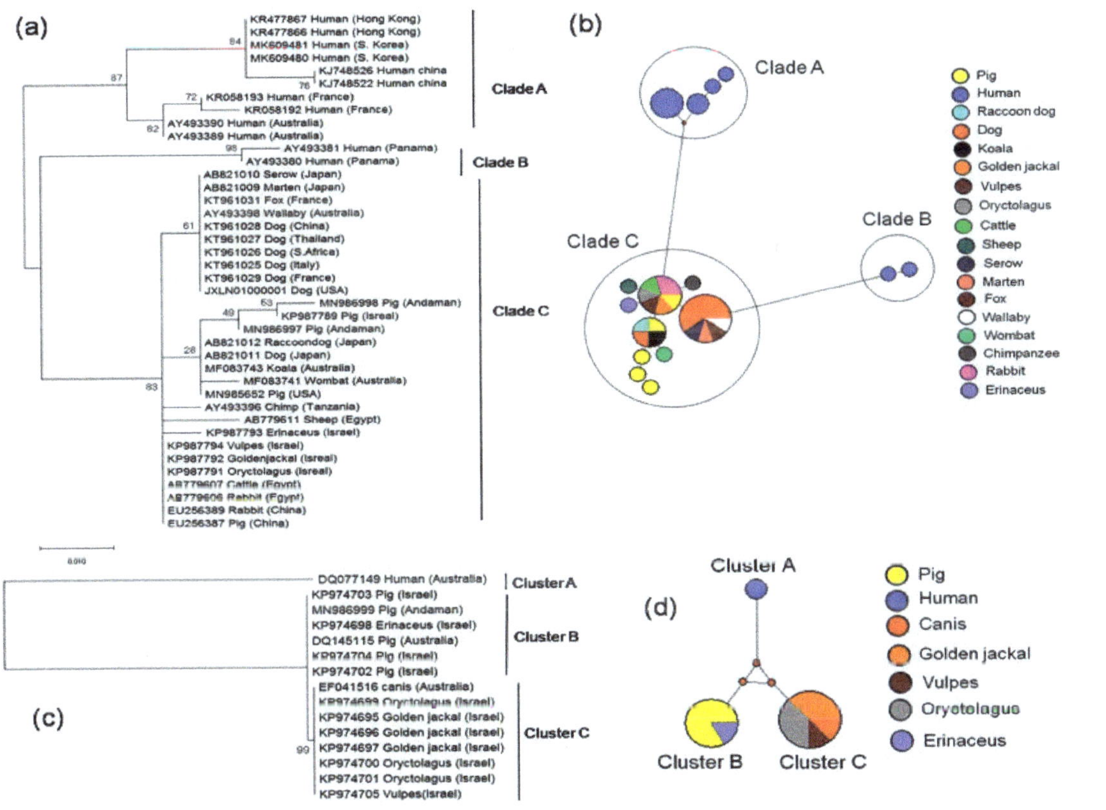

Figure 2. Evolutionary relationship of different isolates of *S. scabiei*. (**a**) COX1 based phylogenetic tree, (**b**) COX1 based network profile, (**c**) VSSC based phylogenetic tree, (**d**) VSSC-based network profile. Phylogenetic tree was constructed based on maximum likelihood method using Tamura–Nei model [41] implemented in MEGAX following 1000 bootstrap replications. Network was drawn in Network 10 with default settings [42].

Phylogenetic tree based on VSSC sequences showed three host-specific distinct clusters, one for human isolate (Cluster A) and the other two for animal isolates (Figure 2c). Within animal isolates, pig and erinaceus isolates formed one cluster (Cluster B) whereas oryctolagus, golden jackal, vulpes, and canis isolates formed another cluster (Cluster C). Pig isolates of Andaman belonged to Cluster B with pig isolates from Israel, Australia, and erinaceus isolate from Israel. The VSSC based network tree is presented in Figure 2d and three clearly defined clusters were depicted.

3.4. Serum Biochemical Parameters in Crusted Scabies

A significant decrease in plasma, total protein, albumin, and glucose, and significant increase in globulin, ASL, ALT, CK, LDL, and ALP in infested group as compared to those of control group was observed (Figure 3). Moreover, the ration of albumin and globulin (A:G) in infested group (0.6359 ± 0.048) was decreased than that of control group (1.121 ± 0.066).

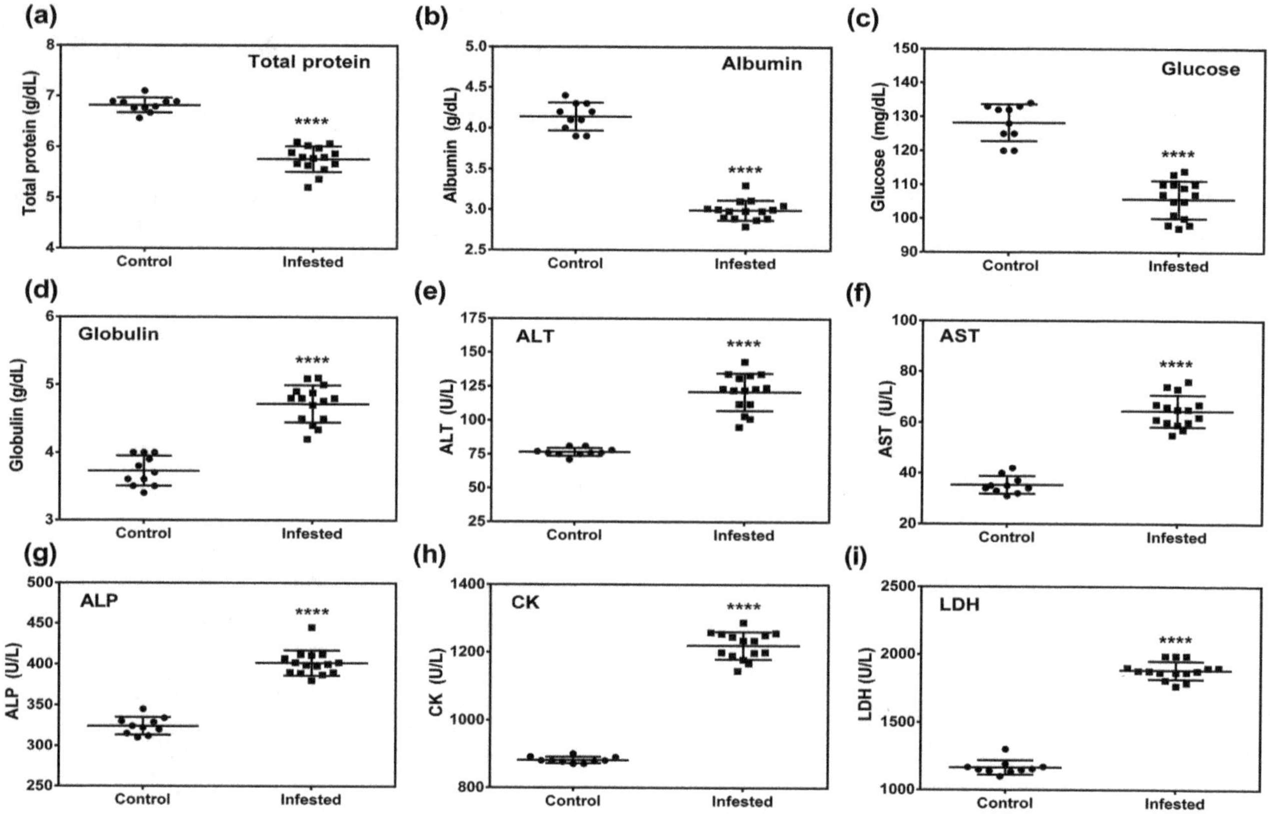

Figure 3. Effect of crusted scabieson serum biochemical parameters in a porcine model. (**a**) Serum total protein, (**b**) serum albumin, (**c**) serum glucose, (**d**) serum globulin, (**e**) alanine aminotransferase (ALT), (**f**) aspartate aminotransferase (AST), (**g**) alkaline phosphatase (ALP), (**h**) creatine kinase (CK), (**i**) lactate dehydrogenase (LDH). Data in scatter plot are shown as mean ± SD. *t*-test was performed to find out significant difference between the two groups. **** denotes $p \leq 0.0001$.

3.5. Crusted Scabies Leads to Dyslipidemia in Pigs

The results of the lipid profile analysis are presented in Figure 4. In the infested group, an atherogenic dyslipidemic profile indicated by elevated levels of total cholesterol, low-density lipoprotein cholesterol (LDL-c) and triglycerides (TG), and a decreased level of high-density lipoprotein cholesterol (HDLc) as compared to control group was observed. This was further supported by higher CRF and AI values in infested animals than those of control animals.

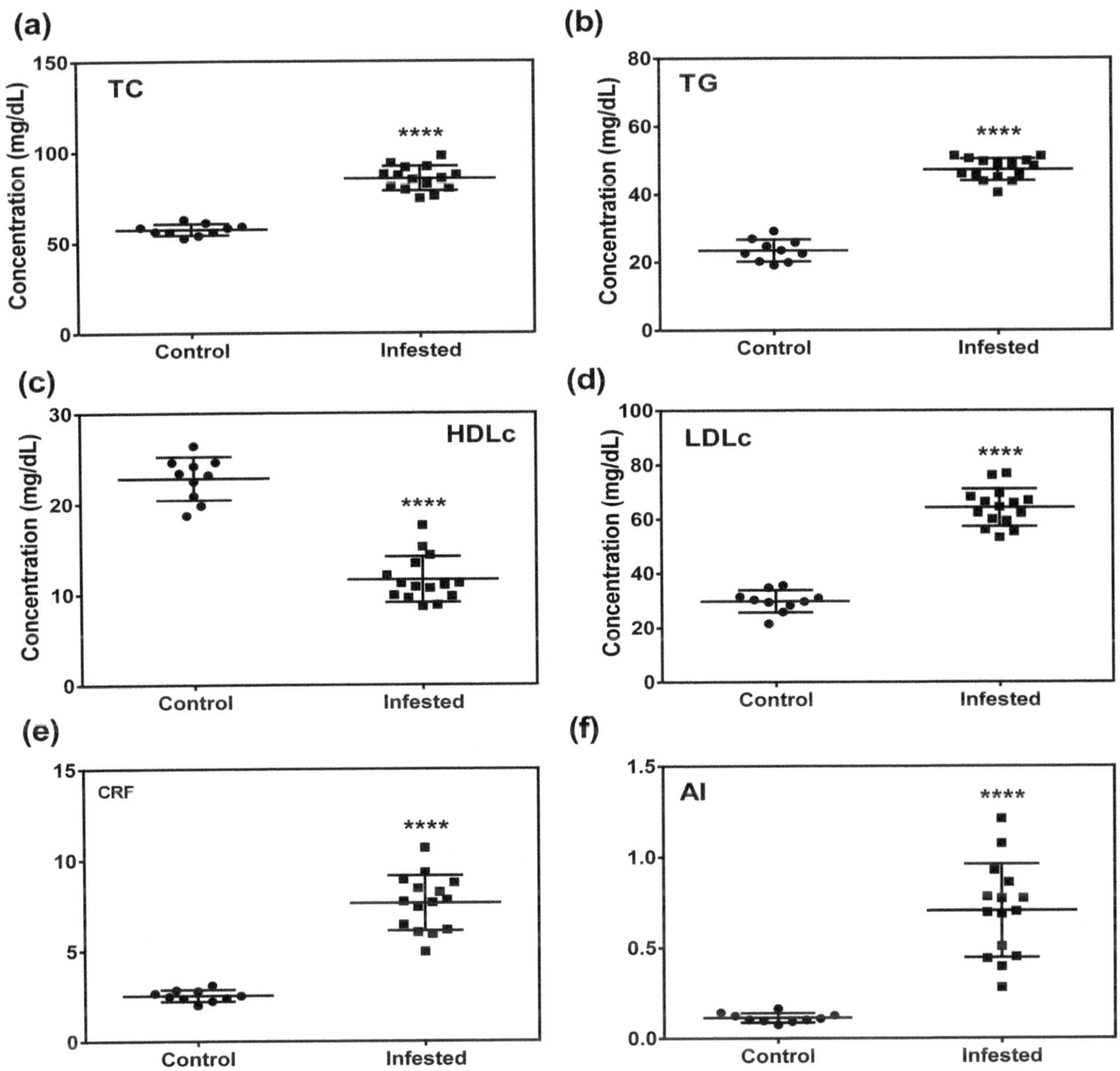

Figure 4. Effect of crusted scabies on serum lipid profile in a porcine model. (**a**) Total cholesterol (TC) concentration, (**b**) triglycerides (TG) concentration, (**c**) high-density lipoprotein cholesterol (HDLc) concentration, (**d**) low-density lipoprotein cholesterol (LDLc) concentration, (**e**) cardiac risk factor (CRF), (**f**) atherogenic index (AI). Data in scatter plot are shown as mean ± SD. *t* test was performed to find out significant difference between the two groups. **** denotes $p \leq 0.0001$.

3.6. Crusted Scabies Induces Oxidative Stress

To investigate the effect of *S. scabiei* infestation on oxidant/antioxidant balance in serum, the markers of oxidative stress such as total antioxidant activity (T-AOC), total nitric oxide (TNO) concentration, levels of lipid peroxides, and malonyldialdehyde (MDA) as well as the levels of antioxidant enzymes; superoxide dismutase (SOD), glutathione-S-transferase (GSH) and catalase were determined and compared to control animals (Figure 5). The infested group showed significantly higher serum total nitric oxide (TNO) concentration than the control group. Total antioxidant activity (T-AOC) in the infested group was significantly lower than that of control group. Activity of catalase, SOD, and concentration of GSH in infested animals decreased significantly as compared to those of control animals. On the other hand, MDA concentration in the infested group was found significantly higher than its corresponding value in the control group (Figure 5).

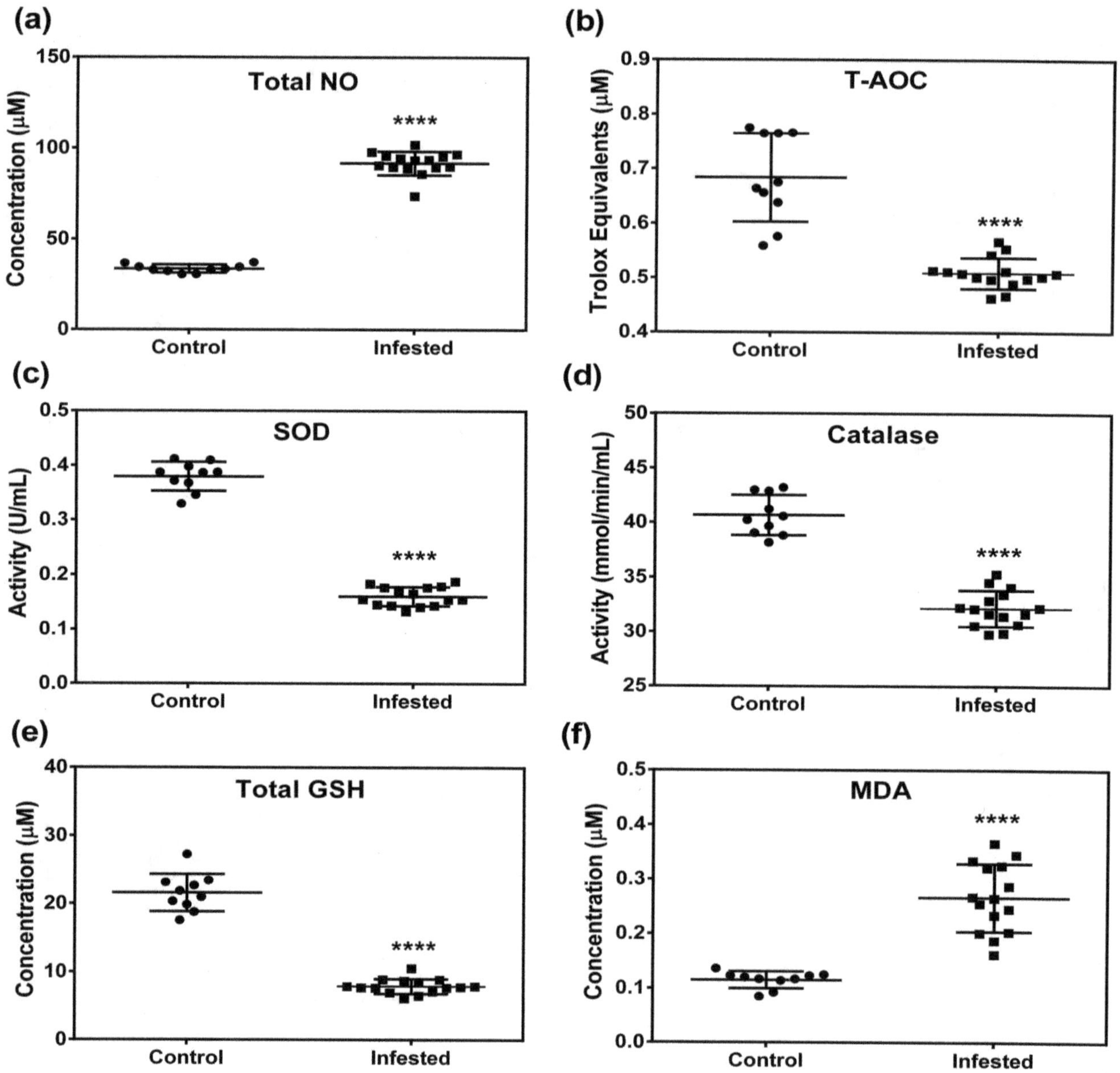

Figure 5. Effect of crusted scabies on antioxidant profiles and oxidative stress indicator in a porcine model. (**a**) Total nitric oxide (NO) concentration, (**b**) total antioxidant capacity (T-AOC), (**c**) superoxide dismutase (SOD) activity, (**d**) catalase activity, (**e**) glutathione-S-transferase (GSH) concentration, (**f**) malonyldialdehyde (MDA) concentration. Data in scatter plot are shown as mean ± SD. *t*-test was performed to find out significant difference between the two groups. **** denotes $p \leq 0.0001$.

3.7. Crusted Scabies Is Associated with Stress

To investigate whether *S. scabiei* infestation leads to stress in host animals, level of stress biomarkers such as serum cortisol concentration and serum levels of four heat shock proteins (HSP20, HSP40, HSP70, and HSP90) in control and infested animals were analyzed. Serum cortisol concentration in infested group was found significantly higher than that of control group (Figure 6).

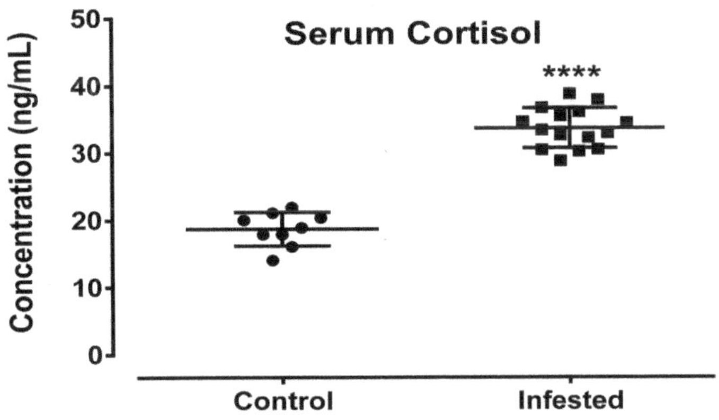

Figure 6. Effect of crusted scabieson serum cortisol concentration in a porcine model. Data in scatter plot are shown as mean ± SD. *t*-test was performed to find out significant difference between the two groups. **** denotes $p \leq 0.0001$.

HSP20, HSP70, and HSP90 were up-regulated in infested animals compared with the control animals. On the other hand, no significant change in HSP40 level between control and infested animals was detected (Figure 7).

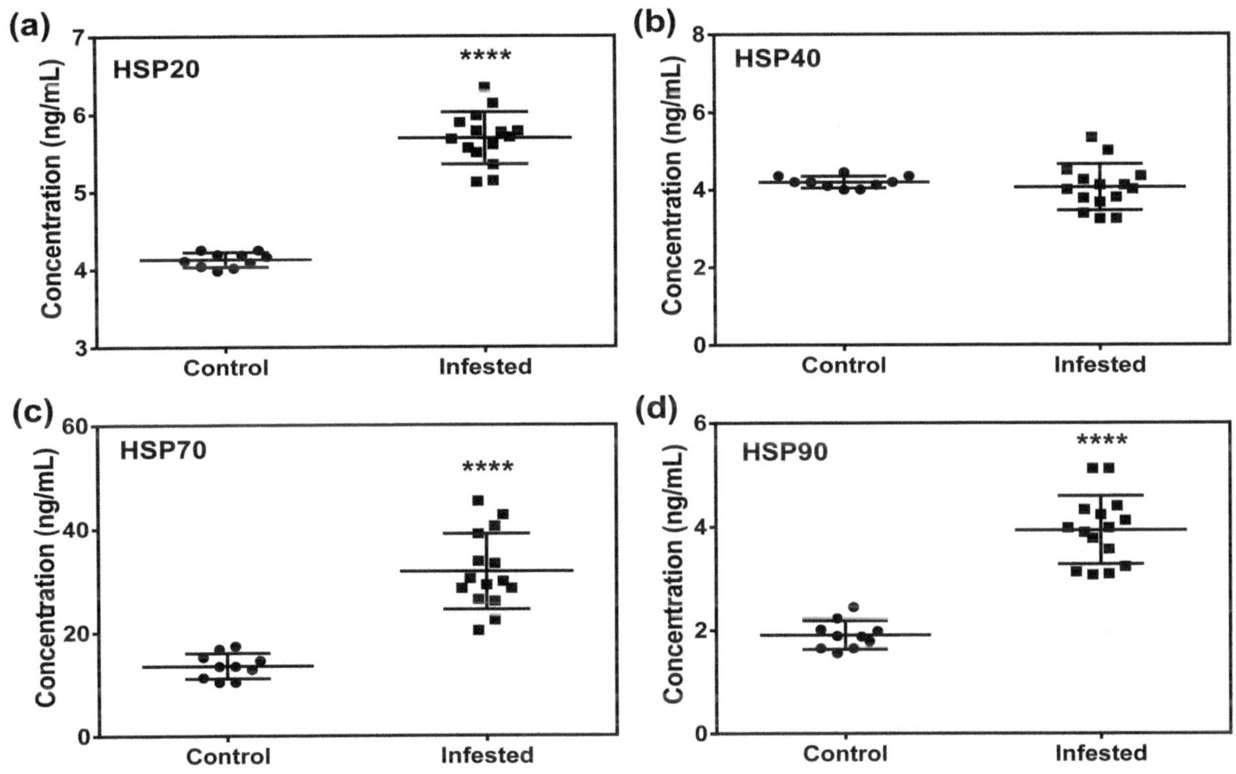

Figure 7. Effect of crusted scabies on serum heat shock proteins (HSPs) concentration in a porcine model. (**a**) HSP20, (**b**) HSP40, (**c**) HSP70, and (**d**) HSP90.Data in scatter plot are shown as mean ± SD. *t*-test was performed to find out significant difference between the two groups. **** denotes $p \leq 0.0001$.

3.8. Crusted Scabies Up-Regulates Serum Levels of Apoptotic Markers

Serum concentrations of all three apoptotic markers (Caspase 3, 7, and 8) in infested and control animals were recorded. Up-regulation of all three apoptotic markers was detected in infested group as compared to control group (Figure 8).

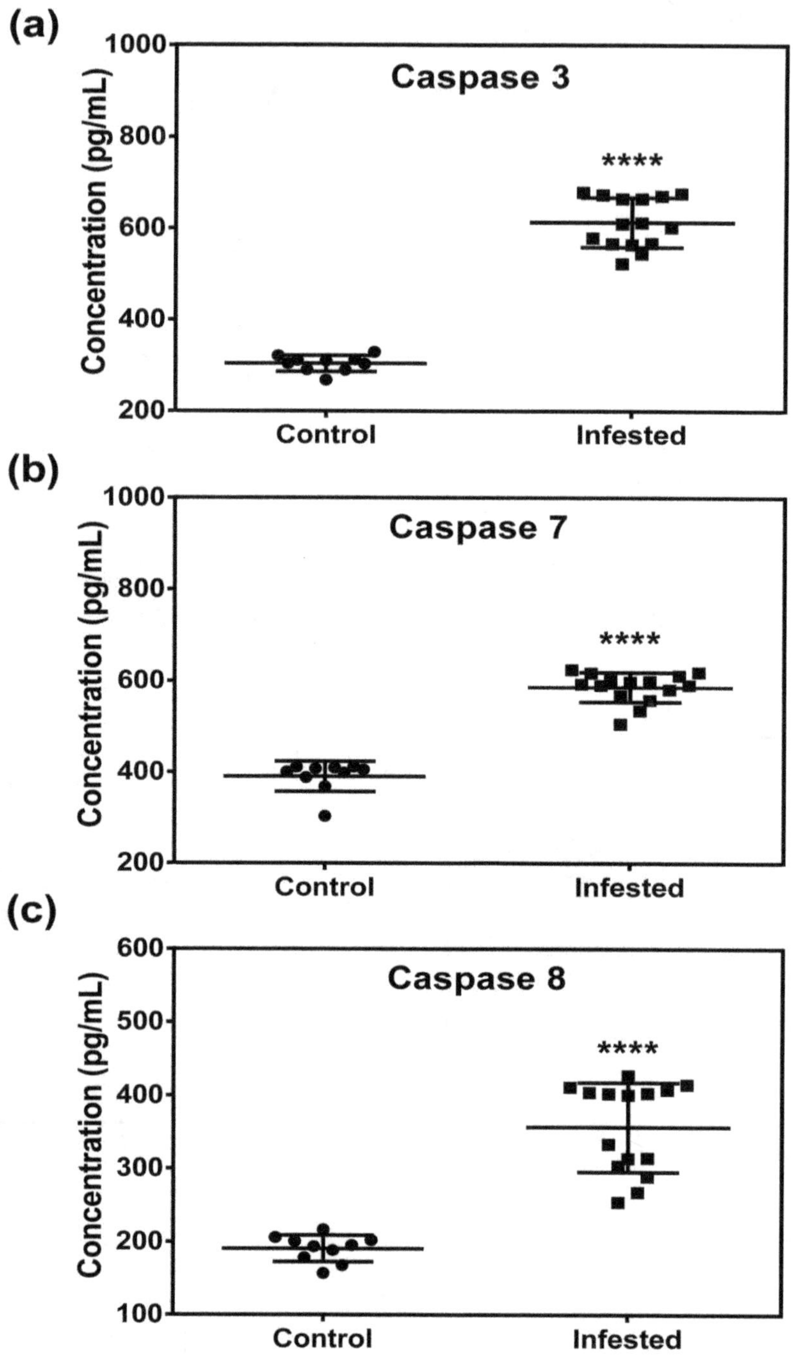

Figure 8. Effect of crusted scabieson serum levels of apoptotic markers in a porcine model. (**a**) Caspase 3, (**b**) caspase 7, (**c**) caspase 8. Data in scatter plot are shown as mean ± SD. *t*-test was performed to find out significant difference between the two groups. **** denotes $p \leq 0.0001$.

3.9. Crusted Scabies Alters Immune Response

Effect of *S. scabiei* infestation on the concentration of immunoglobulins and the level of cytokines were evaluated. Significantly higher concentrations of serum IgA, IgG, and IgM were detected in the infested group as compared to those of the control group (Figure 9a–c). Up-regulation of pro-inflammatory cytokines (IL-2, IL-6, IL-12, IL-1β, and IFN-γ) and anti-inflammatory cytokine IL-4 were detected in the infested group than the control group (Figure 9d–j). On the other hand, no significant difference in IL-8 concentration between the two groups was detected (Figure 9g).

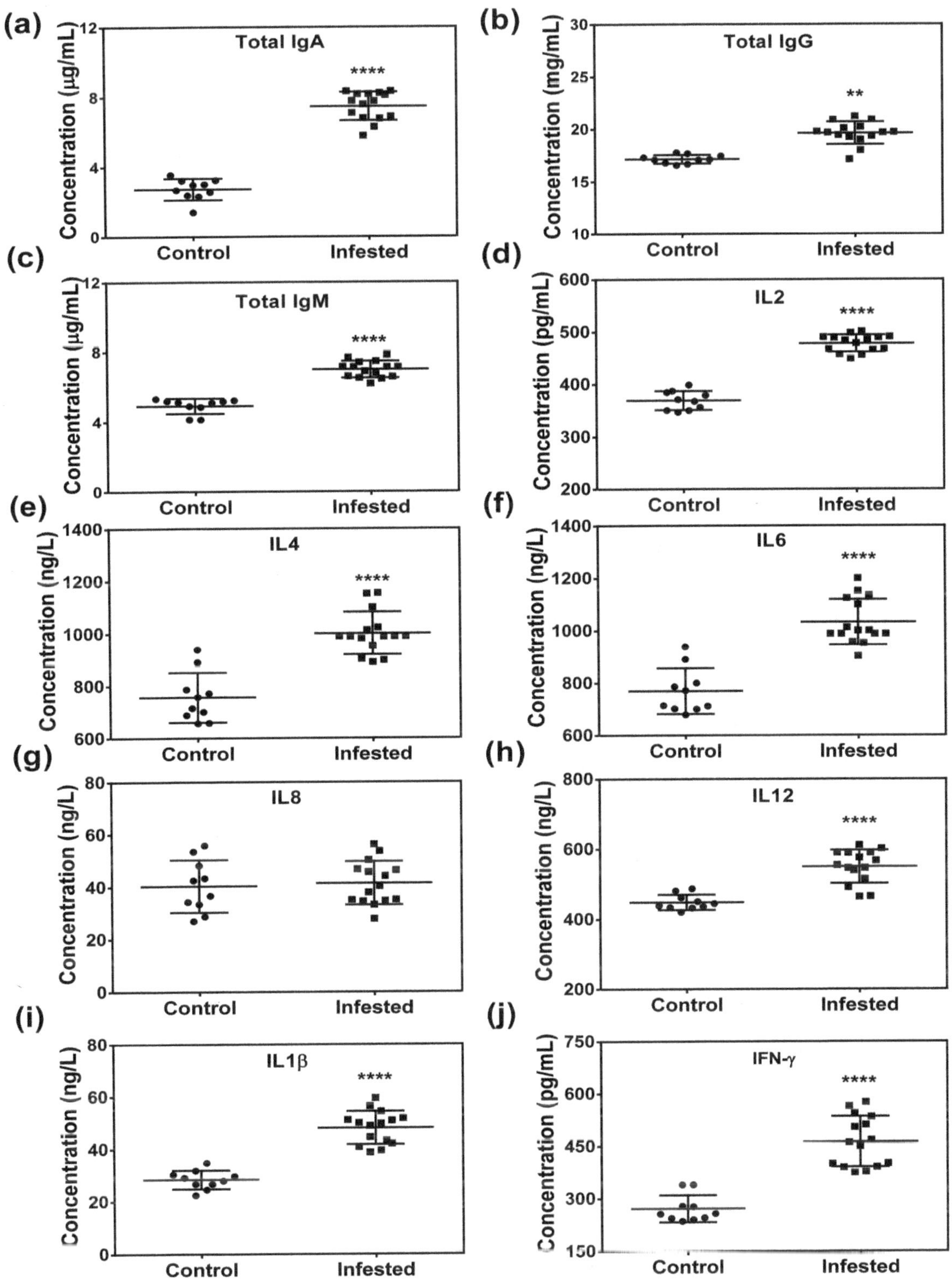

Figure 9. Effect of crusted scabieson total serum immunoglobulins and cytokine response in a porcine model. (**a**) Total IgA, (**b**) total IgG, (**c**) total IgM, (**d**) IL-2, (**e**) IL-4, (**f**) IL-6, (**g**) IL-8, (**h**) IL-12, (**i**) IL-1β, and (**j**) IFN-γ. Data in scatter plot are shown as mean ± SD. *t*-test was performed to find out significant difference between the two groups. ** denotes $p \leq 0.01$, **** denotes $p \leq 0.0001$.

3.10. Histopathology

Parakeratotic hyperkeratosis characterized by thickening of the stratum corneum and the presence of nuclei was observed. Mite with its exoskeleton and remnants were detected in the tunnel of stratum corneum of the epidermis and appeared as a cleft in the upper epidermis. Epidermis exhibited acanthosis and spongiosis associated with dense eosinophilic dermal infiltrate. Superficial perivascular or diffuse infiltrate of lymphocytes and histiocytes, accompanied by neutrophils and eosinophils were evident in the dermis. There was psoriasiform hyperplasia characterized by epidermal projections into the dermis for interdigitaion with dermal papillae. Excessive production of squames suggested crust formation (Figure 10).

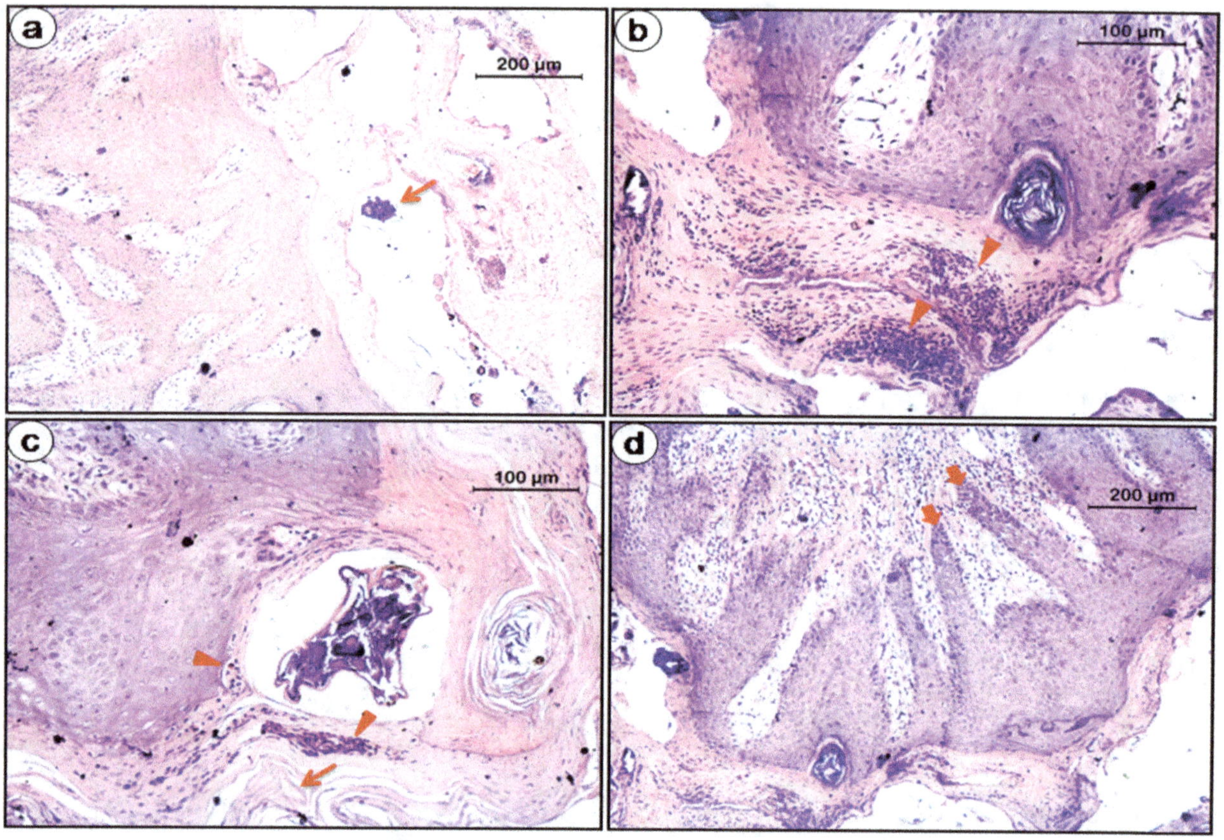

Figure 10. Histopathology of infested skin (**a**) Mite (arrow) with its exoskeleton and remnants prevailed in the tunnel of stratum cornium of epidermis (original magnification 100×, scale bar: 200 μm), (**b**,**c**) Parakeratotic hyperkeratosis characterized by upsurge in the thickness of the stratum corneum and excessive production of squames (arrow) followed by infiltration (arrow head) into epidermis suggested crust formation. There was infiltration of cells especially eosinophils (arrow head) into epidermis and dermal vascular area causing dermatitis (original magnification 200×, scale bar: 100 μm), (**d**) Psoriasiform hyperplasia: Note the epidermal projections (block arrow) into the dermis for interdigitaion with dermal papillae (original magnification 100×, scale bar: 200 μm).

4. Discussion

Scabies is considered a disease of resource-poor communities of underdeveloped and developing countries and a neglected tropical disease [46]. Wide host range and presence of different varieties necessitate differential identification for epidemiological study and for designing eradication strategy. *S. scabiei* infestation in multiple hosts including humans, companion animals, farm animals, lab animals, and wild animals throughout the globe points toward pathogen dispersal and spillover [47,48]. Bidirectional interactions among human, animals, pathogen, and environment might be the underlying reason behind its multi-host adaptation [49]. As morphological and serological tests are not much successful at variety level identification, molecular markers have emerged as alternative differential diagnostic tools. Mitochondrial cytochrome C oxidase subunit I gene (COX1) is a well-established universal marker for species identification due to its high variability [50,51] and is being used extensively for DNA bar-coding of medically important parasites [52]. Erster et al. [34] used nuclear marker

VSSC for genetic characterization of *S. scabiei* from multiple hosts in Israel. In the present study, we used COX1 and VSSC markers for molecular characterization of the *S. scabiei* isolated from pig host. COX1 based phylogenetic tree (Figure 2a) indicated that isolates under animal clade (Clade C) were phylogenetically closer to Clade B (human isolates from Panama) than Clade A (human isolates from Hong Kong, South Korea, China, France, and Australia). In general, human isolates of *S. scabiei* are heterogeneous in nature, and proximity of Clade B and Clade C may be due to low gene flow between mites of those groups [53]. COX1 and VSSC based phylogenetic study could not distinguish host or geographical specific isolates belonging to animal origin. Absence of host-specific cluster among animal isolates argues against the hypothesis of delineating *S. scabiei* as per host origin and provides support to the hypothesis that *S. scabiei* from different hosts and different geographical location arose from a single speciation event [16,54,55]. Evolution of different varieties in different hosts might be due to mitochondrial capture or selective sweep phenomenon which is considered as the driving force behind uniparental inheritance [56]. This hypothesis has been proposed as the adaptation of *Sarcoptes* in different marsupials in Australia [48]. Moreover, parasites with low independent dispersal capacities face strong population bottlenecks; under such situations they lower their genetic diversity to maintain their adaptive potential [57,58]. This might explain the low genetic diversity in *S. scabiei* among animal isolates.

S. scabiei is a contagious disease with a broad host range of more than 100 species and its effects across species are generally conserved [59]. Therefore, it is reasonable to assume that understanding the changes in one host may have significance in other hosts [60]. In recent years, pigs have gained popularity as a biomedical model in translational research due to its anatomical and physiological similarity with humans [61,62]. Close resemblance between human and pig in clinical manifestation and disease progression of *S. scabiei* [63,64] underscore the importance of porcine model in understanding host-parasite interactions of scabies/mange. The present study showed marked changes in serum biochemical parameters, lipid profiles, stress parameters, oxidant/antioxidant balance, and immune parameters following crusted scabies in a porcine model.

Increased ALT, AST, ALP, LDH, CK, and decreased albumin and glucose levels in infested animals indicate organ damage, especially compromised liver function [65]. Oxidative stress has been associated with cell necrosis and apoptosis through activation of several cell signaling pathways such as JNK, mitogen-activated protein kinase (MAPK) leading to cellular and organ damage [66,67]. It is a well-established fact that oxidative stress causes liver injury [68] as the liver is a major target organ of ROS [69]. Moreover, free radicals, especially ROS catalyze the oxidation of LDL to generate oxidized LDL and oxidized LDL also promotes cellular apoptosis in different organs [67,70]. In the present study, crusted scabies induced oxidative stress in pigs which might have detrimental effects on organs including the liver. Oxidative stress-induced organ damage might explain elevated levels of AST, ALT, and alkaline phosphatase. Alteration in the biochemical parameters was also reported in sarcoptic mange affected goats and dogs [37,38,71]. As the liver is the major organ for albumin synthesis and glucose generation through gluconeogenesis and glucogenolysis [72], impaired liver function may attribute low levels of glucose and albumin in infested animals. In addition, high ROS has been reported to impair insulin signaling [73,74] causing an increase in insulin secretion; which might be another reason for low glucose concentration in infested animals. On the contrary, up regulation in globulin production in infested animals might be due to the production of antibodies against *S. scabiei* antigens [38]. Low glucose and albumin and high globulin were also reported in Sarcoptes-infested goats [37] and dogs [38].

Abnormal blood lipid metabolites including elevated TC, LDLc, and TG were detected in infested animals than control animals. Imbalance in lipid metabolites is considered to be a predisposing cause of atherosclerosis and cardiovascular disorders [75]. In the present study, atherogenic dyslipidemia associated with high CRF and AI values in infested animals is an indicator of their susceptibility towards cardiovascular diseases. Imbalance in lipid metabolism is associated with many dermatological disorders especially chronic inflammatory skin diseases such as psoriasis, litchen planus, granuloma annulare, and histiocytosis [76]. Chronic inflammation in animals with crusted scabies may explain the abnormal lipid profiles. Moreover, oxidative stress which was also observed in the present study induced production of TNF-Alpha by Kupffer cells, which might induce inflammation [68]. Increased levels of pro-inflammatory cytokines following infestation might be the underlying cause behind dyslipidemia [76]. Increased serum levels of pro-inflammatory cytokines such as IL-2, IL-6, IL-12, IL-1β, and IFN-γ in infested animals were detected in the present study. Pro-inflammatory cytokines such as IL-6, IFN-γ inhibit the activity of lipoprotein lipase (LPL) [77] which hampers the clearance of VLDL and LDL cholesterol [78,79] leading to their increased concentration in blood. Moreover, crusted scabies induced oxidative stress in animals, and under oxidative stress, ROS induced activation of atherogenic genes via NF-kappa B [67] may further explain the atherogenic dyslipidemia in infested animals. In addition, alopecia due to infestation results in disruption of pelt-environment interface which in turn hampers thermoregulation as excessive heat loss to the environment occurs through the skin. This creates a negative energy balance to the host [60]. Mobilization of fat from fat stores to meet the energy deficiency may induce imbalance in lipid profile. An imbalance in fatty acid composition in adipose tissue with up-regulated omega-6 acids and down-regulated omega-3 acids in *S. scabiei* infested wombat host was reported [60]. The results of the study indicate that crusted scabies may shift lipid profile towards atherogenic dyslipidemia with high susceptibility towards cardiovascular disorder.

We determined the serum concentration of cortisol which is considered a biomarker of stress. The study found a significant increase in serum cortisol concentration in infested animals than control animals which indicated that infestation triggered stress response. Hypothalamic-pituitary-adrenal (HPA) axis, an important hormonal regulator of stress, is thought to be involved in the production of cortisol hormone [80]. In stressful conditions, activation of HPA axis followed by elevated plasma cortisol level is an adaptive response of the host [81]. HSPs are constitutively produced in normal physiological conditions whereas stress of any kind including environmental stress, viral infection, glucose deprivation, exposure of toxins, and oxidative stress induce over-expression of HSPs or cell-stress proteins [82]. HSPs are a classic example of proteins with 'moonlighting functions' [83] as they are involved in a number of physiological functions. Besides acting as chaperone and protein folding, involvement of HSPs in immune function such as antigen processing and presentation, expression of innate receptors and stimulation of innate immunity is well documented [84]. Moreover, HSPs, especially HSP70 and 27 play vital roles in stress-induced DNA repair by modulating DNA-repair enzymes, thus maintaining genome integrity [84]. Stress up-regulates the intracellular production of HSPs and they are released into the circulation following a non-classical secretion pathway [85]. In the present study, crusted scabies induced cellular and oxidative stress which in turn might have stimulated over-expression of HSPs. Thus, HSP orchestrated activation of heat shock response is an adaptation mechanism under stress [86]. Oxidative stress shifts the intracellular environment towards the oxidative state which in turn disturbs the protein native conformation and proteins lose their folded structure [86]. HSPs act as sensors to cellular redox changes both in prokaryotes and in eukaryotes; then give signals for activation of the heat stress response [86]. HSP70 and HSP90 act as the primary sensors of protein misfolding. Moreover, HSP27 has been reported to act as an antioxidant by preventing oxidation of glutathione under oxidative stress [87]. HSP70 and HSP90 act as anti-apoptotic proteins; they exert their role by binding to apoptosis protease activity factor 1 (Apaf-1) blocking downstream cascades of apoptosis pathway [88,89]. In the present study, the infested animals under oxidative stress might have induced cellular apoptosis. This is supported by the up-regulation of serum levels of apoptotic markers in infested animals. The up-regulation of HSPs in infested animals might be an adaptation mechanism to prevent cellular apoptosis.

Oxidative stress has been reported to be involved in the pathogenesis of several diseases including parasitic infections [90]. Cellular metabolism produces reactive oxygen species (ROS) and reactive nitrogen species (RNS) [91]. At a low to moderate level, they are involved in several physiological functions including cell signaling as well as immune functions [92]. On the contrary, at a high level, they cause damage to molecules including lipids, proteins, lipoproteins, and nucleic acids starting a chain reaction of free radical formation leading to a condition known as oxidative stress [93,94]. Therefore, tight regulation in production of ROS and RNS and delicate balance between beneficial and detrimental effects is vital for cellular homeostasis. Under oxidative stress, the antioxidant defense system elicits several antioxidant enzymes to fight against free radicals and maintain homeostasis. Superoxide dismutase, catalase, and glutathione peroxidase act as first-line defense antioxidants to suppress or prevent the formation of reactive species in cells [95]. SOD catalyzed the conversion of O_2^- into H_2O_2 which is further reduced to H_2O and O_2 by either catalase or glutathione peroxidase [96]. In the present study, it was observed that crusted scabies caused an increase in the production of serum total NO in pigs. Though we did not measure ROS, oxidative stress induction in infested animals was evident from the reduction of total antioxidant capacity, activity of catalase, SOD, and concentration of GSH as well as an increase in MDA concentration as compared to control animals. The down-regulation of T-AOC and antioxidant enzymes indicate that they have been over-consumed to tackle oxidative stress [97]. The results of our study are in agreement with the report of Beighet al. [98], in which decreased catalase and GSH in dogs suffering from dermatophytosis was reported. A decrease in antioxidant enzyme activities was also reported in buffaloes infested by sarcoptic mange [99] and in sheep, which was suffering from psoroptic mange [100]. Increased MDA concentration in infested animals indicated oxidative injury. Cell membranes with a rich store of polyunsaturated fatty acids are excellent targets for free radical attacks [101] and oxidation of lipid molecules induce production of MDA [102]. So, MDA, the end product of lipid peroxidation, is considered as a hallmark of oxidative damage [103]. In the present study, increased MDA concentration in infested animals might be associated with cellular damage. An increase in skin MDA in *S. scabiei* infested dogs were reported by Nwufoh et al. [104].

S. scabiei infestation is associated with modulation of various parameters of host immune responses; humoral, adaptive, and inflammatory immune responses [31,33]. IgA, IgG, and IgM are the major immunoglobulins associated with humoral immunity. IgM is produced at the early stage of antibody response against a foreign antigen. IgG, being the most abundant antibody in blood and extracellular fluid, is involved in systemic immune response. IgA is generally associated with mucosal immunity and primarily found in secretions [105]. In the present study, up-regulation of total IgA, IgG, and IgM in infested pigs than the control group was observed. Elevated levels of immuniglobulins in infested animals indicated that mite had elicited antibody-mediated immune response against mite antigens although it was not possible to know whether or not the antibody response was *S. scabiei* specific. Up-regulation of total IgG might be a consequence of secondary bacterial infection which is very common in scabies infestation. Increased IgG in *S. scabiei* infested rabbits, dogs [21,106], and human [107] was reported. Elevated levels of circulatory IgA were reported in human crusted scabies [107].

We further assessed the systemic inflammatory response of the animals by determining serum levels of pro-inflammatory cytokines including IL-1β, IL-2, IL-6, IL-12, and IFN-γ and anti-inflammatory cytokine IL-4. Cytokines play key roles in the host immune and inflammatory responses as well as in the maintenance of tissue integrity [108]. The present study recorded dysregulation of cytokine balance which might be due to modulation of immunity by *S. scabiei* released antigens. Th1 and Th2 are the two major subpopulations of T helper cells and parasitic infections are associated with either Th1 or Th2 polarized immune response [109]. IL-2, TNF-β, and IFN-γ are Th1 cells specific cytokines whereas Th2 cells release IL-4, IL-5, IL-10, and IL-13 as signature cytokines [110]. Naïve helper T cells (Th0) can be differentiated to either Th1 or Th2 based on distinct activation pathways; cytokines such as IFN-γ andIL-12 activates Th0 to Th1 cells, otherwise, IL-10 and IL-4 are crucial stimulatory cytokines for Th2 cell polarization [111]. Intricate balance among different cytokines is crucial for homeostasis of mammalian species and imbalance may pose threat to health [112]. In the present study, *S. scabiei* infestation was associated with up-regulation of IL-2, IFN-γ, IL-1β, and IL-4 indicating both Th1 and Th2 response. The most probable cause of the mixed Th1/Th2 response might be dysregulation of cytokine balance due to modulation of immunity by *S. scabiei* released antigens or changes of cytokine levels after a chronic infection. Th1 immune response is generally associated with protection in most infectious diseases whereas Th2 immune response elicits high titers of antibody production and cell-mediated inflammation [113]. Moreover, allergic inflammatory diseases are dominated by Th2 immune response [6]. Induction of mixed Th1/Th2 immune response in the current study indicates that the immune response to mange infestation is complex and local immune response analysis is necessary for a better understanding of the disease. Th2 response had been described as a predominant immune response in crusted scabies and other allergic inflammatory disorders [6]. Bioactive compounds in arthropod saliva trigger different immune response to host. Low molecular weight salivary components cannot act as antigen but can bind to skin proteins as haptens and stimulate Th1 response. Some salivary antigens may cause basophil hypersensitivity (Th1 response) by binding to epidermal langerhans cells. Salivary antigens also may trigger Th2 response in association with IgE production and type I hypersensitivity [107].

The histopathological findings in the study mimic the classical narrative of sarcoptic mange in mammalian species [3]. Antigenic materials including excretion and secretions of mites trigger hypersensitivity reactions in the skin [114] which might be the reason behind eosinophilia observed in the infested animals. Our observations are consistent with those in vulpes [115], racoon dog [116], wombats [117] and Iberian ibex [118].

5. Conclusions

This communication is the first report on genetic characterization of *S. scabiei* from India. Mitochondrial (COX1) or nuclear (VSSC) based markers could not distinguish *S. scabiei* at a variety level especially for animal isolates which suggests that delineating varieties based on host origin is not warranted. The study contributes to the rich pool of knowledge on the consequences of crusted scabies on host physiology. We could establish a new connection showing that mange infestation results in an atherogenic dyslipidemia in the host.

Author Contributions: Conceptualization, A.K.D. and S.S.; methodology, A.K.D., S.S., P.P., S.M., S.K.R., G.S. and K.M.; software, A.K.D. and S.B.; validation, D.M. and A.K.; formal analysis, A.K.D. and A.K.B.; investigation, A.K.T., D.B., G.S., and A.K.D.; resources, A.K.D., D.B. and A.K.; data curation, A.K.D.; writing—original draft preparation, A.K.D.; writing—review and editing, D.B.; visualization, D.B.; supervision, S.B.; project administration, A.K.D.; funding acquisition, A.K.D. All authors have read and agreed to the published version of the manuscript.

Acknowledgments: The authors acknowledge the Director, ICAR-Central Island Agricultural Research Institute (CIARI), Port Blair, Andaman and Nicobar Islands, India for providing all the necessary facilities to carry out the present study.

References

1. Heukelbach, J.; Wilcke, T.; Winter, B.; Feldmeier, H. Epidemiology and morbidity of scabies and *pediculosis capitis* in resource-poor communities in Brazil. *Br. J. Dermatol.* **2005**, *153*, 150–156. [CrossRef] [PubMed]
2. Alasaad, S.; Rossi, L.; Heukelbach, J.; Pérez, J.M.; Hamarsheh, O.; Otiende, M.; Zhu, X.Q. The neglected navigating web of the incomprehensibly emerging and re-emerging *Sarcoptes* mite. *Infect. Genet. Evol.* **2013**, *17*, 253–259. [CrossRef] [PubMed]

3. Bornstein, S.; Morner, T.; Samuel, W.M. Sarcoptesscabiei and sarcoptic mange. In *Parasitic Diseases of Wild Mammals*, 2nd ed.; Samuel, W.M., Pybus, M.J., Kocan, A.A., Eds.; Manson Publishing: London, UK, 2001; pp. 107–119.
4. Walton, S.F.; Currie, B.J. Problems in diagnosing scabies, a global disease in human and animal populations. *Clin. Microbiol. Rev.* **2007**, *20*, 268–279. [CrossRef] [PubMed]
5. Dagleish, M.P.; Ali, Q.; Powell, R.K.; Butz, D.; Woodford, M.H. Fatal *Sarcoptesscabiei* infection of blue sheep (*Pseudoisnayaur*) in Pakistan. *J. Wildl. Dis.* **2007**, *43*, 512–517. [CrossRef] [PubMed]
6. Bhat, S.A.; Mounsey, K.E.; Liu, X.; Walton, S.F. Host immune responses to the itch mite, *Sarcoptesscabiei*, in humans. *Parasites Vectors* **2017**, *10*, 385. [CrossRef] [PubMed]
7. Hengge, U.R.; Currie, B.J.; Jäger, G.; Lupi, O.; Schwartz, R.A. Scabies: A ubiquitous neglected skin disease. *Lancet Infect. Dis.* **2006**, *6*, 769–779. [CrossRef]
8. Terry, B.C.; Kanjah, F.; Sahr, F.; Kortequee, S.; Dukulay, I.; Gbakima, A.A. *Sarcoptesscabiei* infestation among children in a displacement camp in Sierra Leone. *Public Health* **2001**, *115*, 208–211. [CrossRef]
9. Carapetis, J.R.; Connors, C.; Yarmirr, D.; Krause, V.; Currie, B.J. Success of a scabies control program in an Australian aboriginal community. *Pediatr. Infect. Dis. J.* **1997**, *16*, 494–499. [CrossRef]
10. Andrews, R.M.; McCarthy, J.; Carapetis, J.R.; Currie, B.J. Skin disorders, including pyoderma, scabies, and tinea infections. *Pediatr. Clin. N. Am.* **2009**, *56*, 1421–1440. [CrossRef]
11. Currie, B.J.; McCarthy, J.S. Permethrin and ivermectin for scabies. *N. Engl. J. Med.* **2010**, *362*, 717–725. [CrossRef]
12. Soulsby, E.J.L. *Helminths, Arthropods and Protozoa of Domesticated Animals*, 7th ed.; Bailliere Tindall: London, UK, 1982.
13. Walton, S.F.; Dougall, A.; Pizzutto, S.; Holt, D.; Taplin, D.; Arlian, L.G.; Morgan, M.; Currie, B.J.; Kemp, D.J. Genetic epidemiology of *Sarcoptesscabiei* (Acari: Sarcoptidae) in northern Australia. *Int. J. Parasitol.* **2004**, *34*, 839–849. [CrossRef] [PubMed]
14. Daszak, P.; Cunningham, A.A.; Hyatt, A.D. Emerging infectious diseases of wildlife—Threats to biodiversity and human health. *Science* **2000**, *287*, 443–449. [CrossRef] [PubMed]
15. Alasaad, S.; Oleaga, Á.; Casais, R.; Rossi, L.; Min, A.M.; Soriguer, R.C.; Gortázar, C. Temporal stability in the genetic structure of *Sarcoptesscabiei* under the host-taxon law: Empirical evidences from wildlife-derived *Sarcoptes* mite in Asturias, Spain. *Parasites Vectors* **2011**, *4*, 151. [CrossRef] [PubMed]
16. Berrilli, F.; D'Amelio, S.; Rossi, L. Ribosomal and mitochondrial DNA sequence variation in *Sarcoptes* mites from different hosts and geographical regions. *Parasitol. Res.* **2002**, *88*, 772–777. [CrossRef] [PubMed]
17. Menzano, A.; Rambozzi, L.; Rossi, L. Outbreak of scabies in human beings, acquired from chamois (*Rupicaprarupicapra*). *Vet. Rec.* **2004**, *155*, 568. [CrossRef]
18. Wallgren, P.; Bornstein, S. The spread of porcine sarcoptic mange during the fattening period revealed by development of antibodies to *Sarcoptesscabiei*. *Vet. Parasitol.* **1997**, *73*, 315–324. [CrossRef]
19. Fain, A. Epidemiological problems of scabies. *Int. J. Dermatol.* **1978**, *17*, 20–30. [CrossRef]
20. Alasaad, S.; Soglia, D.; Spalenza, V.; Maione, S.; Soriguer, R.C.; Pérez, J.M.; Rasero, R.; Degiorgis, M.P.; Nimmervoll, H.; Zhu, X.Q.; et al. Is ITS-2 rDNA suitable marker for genetic characterization of *Sarcoptes* mites from different wild animals in different geographic areas? *Vet. Parasitol.* **2009**, *159*, 181–185. [CrossRef]
21. Arlian, L.G.; Morgan, M.S.; Arends, J.J. Immunologic cross-reactivity among various strains of *Sarcoptesscabiei*. *J. Parasitol.* **1996**, *82*, 66–72. [CrossRef]
22. Garcia, R.; Piche, C.; Davies, P.; Gross, S. Prevalence of sarcoptic mange mites and dermatitis in slaughter pigs in North America and Western Europe. In Proceedings of the 13th Conference of the International Pig Veterinary Society, Bangkok, Thailand, 26–30 June 1994; p. 250. Available online: https://agris.fao.org/agris-search/search.do?recordID=TH2000001208 (accessed on 5 October 2020).
23. Jensen, J.C.; Nielsen, L.H.; Arnason, T.; Cracknell, V. Elimination of mange mites *Sarcoptesscabiei* var. suis from two naturally infested Danish sow herds using a single injection regime with doramectin. *Acta Vet. Scand.* **2002**, *43*, 75–84. [CrossRef]
24. Davies, P.R. Sarcoptic mange and production performance of swine: A review of the literature and studies of associations between mite infestation, growth rate and measures of mange severity in growing pigs. *Vet. Parasitol.* **1995**, *60*, 249–264. [CrossRef]
25. Arends, J.J.; Stanislaw, C.M.; Gerdon, D. Effects of sarcoptic mange on lactating swine and growing pigs. *J. Anim. Sci.* **1990**, *68*, 1495–1499. [CrossRef] [PubMed]

26. Henken, A.M.; Verstegen, M.W.A.; Van Der Hel, W.; Boon, J.H.A. Pilot study of parasite worry and restlessness caused by sarcoptic mange in swine. In Proceedings of the 10th Conference of the International Pig Veterinary Society, Rio de Janerio, Brazil, 14–17 August 1988.
27. Grahofer, A.; Bannoehr, J.; Nathues, H.; Roosje, P. *Sarcoptes* infestation in two miniature pigs with zoonotic transmission—A case report. *BMC Vet. Res.* **2018**, *14*, 91. [CrossRef] [PubMed]
28. Sokolova, T.V.; Lange, A.B. Parazito-khoziainnaiaspetsifichnost' chesotochnogozudnia *Sarcoptesscabiei* (Acariformes: Sarcoptidae) chelovekaizhivotnykh (obzorliteratury) [The parasite-host specificity of the itch mite *Sarcoptesscabiei* (Acariformes: Sarcoptidae) in man and animals (a review of the literature)]. *Parazitologiia* **1992**, *26*, 97–104.
29. Chakrabarti, A. Pig handler's itch. *Int. J. Dermatol.* **1990**, *29*, 205–206. [CrossRef]
30. Laha, R. Sarcoptic mange infestation in pigs: An overview. *J. Parasit. Dis.* **2015**, *39*, 596–603. [CrossRef]
31. Morgan, M.S.; Arlian, L.G.; Markey, M.P. *Sarcoptesscabiei* mites modulate gene expression in human skin equivalents. *PLoS ONE* **2013**, *8*, e71143. [CrossRef]
32. Mullins, J.S.; Arlian, L.G.; Morgan, M.S. Extracts of *Sarcoptesscabiei* De Geer down-modulate secretion of IL-8 by skin keratinocytes and fibroblasts and of GM-CSF by fibroblasts in the presence of proinflammatory cytokines. *J. Med. Entomol.* **2009**, *46*, 845–851. [CrossRef]
33. Cote, N.M.; Jaworski, D.C.; Wasala, N.B.; Morgan, M.S.; Arlian, L.G. Identification and expression of macrophage migration inhibitory factor in *Sarcoptesscabiei*. *Exp. Parasitol.* **2013**, *135*, 175–181. [CrossRef]
34. Erster, O.; Roth, A.; Pozzi, P.S.; Bouznach, A.; Shkap, V. First detection of *Sarcoptesscabiei* from domesticated pig (*Sus scrofa*) and genetic characterization of *S. scabiei* from pet, farm and wild hosts in Israel. *Exp. Appl. Acarol.* **2015**, *66*, 605–612. [CrossRef]
35. Morgan, M.S.; Arlian, L.G. Response of human skin equivalents to *Sarcoptesscabiei*. *J. Med. Entomol.* **2010**, *47*, 877–883. [CrossRef] [PubMed]
36. Lalli, P.N.; Morgan, M.S.; Arlian, L.G. Skewed Th1/Th2 immune response to *Sarcoptesscabiei*. *J. Parasitol.* **2004**, *90*, 711–714. [CrossRef] [PubMed]
37. De, U.K.; Dey, S. Evaluation of organ function and oxidant/antioxidant status in goats with sarcoptic mange. *Trop. Anim. Health Prod.* **2010**, *42*, 1663–1668. [CrossRef] [PubMed]
38. Beigh, S.A.; Soodan, J.S.; Bhat, A.M. Sarcoptic mange in dogs: Its effect on liver, oxidative stress, trace minerals and vitamins. *Vet. Parasitol.* **2016**, *227*, 30–34. [CrossRef]
39. Thompson, J.D.; Higgins, D.G.; Gibson, T.J. CLUSTAL W: Improving the sensitivity of progressive multiple sequence alignment through sequence weighting, position-specific gap penalties and weight matrix choice. *Nucleic Acids Res.* **1994**, *22*, 4673–4680. [CrossRef] [PubMed]
40. Kumar, S.; Stecher, G.; Li, M.; Knyaz, C.; Tamura, K. MEGA X: Molecular Evolutionary Genetics Analysis across Computing Platforms. *Mol. Biol. Evol.* **2018**, *35*, 1547–1549. [CrossRef]
41. Tamura, K.; Nei, M. Estimation of the number of nucleotide substitutions in the control region of mitochondrial DNA in humans and chimpanzees. *Mol. Biol. Evol.* **1993**, *10*, 512–526. [CrossRef]
42. Bandelt, H.J.; Forster, P.; Röhl, A. Median-joining networks for inferring intraspecific phylogenies. *Mol. Biol. Evol.* **1999**, *16*, 37–48. [CrossRef]
43. Yu, I.T.; Ju, C.C.; Lin, J.; Wu, H.L.; Yen, H.T. Effects of probiotics and selenium combination on the immune and blood cholesterol concentration of pigs. *J. Anim. Feed Sci.* **2004**, *13*, 625–634. [CrossRef]
44. Marbut, M.M.; Majeed, B.M.; Rahim, S.M.; Yuusif, M.Y. Estimation of malondialdehyde as oxidative factor and glutathione as early detectors of hypertensive pregnant women. *Tikrit Med. J.* **2009**, *15*, 63–69.
45. Campbell, J.M.; Crenshaw, J.D.; Polo, J. The biological stress of early weaned piglets. *J. Anim. Sci. Biotechnol.* **2013**, *4*, 19. [CrossRef] [PubMed]
46. Steer, A. Scabies Joins the List of WHO Neglected Tropical Diseases. Lancet Global Health Blog. Global Health Blogs. 2014. Available online: http://globalhealth.thelancet.com/2014/07/07/scabies-joins-list-who-neglected-tropical-diseases (accessed on 3 October 2020).
47. Mounsey, K.E.; McCarthy, J.S.; Walton, S.F. Scratching the itch: New tools to advance understanding of scabies. *Trends Parasitol.* **2013**, *29*, 35–42. [CrossRef] [PubMed]
48. Fraser, T.A.; Shao, R.; Fountain-Jones, N.M.; Charleston, M.; Martin, A.; Whiteley, P.; Holme, R.; Carver, S.; Polkinghorne, A. Mitochondrial genome sequencing reveals potential origins of the scabies mite *Sarcoptesscabiei* infesting two iconic Australian marsupials. *BMC Evol. Biol.* **2017**, *17*, 233. [CrossRef]

49. Alexander, K.A.; Carlson, C.J.; Lewis, B.L.; Getz, W.M.; Marathe, M.V.; Eubank, S.G.; Sanderson, C.E.; Blackburn, J.K. The Ecology of pathogen spillover and disease emergence at the human-wildlife-environment interface. In *The Connections between Ecology and Infectious Disease*; Advances in Environmental Microbiology; Hurst, C., Ed.; Springer: Cham, Switzerland, 2018; Volume 5, pp. 267–298.
50. Mandal, S.D.; Chhakchhuak, L.; Gurusubramanian, G.; Kumar, N.S. Mitochondrial markers for identification and phylogenetic studies in insects—A Review. *DNA Barcodes* **2014**, *2*, 1–9. [CrossRef]
51. Pentinsaari, M.; Salmela, H.; Mutanen, M.; Roslin, T. Molecular evolution of a widely-adopted taxonomic marker (COI) across the animal tree of life. *Sci. Rep.* **2016**, *6*, 35275. [CrossRef] [PubMed]
52. Ondrejicka, D.A.; Locke, S.A.; Morey, K.; Borisenko, A.V.; Hanner, R.H. Status and prospects of DNA barcoding in medically important parasites and vectors. *Trends Parasitol.* **2014**, *30*, 582–591. [CrossRef]
53. Andriantsoanirina, V.; Ariey, F.; Izri, A.; Bernigaud, C.; Fang, F.; Charrel, R.; Foulet, F.; Botterel, F.; Guillot, J.; Chosidow, O.; et al. *Sarcoptesscabiei* mites in humans are distributed into three genetically distinct clades. *Clin. Microbiol. Infect.* **2015**, *21*, 1107–1114. [CrossRef]
54. Zahler, M.; Essig, A.; Gothe, R.; Rinder, H. Molecular analyses suggest monospecificity of the genus *Sarcoptes* (Acari: Sarcoptidae). *Int. J. Parasitol.* **1999**, *29*, 759–766. [CrossRef]
55. Gu, X.B.; Yang, G.Y. A study on the genetic relationship of mites in the genus *Sarcoptes* (Acari: Sarcoptidae) in China. *Int. J. Acarol.* **2008**, *34*, 183–190. [CrossRef]
56. Christie, J.R.; Beekman, M. Selective sweeps of mitochondrial DNA can drive the evolution of uniparental inheritance. *Evolution* **2017**, *71*, 2090–2099. [CrossRef]
57. Gandon, S. Local adaptation and the geometry of host–parasite coevolution. *Ecol. Lett.* **2002**, *5*, 246–256. [CrossRef]
58. Appelgren, A.S.C.; Saladin, V.; Richner, H.; Doligez, B.; McCoy, K.D. Gene flow and adaptive potential in a generalist ectoparasite. *BMC Evol. Biol.* **2018**, *18*, 99. [CrossRef] [PubMed]
59. Arlian, L.G.; Morgan, M.S. A review of *Sarcoptesscabiei*: Past, present and future. *Parasites Vectors* **2017**, *10*, 297. [CrossRef] [PubMed]
60. Martin, A.M.; Fraser, T.A.; Lesku, J.A.; Simpson, K.; Roberts, G.L.; Garvey, J.; Polkinghorne, A.; Burridge, C.P.; Carver, S. The cascading pathogenic consequences of *Sarcoptesscabiei* infection that manifest in host disease. *R. Soc. Open Sci.* **2018**, *5*, 180018. [CrossRef] [PubMed]
61. Prather, R.S.; Walters, E.M.; Wells, K.D. Swine in Biomedical Research 2014. *Lab Anim.* **2014**, *44*, 9. [CrossRef]
62. Monticello, T.M.; Haschek, W.M. Swine in translational research and drug development. *Toxicol. Pathol.* **2016**, *44*, 297–298. [CrossRef]
63. Mounsey, K.; Ho, M.F.; Kelly, A.; Willis, C.; Pasay, C.; Kemp, D.J.; McCarthy, J.S.; Fischer, K. A tractable experimental model for study of human and animal scabies. *PLoS Negl. Trop. Dis.* **2010**, *4*, e756. [CrossRef]
64. Rampton, M.; Walton, S.F.; Holt, D.C.; Pasay, C.; Kelly, A.; Currie, B.J.; McCarthy, J.S.; Mounsey, K.E. Antibody responses to *Sarcoptesscabiei* apolipoprotein in a porcine model: Relevance to immunodiagnosis of recent infection. *PLoS ONE* **2013**, *8*, e65354. [CrossRef]
65. Giannini, E.G.; Testa, R.; Savarino, V. Liver enzyme alteration: A guide for clinicians. *CMAJ* **2005**, *172*, 367–379. [CrossRef]
66. Quinn, M.T.; Parthasarathy, S.; Fong, L.G.; Steinberg, D. Oxidatively modified low density lipoproteins: A potential role in recruitment and retention of monocyte/macrophages during atherogenesis. *Proc. Natl. Acad. Sci. USA* **1987**, *84*, 2995–2998. [CrossRef]
67. Ogura, S.; Shimosawa, T. Oxidative stress and organ damages. *Curr. Hypertens Rep.* **2014**, *16*, 452. [CrossRef] [PubMed]
68. Li, S.; Tan, H.Y.; Wang, N.; Zhang, Z.; Lao, L.; Wong, C.; Feng, Y. The role of oxidative stress and antioxidants in liver diseases. *Int. J. Mol. Sci.* **2015**, *16*, 26087–26124. [CrossRef] [PubMed]
69. Sánchez-Valle, V.; Chávez-Tapia, N.C.; Uribe, M.; Méndez-Sánchez, N. Role of oxidative stress and molecular changes in liver fibrosis: A review. *Curr. Med. Chem.* **2012**, *19*, 4850–4860. [CrossRef] [PubMed]
70. Ogura, S.; Kakino, A.; Sato, Y.; Fujita, Y.; Iwamoto, S.; Otsui, K.; Yoshimoto, R.; Sawamura, T. Lox-1: The multifunctional receptor underlying cardiovascular dysfunction. *Circ. J.* **2009**, *73*, 1993–1999. [CrossRef] [PubMed]
71. Sharma, S.K.; Soodan, J.S.; Sharma, N. Haemato-biochemical alterations in canine dermatitis. *Indian Vet. J.* **2011**, *88*, 56–58.

72. Han, H.S.; Kang, G.; Kim, J.S.; Choi, B.H.; Koo, S.H. Regulation of glucose metabolism from a liver-centric perspective. *Exp. Mol. Med.* **2016**, *48*, e218. [CrossRef] [PubMed]
73. Ogihara, T.; Asano, T.; Katagiri, H.; Sakoda, H.; Anai, M.; Shojima, N.; Ono, H.; Fujishiro, M.; Kushiyama, A.; Fukushima, Y.; et al. Oxidative stress induces insulin resistance by activating the nuclear factor-kappa B pathway and disrupting normal subcellular distribution of phosphatidylinositol 3-kinase. *Diabetologia* **2004**, *47*, 794–805. [CrossRef]
74. Fridlyand, L.E.; Philipson, L.H. Reactive species and early manifestation of insulin resistance in type 2 diabetes. *Diabetes Obes. Metab.* **2006**, *8*, 136–145. [CrossRef]
75. Misra, A.; Luthra, K.; Vikram, N.K. Dyslipidemia in Asian Indians: Determinants and significance. *J. Assoc. Physicians India* **2004**, *52*, 137–142.
76. Shenoy, C.; Shenoy, M.M.; Rao, G.K. Dyslipidemia in dermatological disorders. *N. Am. J. Med. Sci.* **2015**, *7*, 421–428. [CrossRef]
77. Hahn, B.H.; Grossman, J.; Chen, W.; McMahon, M. The pathogenesis of atherosclerosis in autoimmune rheumatic diseases: Roles of inflammation and dyslipidemia. *J. Autoimmun.* **2007**, *28*, 69–75. [CrossRef] [PubMed]
78. Kobashigawa, J.A.; Kasiske, B.L. Hyperlipidemia in solid organ transplantation. *Transplantation* **1997**, *63*, 331–338. [CrossRef] [PubMed]
79. Derfler, K.; Hayde, M.; Heinz, G.; Hirschl, M.M.; Steger, G.; Hauser, A.C.; Balcke, P.; Widhalm, K. Decreased postheparin lipolytic activity in renal transplant recipients with cyclosporin A. *Kidney Int.* **1991**, *40*, 720–727. [CrossRef] [PubMed]
80. Stephens, M.A.; Wand, G. Stress and the HPA axis: Role of glucocorticoids in alcohol dependence. *Alcohol Res.* **2012**, *34*, 468–483.
81. Li, L.A.; Yang, J.J.; Li, Y.; Lv, L.; Xie, J.J.; Du, G.M.; Jin, T.M.; Qin, S.Y.; Jiao, X.L. Effect of weaning age on cortisol release in piglets. *Genet. Mol. Res.* **2016**, *15*, 1–10. [CrossRef]
82. Pockley, A.G.; Henderson, B. Extracellular cell stress (heat shock) proteins-immune responses and disease: An overview. *Philos. Trans. R. Soc. Lond. B Biol. Sci.* **2018**, *373*, 20160522. [CrossRef]
83. Campbell, R.M.; Scanes, C.G. Endocrine peptides 'moonlighting' as immune modulators: Roles for somatostatin and GH-releasing factor. *J. Endocrinol.* **1995**, *147*, 383–396. [CrossRef]
84. Bolhassani, A.; Agi, E. Heat shock proteins in infection. *Clin. Chim. Acta* **2019**, *498*, 90–100. [CrossRef]
85. Pockley, A.G.; Bulmer, J.; Hanks, B.M.; Wright, B.H. Identification of human heat shock protein 60 (Hsp60) and anti-Hsp60 antibodies in the peripheral circulation of normal individuals. *Cell Stress Chaperones* **1999**, *4*, 29–35. [CrossRef]
86. Kalmar, B.; Greensmith, L. Induction of heat shock proteins for protection against oxidative stress. *Adv. Drug Deliv. Rev.* **2009**, *61*, 310–318. [CrossRef]
87. Arrigo, A.P. The cellular "networking" of mammalian Hsp27 and its functions in the control of protein folding, redox state and apoptosis. *Adv. Exp. Med. Biol.* **2007**, *594*, 14–26. [CrossRef] [PubMed]
88. Yuan, J.; Murrell, G.A.; Trickett, A.; Wang, M.X. Involvement of cytochrome c release and caspase-3 activation in the oxidative stress-induced apoptosis in human tendon fibroblasts. *Biochim. Biophys. Acta* **2003**, *1641*, 35–41. [CrossRef]
89. Annunziato, L.; Amoroso, S.; Pannaccione, A.; Cataldi, M.; Pignataro, G.; D'Alessio, A.; Sirabella, R.; Secondo, A.; Sibaud, L.; Di Renzo, G.F. Apoptosis induced in neuronal cells by oxidative stress: Role played by caspases and intracellular calcium ions. *Toxicol. Lett.* **2003**, *139*, 125–133. [CrossRef]
90. Ellah, M.R.A. Involvement of free radicals in parasitic infestations. *J. Appl. Anim. Res.* **2013**, *41*, 69–76. [CrossRef]
91. Birben, E.; Sahiner, U.M.; Sackesen, C.; Erzurum, S.; Kalayci, O. Oxidative stress and antioxidant defense. *World Allergy Organ.* **2012**, *5*, 9–19. [CrossRef]
92. Valko, M.; Leibfritz, D.; Moncol, J.; Cronin, M.T.D.; Mazur, M.; Telser, J. Free radicals and antioxidants in normal physiological functions and human disease. *Int. J. Biochem. Cell Biol.* **2007**, *39*, 44–84. [CrossRef]
93. Nordberg, J.; Arnér, E.S.J. Reactive oxygen species, antioxidants, and the mammalian thioredoxin system. *Free Radic. Biol. Med.* **2001**, *31*, 1287–1312. [CrossRef]
94. Phaniendra, A.; Jestadi, D.B.; Periyasamy, L. Free Radicals: Properties, sources, targets, and their implication in various diseases. *Indian J. Clin. Biochem.* **2015**, *30*, 11–26. [CrossRef]

95. Kurutas, E.B. The importance of antioxidants which play the role in cellular response against oxidative/nitrosative stress: Current state. *Nutr. J.* **2016**, *15*, 71. [CrossRef]
96. Griendling, K.K.; FitzGerald, G.A. Oxidative stress and cardiovascular injury: Part I: Basic mechanisms and in vivo monitoring of ROS. *Circulation* **2003**, *108*, 1912–1916. [CrossRef]
97. Beigh, S.A.; Soodan, J.S.; Nazki, S.; Khan, A.M. Oxidative stress, hematobiochemical parameters, trace elements and vitamins in dogs with zinc responsive dermatosis. *VeterinarskiArhiv* **2014**, *84*, 591–600.
98. Beigh, S.A.; Soodan, J.S.; Singh, R.; Khan, A.M.; Dar, M.A. Evaluation of trace elements, oxidant/antioxidative status, vitamin C and β-carotene in dogs with dermatophytosis. *Mycoses* **2014**, *57*, 358–365. [CrossRef]
99. Dimri, U.; Sharma, M.C.; Swarup, D.; Ranjan, R.; Kataria, M. Alterations in hepatic lipid peroxides and antioxidant profile in Indian water buffaloes suffering from sarcoptic mange. *Res. Vet. Sci.* **2008**, *85*, 101105. [CrossRef] [PubMed]
100. Dimri, U.; Sharma, M.C.; Yamdagni, A.; Ranjan, R.; Zama, M.M.S. Psoroptic mange infestation increases oxidative stress and decreases antioxidant status in sheep. *Vet. Parasitol.* **2010**, *68*, 318322. [CrossRef] [PubMed]
101. Brand, A.; Bauer, N.G.; Hallott, A.; Goldbaum, O.; Ghebremeskel, K.; Reifen, R.; Richter-Landsberg, C. Membrane lipid modification by polyunsaturated fatty acids sensitizes oligodendroglial OLN-93 cells against oxidative stress and promotes up-regulation of heme oxygenase-1 (HSP32). *J. Neurochem.* **2010**, *113*, 465–476. [CrossRef] [PubMed]
102. Ardestani, A.; Yazdanparast, R. Antioxidant and free radical scavenging potential of *Achillea santolina* extracts. *Food Chem.* **2007**, *104*, 21–29. [CrossRef]
103. DelRio, D.; Stewart, A.J.; Pellegrini, N. A review of recent studies on malondialdehyde as toxic molecule and biological marker of oxidative stress. *Nutr. Metab. Cardiovasc. Dis.* **2005**, *15*, 316–328. [CrossRef]
104. Nwufoh, O.C.; Sadiq, N.A.; Emikpe, B.O.; Omobowale, T. Assessment of cutaneous and serum oxidative stress changes in dogs infested with *Sarcoptesscabiei* var. *Canis. Acta Vet. Eurasia* **2020**, *46*, 1–6. [CrossRef]
105. Luo, Q.; Cui, H.; Peng, X.; Fang, J.; Zuo, Z.; Deng, J.; Liu, J.; Deng, Y. Intestinal IgA+ cell numbers as well as IgA, IgG, and IgM contents correlate with mucosal humoral immunity of broilers during supplementation with high fluorine in the diets. *Biol. Trace Elem. Res.* **2013**, *154*, 62–72. [CrossRef]
106. Morgan, M.S.; Arlian, L.G. Serum antibody profiles of *Sarcoptesscabiei* infested or immunized rabbits. *Folia Parasitol.* **1994**, *41*, 223–227.
107. Roberts, L.J.; Huffam, S.E.; Walton, S.F.; Currie, B.J. Crusted scabies: Clinical and immunological findings in seventy-eight patients and a review of the literature. *J. Inf. Secur.* **2005**, *50*, 375–381. [CrossRef] [PubMed]
108. Hu, C.H.; Xiao, K.; Luan, Z.S.; Song, J. Early weaning increases intestinal permeability, alters expression of cytokine and tight junction proteins, and activates mitogen-activated protein kinases in pigs. *J. Anim. Sci.* **2013**, *91*, 1094–1101. [CrossRef]
109. Jankovic, D.; Sher, A.; Yap, G. Th1/Th2 effector choice in parasitic infection: Decision making by committee. *Curr. Opin. Immunol.* **2001**, *13*, 403–409. [CrossRef]
110. Romagnani, S. T-cell subsets (Th1 versus Th2). *Ann. Allergy Asthma Immunol.* **2000**, *85*, 9–21. [CrossRef]
111. Kaiko, G.E.; Horvat, J.C.; Beagley, K.W.; Hansbro, P.M. Immunological decision-making: How does the immune system decide to mount a helper T-cell response? *Immunology* **2008**, *123*, 326–338. [CrossRef] [PubMed]
112. Cicchese, J.M.; Evans, S.; Hult, C.; Joslyn, L.R.; Wessler, T.; Millar, J.A.; Marino, S.; Cilfone, N.A.; Mattila, J.T.; Linderman, J.J.; et al. Dynamic balance of pro- and anti-inflammatory signals controls disease and limits pathology. *Immunol. Rev.* **2018**, *285*, 147–167. [CrossRef]
113. Spellberg, B.; Edwards, J.E., Jr. Type 1/Type 2 immunity in infectious diseases. *Clin. Infect. Dis.* **2001**, *32*, 76–102. [CrossRef]
114. Pence, D.B.; Ueckermann, E. Sarcoptic mange in wildlife. *Rev. Sci. Tech. Off. Int. Epizoot.* **2002**, *21*, 385–398. [CrossRef]
115. Nimmervoll, H.; Hoby, S.; Robert, N.; Lommano, E.; Welle, M.; Ryser-Degiorgis, M.P. Pathology of sarcoptic mange in red foxes (*Vulpes vulpes*): Macroscopic and histologic characterization of three disease stages. *J. Wildl. Dis.* **2013**, *49*, 91–102. [CrossRef]
116. Ninomiya, H.; Ogata, M. Sarcoptic mange in free-ranging raccoon dogs (*Nyctereutesprocyonoides*) in Japan. *Vet. Dermatol.* **2005**, *16*, 177–182. [CrossRef]

117. Ryser-Degiorgis, M.P.; Ryser, A.; Bacciarini, L.N.; Angst, C.; Gottstein, B.; Janovsky, M.; Breitenmoser, U. Notoedric and sarcoptic mange in free-ranging lynx from Switzerland. *J. Wildl. Dis.* **2002**, *38*, 228–232. [CrossRef] [PubMed]
118. Espinosa, J.; Ráez-Bravo, A.; López-Olvera, J.R.; Pérez, J.M.; Lavín, S.; Tvarijonaviciute, A.; Cano-Manue, F.J.; Fandos, P.; Soriguer, R.C.; Granados, J.E.; et al. Histopathology, microbiology and the inflammatory process associated with *Sarcoptesscabiei* infection in the Iberian ibex, *Capra pyrenaica*. *Parasites Vectors* **2017**, *10*, 596. [CrossRef] [PubMed]

Anthelmintic Activity of Wormwood (*Artemisia absinthium* L.) and Mallow (*Malva sylvestris* L.) against *Haemonchus contortus* in Sheep

Dominika Mravčáková [1], Michaela Komáromyová [2], Michal Babják [2], Michaela Urda Dolinská [2], Alžbeta Königová [2], Daniel Petrič [1], Klaudia Čobanová [1], Sylwester Ślusarczyk [3], Adam Cieslak [4], Marián Várady [2,*] and Zora Váradyová [1,*]

1 Institute of Animal Physiology, Centre of Biosciences of Slovak Academy of Sciences, 040 01 Košice, Slovakia; mravcakova@saske.sk (D.M.); petric@saske.sk (D.P.); boldik@saske.sk (K.Č.)

2 Institute of Parasitology of Slovak Academy of Sciences, 040 01 Košice, Slovakia; komaromyova@saske.sk (M.K.); babjak@saske.sk (M.B.); dolinska@saske.sk (M.U.D.); konig@saske.sk (A.K.)

3 Department of Pharmaceutical Biology with Botanical Garden of Medicinal Plants, Medical University of Wroclaw, 50-556 Wroclaw, Poland; sylwester.slusarczyk@umed.wroc.pl

4 Department of Animal Nutrition, Poznan University of Life Sciences, 60-637 Poznan, Poland; adam.cieslak@up.poznan.pl

* Correspondence: varady@saske.sk (M.V.); varadyz@saske.sk (Z.V.).

Simple Summary: The gastrointestinal parasitic nematode *Haemonchus contortus* of small ruminants is an important target for chemoprophylaxis. Repeated use of anthelmintics in the form of synthetic drugs increases the risk of residues in food products and the development of anthelmintic resistance. However, the use of combinations of dry traditional medicinal plants as nutraceuticals is an alternative to chemotherapeutics for controlling haemonchosis in ruminants. Therefore, the aim of this study is to determine the effect of dietary supplementation with wormwood, mallow and their mix on parasitological status and inflammatory response in lambs experimentally infected with *H. contortus*. Simultaneously, the present study evaluated by the egg hatch test the in vitro anthelminthic effects of different concentrations (50–1.563 mg/mL) of the aqueous extracts of these plants. Our results revealed that the strong anthelmintic effect of both medicinal plants observed in vitro was not fully confirmed in vivo. This knowledge builds on our previously published findings and highlights that the effect of dry medicinal plants depends on the variety and synergy of plant polyphenols and the combination of bioactive compounds that together have an effect and contribute to a certain pharmacological efficacy.

Abstract: The objective of this study is to evaluate the effect of dry wormwood and mallow on the gastrointestinal parasite of small ruminants *Haemonchus contortus*. Twenty-four experimentally infected lambs were randomly divided into four groups of six animals each: unsupplemented lambs, lambs supplemented with wormwood, lambs supplemented with mallow and animals supplemented with a mix of both plants. Faecal samples from the lambs were collected on day 23, 29, 36, 43, 50, 57, 64 and 75 post-infection for quantification of the number of eggs per gram (EPG). The mix of both plants contained phenolic acids (10.7 g/kg DM) and flavonoids (5.51 g/kg DM). The nematode eggs were collected and in vitro egg hatch test was performed. The aqueous extracts of both plants exhibited strong ovicidal effect on *H. contortus*, with ED50 and ED99 values of 1.40 and 3.76 mg/mL and 2.17 and 5.89 mg/mL, respectively, in the in vitro tests. Despite the great individual differences between the treated lambs in eggs reduction, the mean EPG of the untreated and treated groups did not differ ($p > 0.05$). Our results indicate that using wormwood and mallow as dietary supplements do not have a sufficient effect on lambs infected with *H. contortus*.

Keywords: dietary treatments; plant bioactive compounds; egg counts; UHRMS; *Haemonchus contortus*

1. Introduction

The gastrointestinal nematode (GIN) infection haemonchosis is a prevalent parasitic disease associated with economic losses, lowered productivity, morbidity and mortality. *Haemonchus contortus* is highly prevalent in sheep and goats worldwide and is mainly controlled by chemoprophylaxis through the repeated application of chemotherapeutics with the risk of development of anthelmintic resistance [1].

The screening of traditional medicinal plants containing promising contents of bioactive compounds with anthelmintic activity has great potential as an alternative source of natural anthelmintics and antioxidants that may be sustainable and environmentally acceptable. Various bioactive compounds (i.e., polyphenols, flavonoids, condensed tannins) that possess an anthelmintic effect [2,3] and antibacterial and antioxidant activities have been isolated from wormwood (*Artemisia absinthium* L.) [4,5]. Many authors have reported the antioxidant and antimicrobial properties of wormwood essential oils [6,7] and the anthelmintic activity of the flavonoids quercetin and apigenin [3]. Diets containing dried wormwood as a 5%–10% replacement for rice straw also provide better quality roughage with a considerable content of crude protein [8–10]. The high pharmacological activity of the medicinal plant mallow (*Malva sylvestris* L.), due to the presence of amino acids, flavonoids, mucilages, terpenoids, phenol derivatives, enzymes, coumarins and sterols, is known [11,12]. Mallow has antimicrobial, antifungal and anti-inflammatory properties [13,14].

In traditional medicine, whole plants or mixtures of plants are used rather than isolated compounds, and therefore more research is needed on all types of interaction between plant constituents. The ultra-high-resolution mass spectrometry (UHRMS) analyses of dry medicinal plants or plant mixtures in our recent studies with *H. contortus* [15–17] identified a wide range of bioactive compounds with important pharmacological activities, mainly flavonoids, phenolic acids, diterpenes, and alkaloids. These experiments, which combined chromatographic analyses with the determination of antioxidant capacity, are helpful in identifying plants with consistent concentrations of anthelmintic and antioxidant compounds for in vitro and in vivo studies. Our previous studies showed that medicinal plant mixtures are multicomponent mixes that possess effects via a multitarget additive and synergistic mode [16–18].

Therefore, in the present study, we hypothesize that some medicinal plants from these mixtures are by themselves multicomponent mixes and can elicit effects via pharmacological activity on *H. contortus* infected lambs. The medicinal plants, wormwood and mallow, were chosen based on their previously described best phytotherapeutic properties and anthelmintic activity in vitro [15]. The goal is to determine the effect of dietary supplementation with wormwood and mallow on parasitological status and inflammatory parameters of lambs experimentally infected with *H. contortus*.

2. Material and Methods

2.1. Ethics Statement

All procedures and animals were cared for under European Community guidelines (EU Directive 2010/63/EU). The experimental protocol was approved by the Ethical Committee of the Institute of Parasitology of the Slovak Academy of Sciences, in accordance with national legislation in Slovakia.

2.2. Analysis of Bioactive Compounds

Wormwood and mallow were ground to a fine powder, and 100 mg were extracted three times in 80% MeOH for 30 min at 40 °C. The extracts were evaporated to dryness, dissolved in 2 mL of Milli-Q water (acidified with 0.2% formic acid) and purified by Solid Phase Extraction (SPE) using Oasis HLB 3cc Vac Cartrige (60 mg, Waters Corp., Milford, MA, USA). The cartridges were washed with 0.5% methanol to remove carbohydrates and then washed with 80% methanol to elute phenolics. The phenolic fraction was re-evaporated and dissolved in 1 mL of 80% methanol (acidified with 0.1% formic acid). The sample was then centrifuged (23,000× *g*, 5 min) before spectrometric analysis. All analyses were performed in triplicate for three independent samples and stored in a freezer at −20 °C before analysis. The phenolic acids and flavonoids of the plant materials were analysed by a ultra-high-resolution mass spectrometry (Dionex UltiMate 3000RS, Thermo Scientific, Darmstadt, Germany) system with a charged aerosol detector interfaced with a high-resolution quadrupole time-of-flight mass spectrometer (HR/Q-TOF/MS, Compact, Bruker Daltonik GmbH, Bremen, Germany). The metabolomes of the samples were chromatographically separated, as was described [19]. The flow rate, spectra, operating parameters, collision energy, data calibration and spectra processing were previously described [20]. The amount of the particular phenolic acids in the samples was calculated as the chlorogenic acid (CAS 327-97-9, 3-Caffeoylquinic acid) equivalent, and hyperoside (CAS 482-36-0, quercetin 3-galactoside) was used for calculating the amount of identified flavonoids. Stock solutions of hyperoside and chlorogenic acids were prepared in MeOH, as was described previously [16].

2.3. In Vitro Test

The in vitro egg hatch test (EHT) was performed in order to assess the ovicidal effect of aqueous extracts of wormwood and mallow and compared with the chemotherapeutic effect of thiabendazole anthelmintic drug. The nematode eggs for in vitro EHT were obtained from the untreated UNS group. The concentrations of aqueous extracts used and EHT has been previously described [15].

Chemical tests for the screening of main constituents in the medicinal plants under study were carried out in the aqueous extracts using standard procedures [21,22]. Qualitative phytochemical screening revealed the active compounds mainly tannins, flavonoids, glycosides, saponins, alkaloids, and terpenoids (Table 1).

Table 1. Chemical composition of the aqueous plant extracts.

Plant Species	Tannins	Flavonoids	Glycosides	Saponins	Alkaloids	Terpenoids
A. absinthium	+	-	-	+	-	+
M. sylvestris	+	+	+	-	+	+

(+): the presence of phytochemicals; (-): the absence of phytochemicals.

2.4. Experiment In Vivo

The experiment was conducted on 24 3–4-month-old female lambs (Improved Valachian) with initial body weights of 18.67 ± 0.55 kg. The lambs were housed in common stalls on a sheep farm (Hodkovce, Slovak Republic) with free access to water. After a period of adaptation, all parasite-free lambs were infected by L3 larvae of *H. contortus* MHCo1 strain [16]. The diet of each animal consisted of oats (500 g DM/d) and meadow hay (ad libitum). Four groups of six animals based on their live-weight were established: unsupplemented lambs (UNS), lambs supplemented with stem of *A. absinthium* (ART, 1 g DM/d/lamb), lambs supplemented with flower of *M. sylvestris* (MAL, 15 g DM/d/lamb) and animals

D64 and D75 post-infection for quantification of the eggs per gram (EPG). The detection of strongylid eggs was performed by McMaster technique, as was previously described [23]. The blood sera samples of each animal were obtained from D15, D30, D45 and D70 [18]. Helminthological autopsy were done after 75 days of infection [16].

supplemented with mix of *A. absinthium* and *M. sylvestris* (ARTMAL, 16 g DM/d/lamb). The doses of plant supplements were based on the plant proportions used in our previous study [18]. The dry plants from commercial sources (AGROKARPATY, Plavnica, Slovak Republic) were mixed daily with the oats during the experimental period (75 days, D). The lambs were weighed on D0, D15, D30, D45 and D70. Faecal samples from the rectum of lambs were collected on D23, D29, D36, D43, D50, D57,

2.5. Blood Sera Analysis

Sheep immunoglobulin G (IgG), sheep immunoglobulin A (IgA) and sheep eosinophil peroxidase (EPX) were measured by ELISA kits (MyBioSource Ltd., San Diego, CA, USA). The sensitivity of the IgG, IgA and EPX kits were 0.938 ng/mL, 1.875 ng/mL and 1.0 ng/mL, respectively.

2.6. Statistical Analysis

Statistical analysis was performed using analysis variance (GraphPad Prism 8, GraphPad Software, Inc., San Diego, CA, USA) as repeated-measures mixed models representing the four animal groups (UNS, ART, MAL, ARTMAL) and sampling days. Differences between the animal groups were analysed by a two-way ANOVA with a Bonferroni post hoc test. Differences between the arithmetic EPG means between groups and between worm counts at dissection were analysed by Student's *t*-tests. A logistic regression model was used to determine the ED_{50} and ED_{99} [24].

3. Results

3.1. Bioactive Compounds

The *A. absinthium* contained 6.48 g/kg DM of phenolic acids and 0.35 g/kg DM of flavonoids with greater concentrations of chlorogenic acid (3.42 g/kg DM) and 1,5-dicaffeoylquinic acid (2.12 g/kg DM) (Table 2). The *M. sylvestris* contained 0.65 g/kg DM of phenolic acids and 6.48 g/kg DM of flavonoids with higher concentrations of delphinidin-5-glucoside 3-lathyroside (1.64 g/kg DM), kaempferol-3-O-rutinoside (0.82 g/kg DM), apigenin-o-hex (1.56 g/kg DM) and coumarinic acid (0.47 g/kg DM). The mix of both plants contained 10.7 g/kg DM phenolic acids and 5.51 g/kg DM of flavonoids with greater concentrations of methyl-4-O-beta-d-glucopyranosylcaffeate (2.23 g/kg DM), 1,5-dicaffeoylquinic acid (1.64 g/kg DM), kaempferol-O-Hex (1.40 g/kg DM), apigenin-O-Hex (1.29 g/kg DM) and luteolin-O-Hex (0.70 g/kg DM).

Table 2. Contents of the flavonoids and phenolic acids (g/kg DM) identified in the plants and mix.

No.	RT (min)	λ_{max} (nm)	m/z [M-H]⁻	MS²	MS² Fragments	Formula	Compound	Flavonoids	Phenolic Acids
						Artemisia absinthium			
1	2.80		189.0759	127/0759	171/145/115	$C_8H_{14}O_5$	L-(-)Malic acid diethyl ester		0.22
2	4.10	215.325	353.0877	191/0567	179/161/135	$C_{16}H_{18}O_9$	Chlorogenic acid		3.42
3	7.80		281.1023			$C_{14}H_{18}O_6$	ND	0.01	
4	8.00		367.1031	191/0546	173	$C_{17}H_{20}O_9$	3-O-Feruloylquinic acid		0.08
5	8.90		279.1223	234/1009	261/217/177/199	$C_{15}H_{20}O_5$	Artabsinolide		
6	9.10		325.1283	163	279/235	$C_{16}H_{22}O_7$	ND		0.03
7	9.20		327.1440	279	235	$C_{16}H_{24}O_7$	ND		
8	10.00	289.000	263.1282	201/1271	245/219/149/161/177	$C_{15}H_{20}O_4$	Tanacetin		
9	10.20		281.1386	219/373	263/237/201	$C_{16}H_{24}O_7$	Artabsinolide D		
10	11.00		515.1193	353/0867	191/179/135	$C_{25}H_{24}O_{12}$	1,5-Dicaffeoylquinic acid		2.12
11	11.20		653.1719	345/0595	330/302	$C_{29}H_{34}O_{17}$	Spinacetin 3-rutinoside	0.24	
12	11.40		477.1032	314/0415	357	$C_{22}H_{22}O_{12}$	Isorhamnetin 7-glucoside	0.10	
13	11.70		515.1192	353/0869	173/179/191/155	$C_{25}H_{24}O_{12}$	4,5-Dicaffeoylquinic acid		0.61
14	14.90		507.1502	413/1246	101/324/259	$C_{24}H_{28}O_{12}$	Hedycoryside B		
15	15.00		511.2698	467/2775	405	$C_{30}H_{40}O_7$	Anabsin		
16	15.50		345.1344	301/1433	257/213/187	$C_{19}H_{22}O_6$	Diosbulbin E		
17	15.60		511.2698	245/1175	263/201	$C_{30}H_{40}O_7$	Anabsin		
18	16.50		329.2323	211/1324	229/171/183/139	$C_{18}H_{34}O_5$	Pinellic acid		
						Total flavonoids and phenolic acids		0.35	6.48
						Malva sylvestris			
1	1.60	250.220	517.1195	355/0667	193	$C_{21}H_{26}O_{15}$	Ferullo-O-Hex-O-Hex		0.02
2	1.80	250.301	206.0443	144/0437		$C_{10}H_9NO_4$	ND		0.17
3	7.00	523	757.1846	347/0761	329/261/509	$C_{32}H_{39}O_{21}$	Delphinidin 5-glucoside 3-lathyroside	1.64	
4	7.90	308	163.0381	119/0502		$C_9H_8O_3$	Coumaric acid		0.47
5	8.00	288	465.1046	303/0505	285/275/177	$C_{21}H_{22}O_{12}$	Xeractinol	0.17	
6	8.20	520	449.1094	287/0555	259/243	$C_{21}H_{22}O_{11}$	Cyanidin-O-Hex	0.28	
7	8.50	518	593.1645	431/0982	269/0460	$C_{27}H_{31}O_{15}$	Pelargonidin-O-Hex-O-Hex	0.14	
8	8.70	283	687.1784	507/1142	345/0629/165		ND	0.18	
9	9.00	283	525.1246	345/0815	165/197/139	$C_{23}H_{25}O_{14}$	ND	0.07	
10	9.20	287	303.0498	153/0169	125/217	$C_{15}H_{12}O_7$	ND	0.04	
11	9.50	283	773.1781	507/1124	345/165	$C_{32}H_{38}O_{22}$	ND	0.22	
12	10.00		609.1458	301/0330		$C_{27}H_{31}O_{16}$	Quercetin-3-O-rutinoside	0.40	

Table 2. *Cont.*

No.	RT (min)	λ_{max} (nm)	m/z [M-H]⁻	MS^2	MS^2 Fragments	Formula	Compound	Flavonoids	Phenolic Acids
13	10.20	268.343	447.0928	285/0386		$C_{21}H_{20}O_{11}$	Kaempferol-O-Hex	0.49	
14	10.50	346	505.0981	343/0442		$C_{23}H_{22}O_{13}$	Quercetin 3′-glucoside-7-acetate	0.03	
15	10.90	266.343	593.1504	285/0395		$C_{27}H_{30}O_{15}$	Kaempferol-3-O-rutinoside	0.82	
16	11.10	291.346	433.1124	271/0599	151	$C_{21}H_{22}O_{10}$	Naringenin-O-Hex	0.13	
17	11.25	291	287.0550	259/0596	152/201/243	$C_{15}H_{12}O_6$	Tetrahydroxyflavone	0.30	
18	11.40	268.336	431.0978	269/0435		$C_{21}H_{20}O_{10}$	Apigenin-O-Hex	1.56	
19	15.00	285.340	271.0595	151/0012	177/119	$C_{15}H_{12}O_5$	Naringenin	0.01	
20	15.40		327.2169			$C_{18}H_{32}O_5$	(E)-10-(8-Hydroxyoctanoyloxy)-enoic acid		
21	15.70	215.334	269.0443	151/0016	225	$C_{15}H_{10}O_5$	Trihydroxyflavone	0.02	
					Total flavonoids and phenolic acids			6.50	0.66
					Mix of *A. absinthium* and *M. sylvestris*				
1	4.00	215.325	353.0883	191/0561	173/179	$C_{16}H_{18}O_9$	4-O-Caffeoylquinic acid		0.61
2	4.10	215.325	353.0883	191/0561	179/173	$C_{16}H_{18}O_9$	3-O-Caffeoylquinic acid		0.74
3	5.90	215.287	355.1035	193/0498	149/134	$C_{16}H_{20}O_9$	1-O-2′-Hydroxy-4′-methoxycinnamoyl -b-D-glucose		0.38
4	6.10	215.302	355.1038	149/0598	193/134	$C_{16}H_{20}O_9$	1-O-Feruloylglucose		0.70
5	7.90		161.0225	133/0282		$C_9H_6O_3$	Umbeliferone		0.40
6	8.00		323.0760	161/0221		$C_{15}H_{16}O_8$	Mahaleboside		0.02
7	8.10	225.287	465.1033	303/177	285/0399	$C_{21}H_{22}O_{12}$	Xeractinol	0.04	
8	8.30	520.000	449.1094	287/0555	259/243	$C_{21}H_{22}O_{11}$	Cyanidin-O-Hex	0.03	
9	8.50		367.1025	173/0433	193/155/134	$C_{17}H_{20}O_9$	Feruloylquinic acid		0.25
10	9.00	233.294.318	355.1034	193/0507	149/134	$C_{16}H_{20}O_9$	Methyl-4-O-beta-D-glucopyranosylcaffeate		2.23
11	9.80	255.354	463.0882	301/0337	343	$C_{21}H_{20}O_{12}$	Quercetin O-Hex	0.44	
12	9.90	252.351	609.1472	301/0331	285/0415	$C_{27}H_{30}O_{16}$	Isoquercitrin O-Dhex	0.42	
13	10.30	257,4	447.0920	285/0386		$C_{21}H_{20}O_{11}$	Kaempferol-O-Hex	1.40	
14	10.70	217.291.325	515.1189	353/0877	179/191	$C_{25}H_{24}O_{12}$	3,5-Dicaffeoylquinic acid		0.80
15	10.80		187.0958	125/0968	169	$C_9H_{16}O_4$	ND		
16	10.90	221.329	593.1520	285/0397		$C_{27}H_{30}O_{15}$	Kaempferol-3-O-rutinoside	0.37	
17	11.10	217.291.325	515.1197	353/0869	191/179	$C_{25}H_{24}O_{12}$	1,5-Dicaffeoylquinic acid		1.64
18	11.15	291.346	433.1124	271/0599	151	$C_{21}H_{22}O_{10}$	Naringenin-O-Hex	0.19	

Table 2. *Cont.*

No.	RT (min)	λ_{max} (nm)	*m/z* [M-H]$^-$	MS^2	MS^2 Fragments	Formula	Compound	Flavonoids	Phenolic Acids
19	11.40	266.3	431.0976	269/0434		$C_{21}H_{20}O_{10}$	Apigenin O-Hex	0.56	
20	11.50	268.343	447.0928	285/0386		$C_{21}H_{20}O_{11}$	Luteolin O-Hex	0.70	
21	11.60	266.3	431.0976	269/0434		$C_{21}H_{20}O_{10}$	Apigenin O-Hex	0.73	
22	11.70	215.290.325	515.119	353/0868	173/179/191	$C_{25}H_{24}O_{12}$	4,5-Dicaffeoylquinic acid		0.68
23	12.40	325.0	517.1342	355/1022	353/193/149/161	$C_{25}H_{26}O_{12}$	3-caffeoyl-4-dihydrocaffeoyl quinic acid		0.35
24	12.90	268.320	639.3176	519/2604	476/373/145	$C_{37}H_{44}N_4O_6$	Tris-trans-p-coumaroylspermine		0.50
25	13.10	218.268.339	473.1083	269/0426	413	$C_{23}H_{22}O_{11}$	Apigenin -O-(Hex-Ac)	0.12	
26	13.70	325.0	517.1330	323/0759	353/193/149/161	$C_{25}H_{26}O_{12}$	4-caffeoyl-3-dihydrocaffeoyl quinic acid		0.07
27	14.20	218.268.339	473.1083	269/0426	413	$C_{23}H_{22}O_{11}$	Apigenin -O-(Hex-Ac)	0.22	
28	14.40	266.336	515.1187	269/0444		$C_{25}H_{24}O_{12}$	Formononetin 7-O-glucoside-6″-malonate		0.22
29	15.00	285.340	271.0595	151/0012	177/119	$C_{15}H_{12}O_5$	Naringenin	0.07	
30	15.40		327.2169			$C_{18}H_{32}O_5$	(E)-10-(8-Hydroxyoctanoyloxy)dec-2-enoic acid	0.03	
31	15.70	215.334	269.0443	151/0016	225	$C_{15}H_{10}O_5$	Trihydroxyflavone	0.03	
32	17.10	222.309	785.3554	545/2397	665/502/399/145	$C_{46}H_{50}N_4O_8$	Tetra-trans-p-coumaroylspermine		0.47
33	19.00		373.0914	358/0681	343/329/315	$C_{19}H_{18}O_8$	Dihydroxy—tetramethoxyflavone	0.03	
34	20.30	267.334	559.1069	269/0443	515/1172	$C_{26}H_{24}O_{14}$	Apigenin 7-(2″-acyl-6″maloylglycosyl)	0.13	0.65
					Total flavonoids and phenolic acids			5.51	10.7

No: peak numbers from UV chromatograms; RT: retention time; λ_{max}: wavelengths of maximum absorption in the visible region; MS^2: main ion; ND: not determined.

3.2. In Vitro Test (EHT)

The dose-response relationships of aqueous extracts of *A. absinthium* or *M. sylvestris*, respectively, against *H. contortus* in the egg hatch test (EHT) are shown in Figure 1a,b. Both aqueous plant extracts exhibited a strong ovicidal effect on *H. contortus* in in vitro EHT. The ED_{50} and ED_{99} values were 1.40 and 3.76 mg/mL in *A. absinthium* (Figure 1a) and 2.17 and 5.89 mg/mL in *M. sylvestris* (Figure 1b), respectively. Thiabendazole at a concentration of 1.0 μg/mL has a 100% ovicidal effect.

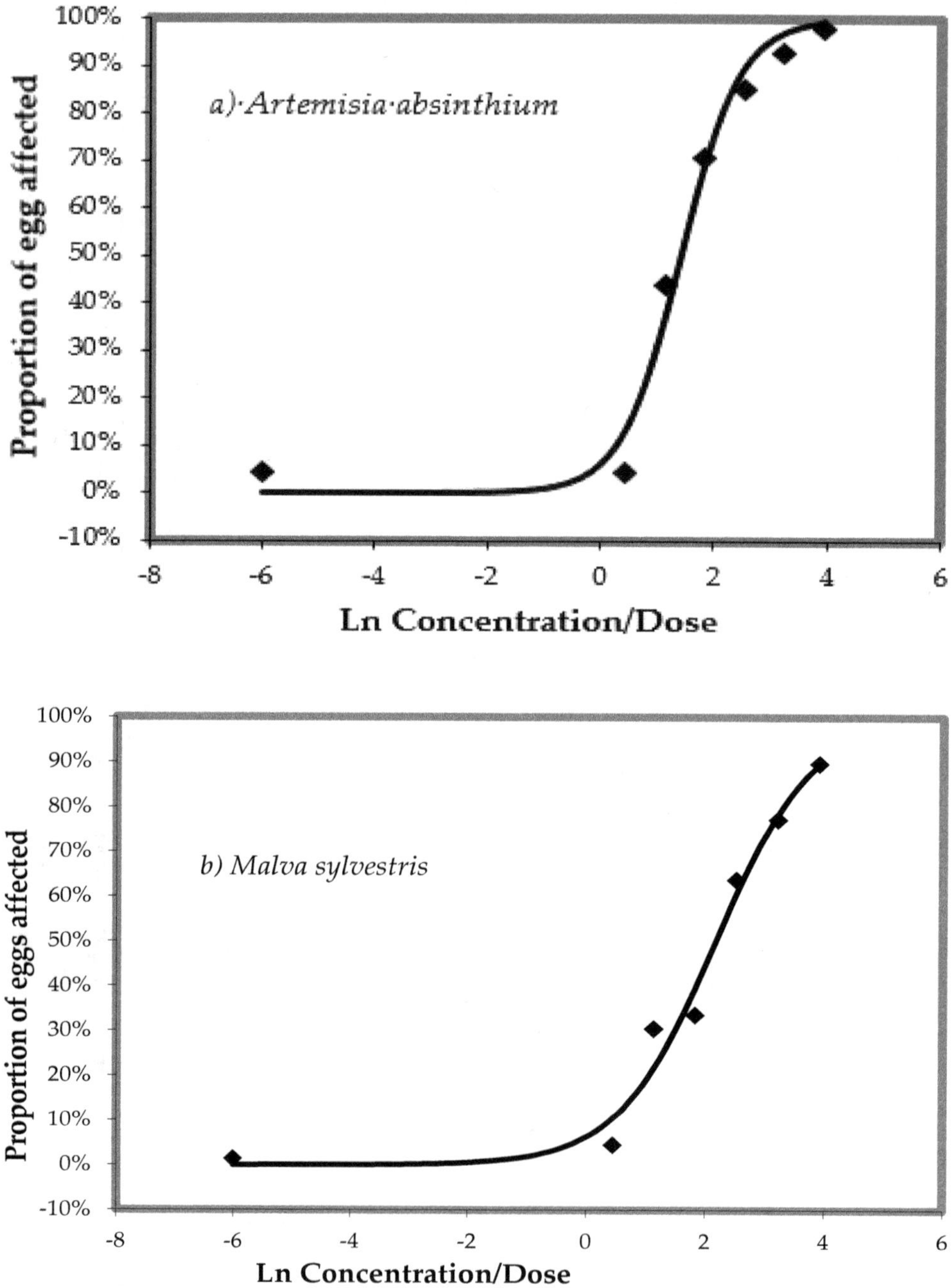

Figure 1. (**a**,**b**) Dose-response relationship of plant aqueous extracts against *Haemonchus contortus* in the egg hatch test (EHT) after 24 h of incubation at 26 °C.

3.3. Parasitological Status

The patterns of egg shedding for UNS, ART, MAL and ARTMAL are shown in Figure 2. Data from D36 were statistically compared and used to determine the reduction in egg output for ART, MAL and ARTMAL relative to UNS. Mean faecal eggs per gram (EPGs) were influenced by time from infection ($p < 0.05$), and for all groups, EPGs increased until D50 or D57, respectively. The EPGs in the lambs treated with MAL, ART and ARTMAL compared with UNS group did not differ ($p > 0.05$). The necropsy on D75 found a numerical decrease ($p > 0.05$) in the abomasal worm counts for the ARTMAL groups compared to the other groups (Figure 3).

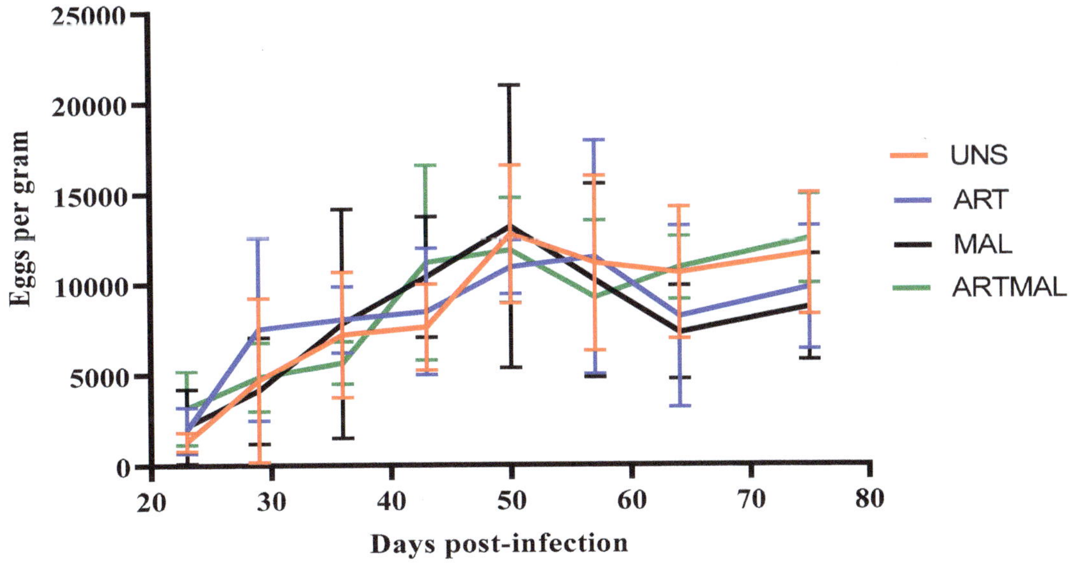

Figure 2. Mean faecal egg counts for the groups of lambs infected with *Haemonchus contortus* (Treatment: $p > 0.05$; time: $p < 0.001$; treatment × time: $p > 0.05$). UNS: unsupplemented; ART: *A. absinthium*; MAL: *M. sylvestris*; ARTMAL: ART plus MAL.

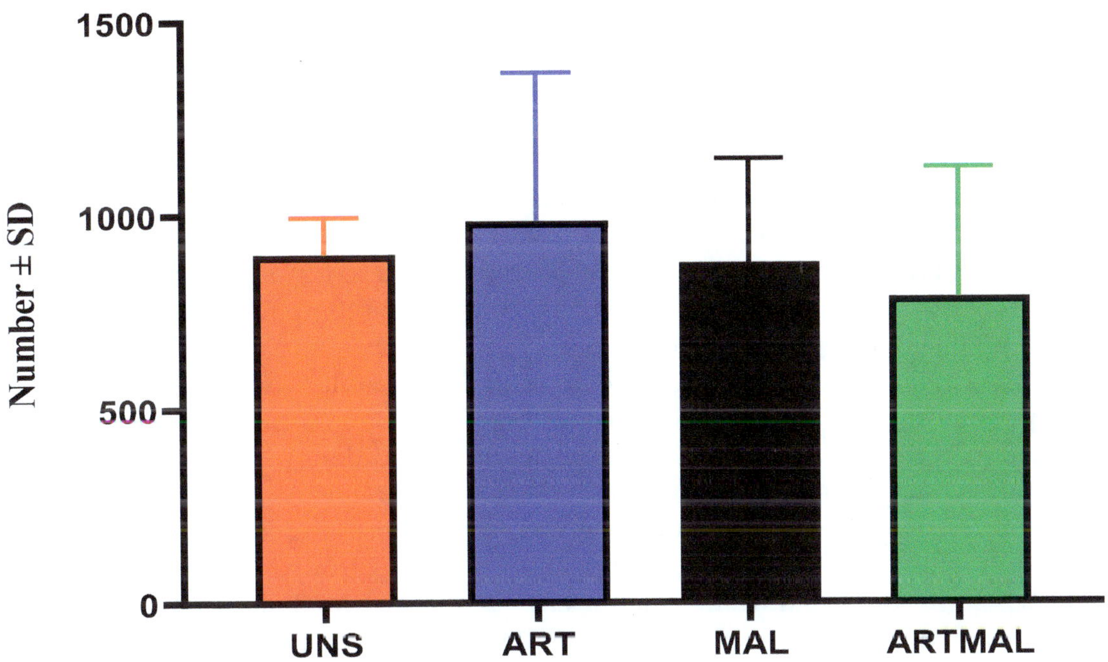

Figure 3. Abomasal worm counts of *Haemonchus contortus* in the lambs of each treatment at the end of the experiment ($p > 0.05$). UNS: unsupplemented; ART: *A. absinthium*; MAL: *M. sylvestris*; ARTMAL: ART plus MAL.

3.4. Inflammatory Response

Table 3 shows the inflammatory IgG, IgA and EPX response. Serum IgG and IgA values were not influenced by treatment, time and treatment × time ($p > 0.05$). Mean serum EPX values ranged in the treated groups from 24.1 to 73.4 ng/mL, and the values were influenced by treatment and time ($p < 0.05$).

Table 3. Inflammatory responses of the experimental groups ($n = 6$).

Item	Day	UNS	ART	MAL	ARTMAL	SD	Significance of Effects		
							Treatment (T)	Time	T × Time
IgG (ng/mL)	15	0.627	2.15	2.31	2.23	2.54	NS	NS	NS
	30	1.03	0.780	0.986	1.61	1.61			
	45	1.33	0.639	0.378	1.04	1.07			
	70	1.16	0.689	3.53	1.39	1.66			
IgA (ng/mL)	15	0.434	1.28	0.811	0.767	0.522	NS	NS	NS
	30	0.825	0.666	0.519	0.589	0.245			
	45	0.529	0.438	0.787	0.485	0.233			
	70	0.813	0.696	0.726	0.626	0.195			
EPX (ng/mL)	15	37.5	66.6	52.2	50.0	17.9	*	*	NS
	30	44.0	36.9	29.4	44.8	13.9			
	45	31.4	38.6	24.1	51.4	17.5			
	70	49.2	33.4	37.8	73.4	21.1			

UNS: unsupplemented; ART: *A. absinthium*; MAL: *M. sylvestris*; ARTMAL: ART plus MAL; EPX: eosinophil peroxidase; NS: not significant; SD: standard deviation. * $p < 0.05$.

4. Discussion

In the present study, phenolic compounds, flavonoids and phenolic acids among them, were detected in wormwood, mallow and a mix of both plants. Phenolic acids, including chlorogenic acid, caffeoylquinic acid derivatives, coumaric acid and methyl 4-O-beta-D-glucopyranosylcaffeate, were identified in a range from 0.65 to 10.7 g/kg DM. Chlorogenic acid and 1,5- and 4,5-dicaffeoylquinic acid possess well-known antibacterial, anthelmintic, anti-inflammatory, and antioxidant biological activities in vitro and in vivo [25,26]. Similarly, coumaric acid in *Senegalia gaumeri* leaf extract compounds has shown potential anthelmintic effects against *H. contortus* larvae [27]. The phenolic acid contents for wormwood and the mix (but not for mallow) were within the range of 3.6 to 57.3 g/kg DM, as was reported for plant mixtures used previously in infected lambs [16,17]. In relation to flavonoids with antioxidant properties, we identified mainly flavones (apigenin and luteolin), flavonols (kaempferol and quercetin) and flavanones (naringenin) [28], which may also have anthelmintic activity [3,29]. However, the total content of flavonoids in wormwood in the present study was lower (0.35 g/kg DM) versus mallow or the mix (6.48 or 5.51 g/kg DM, respectively) or compared to previous studies (9.96 and 29.5 or 41.5 g/kg DM, respectively) [16,17].

It is clear that medicinal plants that have an anthelmintic effect in vitro are often not equally effective in vivo, because there is different bioavailability, pharmacology of host animals, metabolism of bioactive compounds by rumen microflora and experimental conditions [30]. In the present experiment, the aqueous plant extracts of both medicinal plants, *A. absinthium* and *M. sylvestris*, exhibited a strong ovicidal effect on *H. contortus* in vitro, similar to the extracts of the species *Artemisia* against sheep nematodes [31,32]. However, the mean egg outputs of the UNS group compared to ART, MAL and ARTMAL groups showed no significant differences in egg reduction in lambs. Egg production by *H. contortus* females remained high (i.e., thousands EPG) until D50 post-inoculation and then decreased similarly as during the patent period of *H. contortus* in sheep [33]. The rapid reduction in egg excretion after D50 (MAL and ARTMAL) or D57 (ART), respectively, was accompanied by a lower number (not statistically) of adult *H. contortus* worms in the ARTMAL group. No significant differences in egg excretion in the treated groups may have been due to the lower content of plant biologically active compounds, especially flavonoids, compared to our previous studies [16,17]. However, relatively high SD of the means of the treated groups in the present experiment point to a potentially different treatment effect between lambs. This suggests that these plant materials could have an indirect antiparasitic effect and may promote a host's resistance to parasitic infection in the longer term. However, the anthelmintic mechanism of action is unknown. It seems that flavonoids with antioxidant capacity, in particular, contribute to the indirect antiparasitic activity [34,35]. However, not only the content of flavonoids appears to play an important role in the anthelmintic activity of medicinal plants and their mixtures. Our results indicate that wormwood and mallow themselves are not responsible for egg and worm reduction in the lambs but probably acting in synergy with other medicinal plants and their bioactive compounds, as was done in previous mixes [17,18]. The effect of dry medicinal plants on the health of animals depends on the source of the multitarget complex bioactive compounds that work synergistically [36,37] and antagonistically [38]. An increase in the resistance of infected lambs to *H. contortus* infection was shown after the administration of mixtures of dry medicinal plants composed already of 9–13 species [16–18]. However, a generally great contribution to the discovery and development of new drugs is a widely applicable strategy for identifying the combinatory compounds responsible for a certain pharmacological activity of plant medicines followed by in vitro and in vivo validation [39].

Ruminal and intestinal fermentation parameters can be manipulated by supplementing a diet with medicinal plants [40]. No adverse effects of wormwood and mallow on the ruminal fermentation parameters (i.e., pH, ammonia N, methane, gas production, and volatile fatty acids) were found [18]. Mainly, pH and ammonia N can affect the release of phenolic compounds from plant materials and the growth of ruminal microbes for microbial protein synthesis [41,42]. Additionally, phenolic compounds, especially flavonoids, can improve body weight gain, growth and the quality of animal products [43]. In the present experiment, polyphenols as dietary supplements did not significantly affect the body weights or live-weight gains of the infected lambs. Dry medicinal plants in the diets of the infected lambs may [18] or may not have influenced the body weights or live-weight gains, which is consonant with a meta-analysis of gastro-intestinal nematode infection in sheep [44].

Our recent studies [16–18] of lambs infected with the gastrointestinal nematode *H. contortus* showed the potential value of medicinal plant mixtures to decrease egg output and worm numbers in parasitic infections of the digestive tract. However, this effect is probably not a consequence of a direct anthelmintic impact on the viability of nematodes, but an increase in the resistance of lambs to nematode infections. Additionally, a recent study also showed that a complementary vegetable mixture of plants belonging to the *Compositae*, *Cesalpinacae*, *Liliacae*, *Bromeliaceae* and *Labiatae* families used as feed at two different dosages was ineffective against gastrointestinal nematode infection [45]. It seems that mainly a combination of medicinal plants belonging to different botanical families with beneficial bioactive compounds probably contributes to slowing the dynamics of infection. In the present study, because of the low variety and synergy of plant polyphenols and the combination of bioactive compounds of wormwood and mallow, the reduction in parasitic infection intensity in the treated infected lambs was not sufficient during the 75 days of infection compared to previous studies [16–18]. However, it seems that mixtures of dry medicinal plants may affect the host over the longer term. Therefore, more research is needed on combinations of medicinal plants and interactions between compositions of plant mixtures for longer (90-120 days) experimental periods.

5. Conclusions

The data in the present study showed additional new knowledge on the anthelmintic effects of dry medicinal plants as dietary supplements. Our results indicate that using medicinal plants, even those with the best anthelmintic properties in vitro, may not have sufficient effects in vivo on *H. contortus* infected lamb.

Author Contributions: Conceptualization, Z.V., M.V.; Investigation, D.M., Z.V., M.V.; Supervision, M.V.; Formal analysis, D.M., M.K., K.Č., M.B., M.U.D., A.K., D.P., S.Š.; Data Curation, Z.V., M.V., A.C.; Draft Preparation, Z.V.; Writing-Review & Editing, Z.V., M.V. All authors have read and agreed to the published version of the manuscript.

Acknowledgments: The authors are grateful to Valéria Venglovská, Silvia Spišáková, Peter Jerga and Gabriel Benkovský for laboratory and technical assistance.

References

1. Lamb, J.; Elliott, T.; Chambers, M.; Chick, B. Broad spectrum anthelmintic resistance of *Haemonchus contortus* in Northern NSW of Australia. *Vet. Parasitol.* **2017**, *24*, 48–51. [CrossRef]
2. Tariq, K.A.; Chishti, M.Z.; Ahmad, F.; Shawl, A.S. Anthelmintic activity of extracts of *Artemisia absinthium* against ovine nematodes. *Vet. Parasitol.* **2009**, *160*, 83–88. [CrossRef]
3. Akkari, H.; Rtibi, K.; B'chir, F.; Rekik, M.; Darghouth, M.A.; Gharbi, M. In vitro evidence that the pastoral *Artemisia campestris* species exerts an anthelmintic effect on *Haemonchus contortus* from sheep. *Vet. Res. Commun.* **2014**, *38*, 249–255. [CrossRef]
4. Kordali, S.; Kotan, R.; Mavi, A.; Cakir, A.; Ala, A.; Yildirim, A. Determination of the chemical composition and antioxidant activity of the essential oil of *Artemisia dracunculus* and of the antifungal and antibacterial activities of Turkish *Artemisia absinthium, A. dracunculus, Artemisia santonicum* and *Artemisia spicigera* essential oils. *J. Agric. Food Chem.* **2005**, *53*, 9452–9458.
5. Kharoubi, O.; Slimani, M.; Krouf, D.; Seddik, L.; Aoues, A. Role of wormwood (*Artemisia absinthium*) extract on oxidative stress in ameliorating lead induced haematotoxicity. *Afr. J. Tradit. Complement. Altern. Med.* **2008**, *5*, 263–270. [CrossRef]
6. Msaada, K.; Salem, N.; Bachrouch, O.; Bousselmi, S.; Tammar, S.; Alfaify, A.; Al Sane, K.; Ammar, W.B.; Azeiz, S.; Brahim, A.H.; et al. Chemical Composition and Antioxidant and Antimicrobial Activities of Wormwood (*Artemisia absinthium* L.) Essential Oils and Phenolics. *J. Chem.* **2015**, *804658*. [CrossRef]
7. Nguyen, H.T.; Németh Zámboriné, É. Sources of variability of wormwood (*Artemisia absinthium* L.) essential oil. *J. Appl. Res. Med. Aromat. Plants* **2016**, *3*, 143–150. [CrossRef]
8. Kim, J.H.; Kim, C.H.; Ko, Y.D. Influence of dietary addition of dried wormwood (Artemisia sp.) on the performance and carcass characteristics of Hanwoo steers and the nutrient digestibility of sheep. *Asian–Aust. J. Anim. Sci.* **2002**, *15*, 390–395. [CrossRef]
9. Kim, Y.M.; Kim, J.H.; Kim, S.C.; Ha, H.M.; Ko, Y.D.; Kim, C.H. Influence of dietary addition of dried wormwood (Artemisia sp.) on the performance, carcass characteristics and fatty acid composition of muscle tissues of Hanwoo heifers. *Asian–Aust. J. Anim. Sci.* **2002**, *15*, 549–554. [CrossRef]
10. Ko, Y.D.; Kim, J.H.; Adesogan, A.T.; Ha, H.M.; Kim, S.C. The effect of replacing rice straw with dry wormwood (Artemisia sp.) on intake, digestibility, nitrogen balance and ruminal fermentation characteristics in sheep. *Anim. Feed Sci. Technol.* **2006**, *125*, 99–110. [CrossRef]
11. Cutillo, F.; D'Abrosca, B.; Dellagreca, M.; Fiorentino, A.; Zarrelli, A. Terpenoids and phenol derivatives from *Malva silvestris. Phytochemistry* **2006**, *67*, 481–485. [CrossRef] [PubMed]
12. Gasparetto, J.C.; Martins, C.A.; Hayashi, S.S.; Otuky, M.F.; Pontarolo, R. Ethnobotanical and scientific aspects of *Malva sylvestris* L.: A millennial herbal medicine. *J. Pharm. Pharmacol.* **2012**, *64*, 172–189. [CrossRef] [PubMed]
13. Zohra, S.F.; Meriem, B.; Samira, S. Some Extracts of Mallow Plant and its Role in Health. *APCBEE Procedia* **2013**, *5*, 546–550. [CrossRef]
14. Prudente, A.S.; Loddi, A.M.; Duarte, M.R.; Santos, A.R.; Pochapski, M.T.; Pizzolatti, M.G.; Hayashi, S.S.; Campos, F.R.; Pontarolo, R.; Santos, F.A.; et al. Pre-clinical anti-inflammatory aspects of a cuisine and medicinal millennial herb: *Malva sylvestris* L. *Food Chem. Toxicol.* **2013**, *58*, 324–331. [CrossRef]
15. Váradyová, Z.; Pisarčíková, J.; Babják, M.; Hodges, A.; Mravčáková, D.; Kišidayová, S.; Königová, A.; Vadlejch, J.; Várady, M. Ovicidal and larvicidal activity of extracts from medicinal-plants against *Haemonchus contortus. Exp. Parasitol.* **2018**, *195*, 71–77. [CrossRef]
16. Váradyová, Z.; Mravčáková, D.; Babják, M.; Bryszak, M.; Grešáková, Ľ.; Čobanová, K.; Kišidayová, S.; Plachá, I.; Königová, A.; Cieslak, A.; et al. Effects of herbal nutraceuticals and/or zinc against *Haemonchus contortus* in lambs experimentally infected. *BMC Vet. Res.* **2018**, *14*, 78. [CrossRef]
17. Mravčáková, D.; Váradyová, Z.; Kopčáková, A.; Čobanová, K.; Grešáková, Ľ.; Kišidayová, S.; Babják, M.; Urda Dolinská, M.; Dvorožňáková, E.; Königová, A.; et al. Natural chemotherapeutic alternatives for controlling of haemonchosis in sheep. *BMC Vet. Res.* **2019**, *15*, 302. [CrossRef]

18. Váradyová, Z.; Kišidayová, S.; Čobanová, K.; Grešáková, Ľ.; Babják, M.; Königová, A.; Urda Dolinská, M.; Várady, M. The impact of a mixture of medicinal herbs on ruminal fermentation, parasitological status and hematological parameters of the lambs experimentally infected with *Haemonchus contortus*. *Small Rumin. Res.* **2017**, *151*, 124–132. [CrossRef]
19. Rodrigues, M.J.; Matkowski, A.; Ślusarczyk, S.; Magné, C.; Poleze, T.; Pereira, C.; Custódio, L. Sea knotgrass (*Polygonum maritimum* L.) as a potential source of innovative industrial products for skincare applications. *Ind. Crop. Prod.* **2019**, *128*, 391–398. [CrossRef]
20. Rodrigues, M.J.; Monteiro, I.; Placines, C.; Castañeda-Loaiza, V.; Ślusarczyk, S.; Matkowski, A.; Pereira, C.; Pousão-Ferreira, P.; Custódio, L. The irrigation salinity and harvesting affect the growth, chemical profile and biological activities of *Polygonum maritimum* L. *Ind. Crop. Prod.* **2019**, *139*, 111510. [CrossRef]
21. Yadav, R.N.S.; Agarwala, M. Phytochemical analysis of some medicinal plants. *J. Phytol.* **2011**, *3*, 10–14.
22. Jaradat, N.; Hussen, F.; Al Ali, A. Preliminary Phytochemical Screening, Quantitative Estimation of Total Flavonoids, Total Phenols and Antioxidant Activity of *Ephedra alata* Decne. *J. Mater. Environ. Sci.* **2015**, *6*, 1771–1778.
23. Coles, G.C.; Bauer, C.; Borgsteede, F.H.M.; Geerts, S.; Klei, T.R.; Taylor, M.A.; Waller, P.J. World Association for the Advancement of Veterinary Parasitology (W.A.A.V.P) methods for the detection of anthelmintic resistance in nematodes of veterinary importance. *Vet. Parasitol.* **1992**, *44*, 35–44. [CrossRef]
24. Babják, M.; Königová, A.; Urda Dolinská, M.; Vadlejch, J.; Várady, M. Anthelmintic resistance in goat herds—In vivo versus in vitro detection methods. *Vet. Parasitol.* **2018**, *139*, 10–14. [CrossRef] [PubMed]
25. Sato, Y.; Itagaki, S.; Kurokawa, T.; Ogura, J.; Kobayashi, M.; Hirano, T.; Sugawara, M.; Iseki, K. In vitro and in vivo antioxidant properties of chlorogenic acid and caffeic acid. *Int. J. Pharm.* **2011**, *403*, 136–138. [CrossRef] [PubMed]
26. Tajik, N.; Tajik, M.; Mack, I.; Enck, P. The potential effects of chlorogenic acid, the main phenolic components in coffee, on health: A comprehensive review of the literature. *Eur. J. Nutr.* **2017**, *56*, 2215–2244. [CrossRef] [PubMed]
27. Castañeda-Ramírez, G.S.; Torres-Acosta, J.F.J.; Sandoval-Castro, C.A.; Borges-Argáez, R.; Cáceres-Farfán, M.; Mancilla-Montelongo, G.; Mathieu, C. Bio-guided fractionation to identify *Senegalia gaumeri* leaf extract compounds with anthelmintic activity against *Haemonchus contortus* eggs and larvae. *Vet. Parasitol.* **2019**, *270*, 13–19. [CrossRef]
28. Kumar, S.; Pandey, A.K. Chemistry and biological activities of flavonoids: An overview. *Sci. World J.* **2013**, *162750*. [CrossRef]
29. Kozan, E.; Anul, S.A.; Tatli, I.I. In vitro anthelmintic effect of *Vicia pannonica* var. *purpurascens* on trichostrongylosis in sheep. *Exp. Parasitol.* **2013**, *134*, 299–303. [CrossRef]
30. Ferreira, L.E.; Castro, P.M.; Chagas, A.C.; França, S.C.; Beleboni, R.O. In vitro anthelmintic activity of aqueous leaf extract of *Annona muricata* L. (Annonaceae) against *Haemonchus contortus* from sheep. *Exp. Parasitol.* **2013**, *134*, 327–332. [CrossRef]
31. Iqbal, Z.; Lateef, M.; Ashraf, M.; Jabbar, A. Anthelmintic activity of *Artemisia brevifolia* in sheep. *J. Ethnopharmacol.* **2004**, *93*, 265–268. [CrossRef] [PubMed]
32. Irum, S.; Ahmed, H.; Mirza, B.; Donskow-Łysoniewska, K.; Muhammad, A.; Qayyum, M.; Simsek, S. In vitro and in vivo anthelmintic activity of extracts from *Artemisia parviflora* and *A. sieversiana*. *Helminthologia* **2017**, *54*, 218–224. [CrossRef]
33. Borgsteede, H.M.; Couwenberg, T. Changes in LC50 in an in vitro egg development assay during the patent period of *Haemonchus contortus* in sheep. *Res. Vet. Sci.* **1987**, *42*, 413–414. [CrossRef]
34. Akkari, H.; B'chir, F.; Hajaji, S.; Rekik, M.; Sebai, E.; Hamza, H.; Darghouth, M.A.; Gharbi, M. Potential anthelmintic effect of *Capparis spinose* (Capparidaceae) as related to its polyphenolic content and antioxidant activity. *Vet. Med. Czech.* **2016**, *61*, 308–316. [CrossRef]
35. Spiegler, V.; Liebau, E.; Hensel, A. Medicinal plant extracts and plant-derived polyphenols with anthelmintic activity against intestinal nematodes. *Nat. Prod. Rep.* **2017**, *34*, 627–643. [CrossRef] [PubMed]
36. Brusotti, G.; Cesari, I.; Dentamaro, A.; Caccialanza, G.; Massolini, G. Isolation and characterization of bioactive compounds from plant resources: The role of analysis in the ethnopharmacological approach. *J. Pharm. Biomed. Anal.* **2014**, *87*, 218–228. [CrossRef] [PubMed]

37. Klongsiriwet, C.; Quijada, J.; Williams, A.R.; Mueller-Harvey, I.; Williamson, E.M.; Hoste, H. Synergistic inhibition of *Haemonchus contortus* exsheathment by flavonoid monomers and condensed tannins. *Int. J. Parasitol. Drugs Drug Resist.* **2015**, *5*, 127–134. [CrossRef] [PubMed]
38. Xutian, S.; Zhang, J.; Louise, W. New exploration and understanding of traditional Chinese medicine. *Am. J. Chinese Med.* **2009**, *37*, 411–426.
39. Long, F.; Yang, H.; Xu, Y.; Hao, H.; Li, P. A strategy for the identification of combinatorial bioactive compounds contributing to the holistic effect of herbal medicines. *Sci. Rep.* **2015**, *5*, 12361. [CrossRef]
40. Váradyová, Z.; Mravčáková, D.; Holodová, M.; Grešáková, L'.; Pisarčíková, J.; Barszcz, M.; Taciak, M.; Tuśnio, A.; Kišidayová, S.; Čobanová, K. Modulation of ruminal and intestinal fermentation by medicinal plants and zinc from different sources. *J. Anim. Physiol. Anim. Nutr. (Berl)* **2018**, *102*, 1131–1145.
41. Gaillard, B.D.; Richards, G.N. Presence of soluble lignin-carbohydrate complexes in the bovine rumen. *Carbohydr. Res.* **1975**, *42*, 135–145. [CrossRef]
42. Pisulewski, P.M.; Okorie, A.U.; Buttery, P.J.; Haresign, W.; Lewis, D. Ammonia concentration and protein synthesis in the rumen. *J. Sci. Food Agric.* **1981**, *32*, 759–766. [CrossRef] [PubMed]
43. Tufarelli, V.; Casalino, E.; D'Alessandro, A.G.; Laudadio, V. Dietary phenolic compounds: Biochemistry, metabolism and significance in animal and human health. *Curr. Drug Metab.* **2017**, *18*, 905–913. [CrossRef] [PubMed]
44. Mavrot, F.; Hertzberg, H.; Torgerson, P. Effect of gastro-intestinal nematode infection on sheep performance: A systematic review and meta-analysis. *Parasit. Vectors* **2015**, *8*, 557. [CrossRef]
45. Castagna, F.; Palma, E.; Cringoli, G.; Bosco, A.; Nistico, N.; Caligiuri, G.; Britti, D.; Musella, V. Use of complementary natural feed for gastrointestinal nematodes control in sheep: Effectiveness and benefits for animals. *Animals* **2019**, *9*, 1037. [CrossRef]

Permissions

All chapters in this book were first published by MDPI; hereby published with permission under the Creative Commons Attribution License or equivalent. Every chapter published in this book has been scrutinized by our experts. Their significance has been extensively debated. The topics covered herein carry significant findings which will fuel the growth of the discipline. They may even be implemented as practical applications or may be referred to as a beginning point for another development.

The contributors of this book come from diverse backgrounds, making this book a truly international effort. This book will bring forth new frontiers with its revolutionizing research information and detailed analysis of the nascent developments around the world.

We would like to thank all the contributing authors for lending their expertise to make the book truly unique. They have played a crucial role in the development of this book. Without their invaluable contributions this book wouldn't have been possible. They have made vital efforts to compile up to date information on the varied aspects of this subject to make this book a valuable addition to the collection of many professionals and students.

This book was conceptualized with the vision of imparting up-to-date information and advanced data in this field. To ensure the same, a matchless editorial board was set up. Every individual on the board went through rigorous rounds of assessment to prove their worth. After which they invested a large part of their time researching and compiling the most relevant data for our readers.

The editorial board has been involved in producing this book since its inception. They have spent rigorous hours researching and exploring the diverse topics which have resulted in the successful publishing of this book. They have passed on their knowledge of decades through this book. To expedite this challenging task, the publisher supported the team at every step. A small team of assistant editors was also appointed to further simplify the editing procedure and attain best results for the readers.

Apart from the editorial board, the designing team has also invested a significant amount of their time in understanding the subject and creating the most relevant covers. They scrutinized every image to scout for the most suitable representation of the subject and create an appropriate cover for the book.

The publishing team has been an ardent support to the editorial, designing and production team. Their endless efforts to recruit the best for this project, has resulted in the accomplishment of this book. They are a veteran in the field of academics and their pool of knowledge is as vast as their experience in printing. Their expertise and guidance has proved useful at every step. Their uncompromising quality standards have made this book an exceptional effort. Their encouragement from time to time has been an inspiration for everyone.

The publisher and the editorial board hope that this book will prove to be a valuable piece of knowledge for researchers, students, practitioners and scholars across the globe.

List of Contributors

Saeed El-Ashram
College of Life Science and Engineering, Foshan University, 18 Jiangwan street, Foshan 528231, China
Faculty of Science, Kafrelsheikh University, Kafr el-Sheikh, 33516, Egypt

Shawky M. Aboelhadid, Lilian N. Mahrous and Asmaa A. Kamel
Parasitology Department, Faculty of Veterinary Medicine, Beni Suef University, Beni-Suef 62511, Egypt

El-Sayed M. Abdel-Kafy, Shymaa A. Hashem and Eman M. Farghly
Animal Production Research Institute, Agricultural Research Center, Dokki, Giza 12651, Egypt

Marwa A. Ahmed
Department of Pathology, Faculty of Veterinary Medicine, Aswan University, Aswan 24101, Egypt

Ehab Kotb Elmahallawy
Department of Biomedical Sciences, University of León (ULE), 24071 León, Spain
Department of Zoonoses, Faculty of Veterinary Medicine, Sohag University, Sohag 82524, Egypt

Ahmed Gareh
Department of Parasitology, Faculty of Veterinary Medicine, Aswan University, Aswan 24101, Egypt

Abdelbaset Eweda Abdelbaset
National Research Center for Protozoan Diseases, Obihiro University of Agriculture and Veterinary Medicine, Obihiro 080-8555, Japan
Clinical Laboratory Diagnosis, Department of Animal Medicine, Faculty of Veterinary Medicine, Assiut University, Assiut 71515, Egypt

Fatma A. El-Gohary
Department of Hygiene and Zoonoses, Faculty of Veterinary Medicine, Mansoura University, Mansoura 35516, Egypt

Nagwa M. Elhawary
Department of Parasitology, Faculty of Veterinary Medicine, Kafrelsheikh University, Kafr El Sheikh 33511, Egypt

Ahmed K. Dyab
Department of Parasitology, Faculty of Medicine, Assiut University, Assiut 71515, Egypt

Elzahara Elbaz
Department of Internal Medicine and Infectious Diseases, Faculty of Veterinary Medicine, Mansoura University, Mansoura 35516, Egypt

Mostafa F. N. Abushahba
Department of Medicine, Division of Infectious Diseases, School of Medicine, Washington University, St. Louis, MO 63110, USA
Department of Zoonosess, Faculty of Veterinary Medicine, Assiut University, Assiut 71515, Egypt

Maciej Grzybek, Beata Biernat and Joanna Nowicka
Department of Tropical Parasitology, Institute of Maritime and Tropical Medicine, Medical University of Gdansk, Powstania Styczniowego 9B, 81-519 Gdynia, Poland

Mohammed Alsarraf and Anna Bajer
Department of Eco-Epidemiology for Parasitic Diseases, Faculty of Biology, University of Warsaw, 1 Miecznikowa Str, 02-096 Warsaw, Poland

Katarzyna Tołkacz
Department of Eco-Epidemiology for Parasitic Diseases, Faculty of Biology, University of Warsaw, 1 Miecznikowa Str, 02-096 Warsaw, Poland
Department of Antarctic Biology, Institute of Biochemistry and Biophysics, Polish Academy of Sciences, 5A Pawińskiego Str, 02-106 Warsaw, Poland

Tarja Sironen, Sanna Mäki and Antti Vaheri
Department of Virology, University of Helsinki, Haartmaninkatu 3, 00014 Helsinki, Finland

Jolanta Behnke-Borowczyk
Department of Forest Pathology, Poznan University of Life Sciences, Wojska Polskiego 71c, 60-625 Poznan, Poland

Heikki Henttonen
Natural Resources Institute Finland, Latokartanonkaari 9, 00790 Helsinki, Finland

Jerzy M. Behnke
School of Life Sciences, University of Nottingham, University Park, Nottingham NG7 2RD, UK

Amir Steinman, Avital Minderigiu and Ori Arieli
Koret School of Veterinary Medicine, The Robert H. Smith Faculty of Agriculture, Food and Environment, The Hebrew University of Jerusalem, Rehovot 7610001, Israel

Sharon Tirosh-Levy
Koret School of Veterinary Medicine, The Robert H. Smith Faculty of Agriculture, Food and Environment, The Hebrew University of Jerusalem, Rehovot 7610001, Israel
Division of Parasitology, Kimron Veterinary Institute, Bet Dagan 50250, Israel

Igor Savitski, Ludmila Fleiderovitz and Monica Leszkowicz Mazuz
Division of Parasitology, Kimron Veterinary Institute, Bet Dagan 50250, Israel

Nir Edery
Division of Pathology, Kimron Veterinary Institute, Bet Dagan 50250, Israel

Gili Schvartz
Koret School of Veterinary Medicine, The Robert H. Smith Faculty of Agriculture, Food and Environment, The Hebrew University of Jerusalem, Rehovot 7610001, Israel
Division of Virology, Kimron Veterinary Institute, Bet Dagan 50250, Israel

Sándor Hornok and Nóra Takács
Department of Parasitology and Zoology, University of Veterinary Medicine, 1078 Budapest, Hungary

Kristin Mühldorfer and Gábor Á. Czirják
Department of Wildlife Diseases, Leibniz Institute for Zoo and Wildlife Research, 10315 Berlin, Germany

Regina Hofmann-Lehmann and Marina L. Meli
Clinical Laboratory, Department of Clinical Diagnostics and Services, and Center for Clinical Studies, Vetsuisse Faculty, University of Zurich, 8057 Zurich, Switzerland

Miklós Gyuranecz
Institute for Veterinary Medical Research, Centre for Agricultural Research, 1143 Budapest, Hungary

Ester R. Unnsteinsdóttir
Ecology and Consultancy Department, Icelandic Institute of Natural History, 210 Garðabær, Iceland

Alex D. Greenwood
Department of Wildlife Diseases, Leibniz Institute for Zoo and Wildlife Research, 10315 Berlin, Germany
Department of Veterinary Medicine, Freie Universität Berlin, 14163 Berlin, Germany

Tommaso Vezzosi, Stefania Perrucci, Francesca Parisi, Michela Maestrini and Alessandro Poli
Department of Veterinary Sciences, University of Pisa, Viale delle Piagge n. 2, 56124 Pisa, Italy

Simone Morelli and Donato Traversa
Faculty of Veterinary Medicine, University of Teramo, Piano d'Accio, 64100 Teramo, Italy

Giulia Mennuni
Studio Associato Veterinario Razzauti Daolio Anguillesi, 57100 Livorno, Italy

Mohamed S. Ahmed
Department of Pathology, Faculty of Veterinary Medicine, Kafrelsheikh University, Kafrelsheikh 33516, Egypt
Department of Veterinary Pathology, Gifu University, 1-1 Yanagido, Gifu 501-1193, Japan

Reda E. Khalafalla
Department of Parasitology, Faculty of Veterinary Medicine, Kafrelsheikh University, Kafrelsheikh 33516, Egypt

Ashraf Al-Brakati
Department of Human Anatomy, College of Medicine, Taif University, Taif 21944, Saudi Arabia

Tokuma Yanai
Laboratory of Wildlife and Forensic Pathology, Biomedical Science Examination and Research Center, Department of Veterinary Medicine, Faculty of Veterinary Medicine, Okayama University of Science, Okayama 700-0005, Japan

Katarzyna Skrzypek, Jacek Karamon, Małgorzata Samorek-Pieróg, Joanna Dąbrowska, Maciej Kochanowski , Jacek Sroka, Ewa Bilska-Zając and Tomasz Cencek
Department of Parasitology and Invasive Diseases, National Veterinary Research Institute, Partyzantów Avenue 57, 24-100 Puławy, Poland

Ladislav Molnár and Peter Major
Clinic for Birds and Exotic Animals, University of Veterinary Medicine and Pharmacy, 040 01 Košice, Slovakia

Zuzana Vasilková
Institute of Parasitology of the Slovak Academy of Sciences, 040 01 Košice, Slovakia

Martina Tomková
Slovak Hydrometeorological Institute, Ďumbierska 26, 041 17 Košice, Slovakia

Sylwia Koziatek-Sadłowska and Rajmund Sokół
Department of Parasitology and Invasive Diseases, Faculty of Veterinary Medicine, University of Warmia and Mazury in Olsztyn, ul. Oczapowskiego 13, 10-719 Olsztyn, Poland

Doolyawat Kladkempetch
Master's Degree Program in Veterinary Science, Faculty of Veterinary Medicine, Chiang Mai University, Chiang Mai 50100, Thailand

Sahatchai Tangtrongsup
Department of Companion Animal and Wildlife Clinic, Faculty of Veterinary Medicine, Chiang Mai University, Chiang Mai 50100, Thailand
Research Center of Producing and Development of Products and Innovations for Animal Health and Production, Faculty of Veterinary Medicine, Chiang Mai University, Chiang Mai 50100, Thailand

Saruda Tiwananthagorn
Department of Veterinary Biosciences and Veterinary Public Health, Faculty of Veterinary Medicine, Chiang Mai University, Chiang Mai 50100, Thailand
Excellent Center in Veterinary Bioscience, Faculty of Veterinary Medicine, Chiang Mai University, Chiang Mai 50100, Thailand

Adrian Zaragoza-Bastida, Ana Lizet Morales-Ubaldo, Lenin Rangel-López and Nallely Rivero-Pérez
Universidad Autónoma del Estado de Hidalgo, Área Académica de Medicina Veterinaria y Zootecnia, Instituto de Ciencias Agropecuarias, Rancho Universitario Av. Universidad km 1, EX-Hda de Aquetzalpa, Tulancingo, Hidalgo 43600, Mexico

Saudy Consepcion Flores-Aguilar and Liliana Mireya Aguilar-Castro
Universidad Autónoma del Estado de Hidalgo, Área Académica de Biología, Instituto de Ciencias Básicas e Ingeniería. Carretera Pachuca-Tulancingo S/N Int. 22 Colonia Carboneras, Mineral de la Reforma, Hidalgo 42180, Mexico

Benjamín Valladares-Carranza
Facultad de Medicina Veterinaria y Zootecnia Universidad Autónoma del Estado de México, El Cerrillo Piedras Blancas, Toluca 50295, Mexico

Agustín Olmedo-Juárez
Centro Nacional de Investigación Disciplinaria en Salud Animal e Inocuidad (CENID SAI-INIFAP), Carretera Federal Cuernavaca-Cuautla No. 8534 / Col. Progreso, Jiutepec 62550, Morelos, Mexico

Carla E. Rosenfeld-Miranda
Facultad de Ciencias Veterinarias, Universidad Austral de Chile, Isla Teja s/n, Casilla 567, Valdivia, Chile

Aphrodite I. Kalogianni, Ioannis Bossis and Athanasios I. Gelasakis
Laboratory of Anatomy and Physiology of Farm Animals, Department of Animal Science, Agricultural University of Athens (AUA), Iera Odos 75 str., 11855 Athens, Greece

Loukia V. Ekateriniadou
Veterinary Research Institute, ELGO-Demeter, Thermi, 57001 Thessaloniki, Greece

Md Mazharul Islam
Department of Animal Resources, Ministry of Municipality and Environment, Doha, Qatar
School of Laboratory Medicine and Medical Sciences, College of Health Sciences, University of KwaZulu Natal, Durban 4000, South Africa

Elmoubashar Farag, Devendra Bansal and Hamad Al-Rumaihi
Ministry of Public Health, Doha, Qatar

Mohammad Mahmudul Hassan
Faculty of Veterinary Medicine, Chattogram Veterinary and Animal Sciences University, Khulshi, Chattogram 4225, Bangladesh

Salah Al Awaidy
Ministry of Health, PC 113 Muscat, Oman

Abdinasir Abubakar
Infectious Hazard Preparedness (IHP) Unit, WHO Health Emergencies Department (WHE), World Health Organization, Regional Office for the Eastern Mediterranean, Cairo 11371, Egypt

Zilungile Mkhize-Kwitshana
School of Life Sciences, College of Agriculture, Engineering & Science, University of KwaZulu Natal, Durban 40000, South Africa
South African Medical Research Council, Cape Town 7505, South Africa

Ylva Hedberg-Alm
Horse Clinic, University Animal Hospital, Swedish University of Agricultural Sciences, 750 07 Uppsala, Sweden

Johanna Penell
Division of Veterinary Nursing, Department of Clinical Sciences, Swedish University of Agricultural Sciences, 750 07 Uppsala, Sweden

Miia Riihimäki
Equine Medicine Unit, Department of Clinical Sciences, Swedish University of Agricultural Sciences, 750 07 Uppsala, Sweden

Eva Osterman-Lind
National Veterinary Institute, Department of Microbiology, Section for Parasitology diagnostics, 751 89 Uppsala, Sweden

Martin K. Nielsen
Maxwell H. Gluck Equine Research Center, Department of Veterinary Science, University of Kentucky, Lexington, KY 40546, USA

Eva Tydén
Parasitology Unit, Department of Biomedical Science and Veterinary Public Health, Swedish University of Agricultural Sciences, 750 07 Uppsala, Sweden

Hector M. Espiritu, Lovelia L. Mamuad, Seon-ho Kim, Su-jeong Jin, Sang-suk Lee and Yong-il Cho
Department of Animal Science and Technology, Sunchon National University, Suncheon, Jeonnam 57922, Korea

Seok-won Kwon
Woosarang Animal Hospital, Yongin, Gyeonggi 17026, Korea

Reem A. Alajmi
Department of Zoology, College of Science, King Saud University, Riyadh 11451, KSA

Dina M. Metwally
Department of Zoology, College of Science, King Saud University, Riyadh 11451, KSA
Department of Parasitology, Faculty of Veterinary Medicine, Zagazig University, Zagazig 44519, Egypt

Tahani T. Al-Otaibi
Department of Biology, Al-Nairiyah University College, University of Hafr Al-Batin, Hafr Al-Batin 31991, Saudi Arabia

Isra M. Al-Turaiki
Department of Information Technology, College of Computer and Information Sciences, King Saud University, Riyadh 11451, Saudi Arabia

Manal F. El-Khadragy
Department of Biology, Faculty of Science, Princess Nourah Bint Abdelrahman University, Riyadh 84428, Saudi Arabia
Department of Zoology and Entomology, Faculty of Science, Helwan University, Cairo 11795, Egypt

Giuseppe Piegari
Department of Veterinary Medicine and Animal Production, Unit of Pathology, University of Naples Federico II, 80137 Naples, Italy

Lorena Cardillo, Flora Alfano, Lucia Vangone and Giovanna Fusco
Istituto Zooprofilattico Sperimentale del Mezzogiorno, Portici, 81100 Naples, Italy

Valentina Iovane
Department of Pharmacy, University of Salerno, 84084 Fisciano, Italy

Arun Kumar De, Sneha Sawhney, Perumal Ponraj, Sanjay Kumar Ravi, Kangayan Muniswamy, Arvind Kumar Tripathi and Debasis Bhattacharya
Animal Science Division, ICAR-Central Island Agricultural Research Institute, Port Blair 744101, India

Samiran Mondal and Gopal Sarkar
Department of Veterinary Pathology, West Bengal University of Animal and Fishery Sciences, Kolkata 700037, India

Santanu Banik
Department of Animal Genetics and Breeding, ICAR-National Research Centre on Pig, Guwahati 781131, India

Dhruba Malakar
Animal Biotechnology Centre, National Dairy Research Institute, Karnal 132001, India

Ashish Kumar
CTARA, IIT Bombay, Mumbai 400076, India

Asit Kumar Bera
Reservoir and Wetland Fisheries Division, ICAR-Central Inland Fishery Research Institute, Barrackpore, Kolkata 700120, India

Dominika Mravčáková, Daniel Petrič, Klaudia Čobanová and Zora Váradyová
Institute of Animal Physiology, Centre of Biosciences of Slovak Academy of Sciences, 040 01 Košice, Slovakia

Michaela Komáromyová, Michal Babják, Michaela Urda Dolinská, Alžbeta Königová and Marián Várady
Institute of Parasitology of Slovak Academy of Sciences, 040 01 Košice, Slovakia

Sylwester Ślusarczyk
Department of Pharmaceutical Biology with Botanical Garden of Medicinal Plants, Medical University of Wroclaw, 50-556Wroclaw, Poland

Adam Cieslak
Department of Animal Nutrition, Poznan University of Life Sciences, 60-637 Poznan, Poland

Index

www.ingramcontent.com/pod-product-compliance
Lightning Source LLC
LaVergne TN
LVHW080929210926
848485LV00004B/759